Documentation Manual
for Occupational Therapy
Writing SOAP Notes

FOURTH EDITION

Documentation Manual for Occupational Therapy
Writing SOAP Notes
FOURTH EDITION

CRYSTAL A. GATELEY, PhD, OTR/L
ASSOCIATE CHAIR & ASSOCIATE TEACHING PROFESSOR
DEPARTMENT OF OCCUPATIONAL THERAPY
UNIVERSITY OF MISSOURI - SCHOOL OF HEALTH PROFESSIONS
COLUMBIA, MISSOURI

SHERRY BORCHERDING, MA, OTR/L
CLINICAL ASSOCIATE PROFESSOR, RETIRED
UNIVERSITY OF MISSOURI
COLUMBIA, MISSOURI

SLACK
INCORPORATED

www.Healio.com/books

ISBN: 978-1-63091-231-4

Copyright © 2017 by SLACK Incorporated

Instructors: *Documentation Manual for Occupational Therapy: Writing SOAP Notes, Fourth Edition Instructor's Manual* is also available from SLACK Incorporated. Don't miss this important companion to *Documentation Manual for Occupational Therapy: Writing SOAP Notes, Fourth Edition*. To obtain the Instructor's Manual, please visit http://www.efacultylounge.com

Dr. Crystal A. Gateley and *Sherry Borcherding* have no financial or proprietary interest in the materials presented herein.

The procedures and practices described in this publication should be implemented in a manner consistent with the professional standards set for the circumstances that apply in each specific situation. Every effort has been made to confirm the accuracy of the information presented and to correctly relate generally accepted practices. The authors, editors, and publisher cannot accept responsibility for errors or exclusions or for the outcome of the material presented herein. There is no expressed or implied warranty of this book or information imparted by it. Care has been taken to ensure that drug selection and dosages are in accordance with currently accepted/recommended practice. Off-label uses of drugs may be discussed. Due to continuing research, changes in government policy and regulations, and various effects of drug reactions and interactions, it is recommended that the reader carefully review all materials and literature provided for each drug, especially those that are new or not frequently used. Some drugs or devices in this publication have clearance for use in a restricted research setting by the Food and Drug and Administration or FDA. Each professional should determine the FDA status of any drug or device prior to use in their practice.

Any review or mention of specific companies or products is not intended as an endorsement by the author or publisher.

SLACK Incorporated uses a review process to evaluate submitted material. Prior to publication, educators or clinicians provide important feedback on the content that we publish. We welcome feedback on this work.

Published by: SLACK Incorporated
                  6900 Grove Road
                  Thorofare, NJ 08086 USA
                  Telephone: 856-848-1000
                  Fax: 856-848-6091
                  www.Healio.com/books

Contact SLACK Incorporated for more information about other books in this field or about the availability of our books from distributors outside the United States.

Library of Congress Cataloging-in-Publication Data

Names: Gateley, Crystal A., - author. | Borcherding, Sherry, author.
Title: Documentation manual for occupational therapy : writing SOAP notes /
   Crystal A. Gateley, Sherry Borcherding.
Description: Fourth edition. | Thorofare, NJ : SLACK Incorporated, [2017] |
   Preceded by Documentation manual for occupational therapy : writing SOAP
   notes / Crystal A. Gateley, Sherry Borcherding. 3rd ed. c2012. | Includes
   bibliographical references and index.
Identifiers: LCCN 2016025712 (print) | LCCN 2016026325 (ebook) | ISBN
   9781630912314 (paperback : alk. paper) | ISBN 9781630912321 (epub) | ISBN
   9781630912338 (web)
Subjects: | MESH: Forms and Records Control | Occupational Therapy--methods |
   Patient Care Planning | Medical Records | Writing | Handbooks
Classification: LCC RM735.4 (print) | LCC RM735.4 (ebook) | NLM WB 39 | DDC
   615.8/515--dc23
LC record available at https://lccn.loc.gov/2016025712

For permission to reprint material in another publication, contact SLACK Incorporated. Authorization to photocopy items for internal, personal, or academic use is granted by SLACK Incorporated provided that the appropriate fee is paid directly to Copyright Clearance Center. Prior to photocopying items, please contact the Copyright Clearance Center at 222 Rosewood Drive, Danvers, MA 01923 USA; phone: 978-750-8400; website: www.copyright.com; email: info@copyright.com

Printed in the United States of America.

Last digit is print number: 10 9 8 7 6 5 4 3 2 1

DEDICATION

This book is dedicated to all of my past, current, and future OT students who make teaching a wonderful and rewarding experience. It is my hope that this book will serve you in your endeavors to provide compassionate care to your clients and to communicate the benefit of the occupational therapy profession.

Crystal A. Gateley, PhD, OTR/L

This book is dedicated to the occupational therapy students, faculty, and fieldwork instructors who have taught me so much about documentation, and to my grandson, Jan, who carries on the family tradition in occupational therapy.

Sherry Borcherding, MA, OTR/L

Contents

Instructors: *Documentation Manual for Occupational Therapy: Writing SOAP Notes, Fourth Edition Instructor's Manual* is also available from SLACK Incorporated. Don't miss this important companion to *Documentation Manual for Occupational Therapy: Writing SOAP Notes, Fourth Edition*. To obtain the Instructor's Manual, please visit http://www.efacultylounge.com

ACKNOWLEDGMENTS

I would like to thank Sherry Borcherding for teaching me how to document long ago as a student, for her support and encouragement over the past two decades, and for her trust in me to serve as coauthor on this project. I would also like to thank Brien Cummings and the staff at SLACK Incorporated who supported Sherry and me through the revision process.

I am grateful for the support of all of my departmental colleagues at the University of Missouri. It is wonderful to work in a department where faculty members and staff support the educational and professional advancement of their colleagues by taking on extra responsibilities when needed.

A big thank you goes out to the many University of Missouri OT students who have allowed their notes to be used in this book to teach others. I especially want to thank the Classes of 2013, 2014, 2015, 2016, and 2017 that provided helpful suggestions during the revision process. I would like to acknowledge the contributions of Vic Zuccarello, David McSpadden, Shelia Tenny, Joe Sadewhite, Patty Daus, Kathy Nelson, Stephanie Schmidt, Shawna Dunnaway, Michelle Wheeler, Kayla Harmon, and Melanie Cook in helping us make certain that the content of this book is consistent with current occupational therapy practice. I would also like to acknowledge Karthik Rao and Sanjay Patel of Princeton Global Services (PT Practice Pro Software), Karen Bond and Karen Soderquist of Cedaron Medical (AOTA PERFORM Software), and Cheryl Harrington and Bruce vanBerkum (school therapy doc—electronic therapy documentation) for their assistance in providing screenshots of electronic documentation for this textbook.

Most importantly, I would like to thank my husband, Curt, and my two daughters, Katrina and Lauren, whose patience, love, and support continue to be my inspiration in life. When I worked on the last edition of this book, Katrina and Lauren were still in middle and elementary school. Since that time, I have watched them grow into beautiful, intelligent, and accomplished young women. I can't wait to see what life will bring for them over the next few years.

Crystal A. Gateley, PhD, OTR/L

Many people have contributed to the development of this manual. First, I would like to thank Crystal Gateley for joining me as coauthor beginning with the 3rd edition. Her upgrades to the manual have taken it to another level. I would like to thank Diana Baldwin for her patience in teaching me how to teach. Without her nurturing and support, I might have taken another pathway entirely. Thanks to Fred Dittrich for moving me as gracefully and quickly into the Information Age as I could tolerate, and to both Fred Dittrich and Boden Lyon for teaching me video editing. Thanks to Sandy Matsuda for her editing contributions, and for her loving friendship and support. Thanks to Doris O'Hara for bequeathing me the basic course material many years ago, and to Leanna Garrison for being the Format Goddess. Most of all, I would like to thank the occupational therapy classes at the University of Missouri, who allowed their notes to be used to teach others.

Sherry Borcherding, MA, OTR/L

About the Authors

Crystal A. Gateley, PhD, OTR/L is Associate Chair and Associate Teaching Professor at University of Missouri in Columbia, where she has taught since 2009. She teaches a variety of courses across the curriculum including Foundations & Theory in OT, Clinical Pathophysiology, Human Development & Occupations I and II, Level I Fieldwork, and Clinical Reasoning & Documentation.

Crystal graduated Summa Cum Laude from University of Missouri with a BHS in Occupational Therapy and went on to complete a master's and doctorate in Educational Leadership and Policy Analysis (ELPA), also from University of Missouri. Crystal has worked in a variety of occupational therapy practice settings, including acute care, inpatient and outpatient rehabilitation, skilled nursing, home health, outpatient pediatrics, public schools, and sheltered workshops.

Besides teaching, Crystal enjoys attending her daughters' extracurricular events, particularly Southern Boone Lady Eagles soccer and basketball, and frequently volunteers her time to support school and community organizations. She also loves camping, fishing, canoeing, and boating with family and friends.

Sherry Borcherding, MA, OTR/L is retired from the faculty of University of Missouri, where she taught for 15 years. During the time she was on faculty, she taught disability awareness; complementary therapy; clinical ethics; frames of reference; psychopathology; loss and disability; long-term care; wellness; and a three-semester fieldwork sequence designed to develop critical thinking, clinical reasoning, and documentation skills. Two of her courses were designated as campus writing courses and one was credentialed for computer and information proficiency. As a part of the fieldwork and documentation courses, she filmed simulated occupational therapy interventions for student use in class. Twelve of those "movies" are available on www.efacultylounge.com with this edition of the book.

Sherry graduated with honors from Texas Woman's University, Denton, Texas with a BS in occupational therapy and went on to complete her master's in special education with special faculty commendation at George Peabody College, Nashville, Tennessee. Following her staff positions in rehabilitation, home health, and pediatrics, she assumed a number of management roles including Chief Occupational Therapist at East Texas Treatment Center, Kilgore, Texas; Director of Occupational Therapy at Mid-Missouri Mental Health Center, Columbia; and Director of Rehabilitation Services at Transitional Housing Agency, Columbia, Missouri. She has also planned, designed and directed occupational therapy programs at Capital Regional Medical Center, Jefferson City, Missouri and at Charter Behavioral Health Center, Columbia, Missouri.

Sherry is a lifelong learner. Since her retirement, she has further expanded her private practice devoted to complementary and alternative therapies. She is certified in CranioSacral Therapy at the techniques level through Upledger Institute, Palm Beach Gardens, Florida and is attuned as a Reiki master. For leisure, Sherry enjoys music, English country dance, and all kinds of three-dimensional art. Her pottery has appeared in several local shows over the past several years. She volunteers with the Community Emergency Response Team doing logistics.

Documenting the Occupational Therapy Process

Welcome to a new style of writing. The first time you see an experienced occupational therapist make an entry in a health record, you may be tempted to think you will never be able to do it. The technical language alone can be intimidating. Then, there is the amazing attention to detail in the client observation, the insightful assessment, and the plan that just seems to roll off the therapist's fingertips while you are wondering how long it will take you to be able to predict a course of treatment like that.

Professional documentation is a skill, and like any skill, it can be learned. Learning a new skill requires two things: instruction and practice. This manual is designed to provide you with both parts of the process. Information is presented about each part of the documentation process, and the worksheets are designed to let you practice each step as you learn it.

The material presented here grew out of a course on clinical documentation taught to occupational therapy students at the University of Missouri. It has been field-tested to ensure it is understandable and effective in helping you learn both documentation and the clinical reasoning skills underlying the documentation process.

Occupational therapy practitioners use different formats for documentation depending on their practice settings. This manual introduces specific formats for writing occupation-based problem statements and goals. In addition, this manual presents a systematic approach to one form of documentation: the SOAP note. SOAP is an acronym for the four parts of an entry into a health record. The letters stand for *Subjective, Objective, Assessment,* and *Plan.* Although not all practice settings use the SOAP note format, the clinical reasoning skills underlying SOAP note documentation can be adapted to fit the written or electronic documentation requirements of nearly any occupational therapy practice setting.

OUR EVOLVING PROFESSION

The American Occupational Therapy Association (AOTA) represents the interests and concerns of occupational therapy practitioners and students in all aspects of professional practice including provision of quality services, improvement of consumer access to occupational therapy services, and promotion of professional development (AOTA, 2015a). The following statement serves as the overarching vision of our national professional association:

> AOTA advances occupational therapy as the preeminent profession in promoting the health, productivity, and quality of life of individuals and society through the therapeutic application of occupation. (AOTA, 2015a, para. 6)

Furthermore, in April 2016, AOTA released its new Vision 2025 statement to serve as a guide for the occupational therapy profession over the next decade:

> Occupational therapy maximizes health, well-being, and quality of life for all people, populations, and communities through effective solutions that facilitate participation in everyday living. (AOTA, 2016)

Gateley CA, Borcherding S. *Documentation Manual for
Occupational Therapy: Writing SOAP Notes, Fourth Edition (pp 1-6).*
© 2017 SLACK Incorporated

These vision statements serve as a roadmap for all aspects of professional practice, including documentation. Current occupational therapy practice is in many ways determined by which services are reimbursable, and documentation of client care is the vehicle through which those services are communicated. As the profession continues the move toward evidence-based practice in the context of a rapidly changing health care environment, well-documented occupational therapy services are more likely to be recognized and reimbursed as a cost-effective solution for treating and preventing injury and improving health outcomes (Rexe, Lammi, & von Zweck, 2013).

Occupational therapists are challenged with combining the ever-changing knowledge base of the profession with its historical foundations and this visionary roadmap for the future. Leaders in the profession have identified four principles to guide contemporary occupational therapy practice (Boyt Schell, Scaffa, Gillen, & Cohn, 2014):

1. Client-centered practice
2. Occupation-centered practice
3. Evidence-based practice
4. Culturally relevant practice

Clinical documentation in occupational therapy must reflect these principles. Occupational therapists must collaborate with clients during evaluation and intervention to ensure that clients have an active role in their care, and that collaboration should be documented throughout the therapeutic process. The targeted outcome of occupational therapy intervention is enhanced engagement in meaningful occupations, and the documented goals and interventions should have occupation as a central theme. Occupational therapists should document assessments and interventions that represent the best evidence available for addressing a client's specific needs. Finally, occupational therapists should be sensitive to and document cultural differences that affect the evaluation and intervention process.

OUR EVOLVING PROFESSIONAL LANGUAGE

INTERNATIONAL CLASSIFICATION OF FUNCTIONING DISABILITY AND HEALTH

The *International Classification of Functioning, Disability and Health* (World Health Organization [WHO], 2002), known commonly as *ICF*, was published by the WHO to provide a common language and framework for describing health and disability. The ICF is based on a biopsychosocial model that views disability and function as the "outcomes of interactions between health conditions…and contextual factors" (WHO, 2002, p. 9). Health conditions include diseases, disorders, and injuries. Contextual factors include personal factors as well as environmental factors. In this model (Figure 1-1), function is classified at three levels:

1. Body functions and structure
2. Individual activity
3. Participation in society

Figure 1-1. ICF model of disability. (Reprinted with permission from World Health Organization. (2002). *Towards a common language for functioning, disability and health: ICF.* Geneva, Switzerland: Author. Retrieved from http://www.who.int/classifications/icf/training/icfbeginnersguide.pdf.)

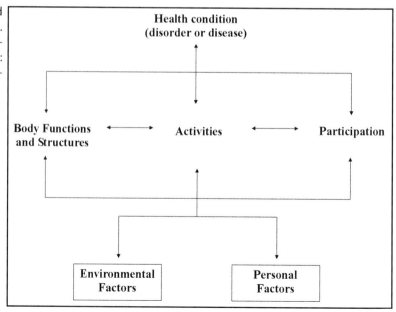

The standard language and global theoretical framework of the ICF can be used for communication across countries, disciplines, and populations (Pettersson, Pettersson, & Frisk, 2012). Furthermore, use of ICF concepts and terminology "can expose occupational therapy to a wider interdisciplinary audience" (Mahaffey & Colaianni, 2012, p. 8). The concepts presented in the ICF are useful to many health professionals, including occupational therapists, in communicating with team members of other disciplines and with external parties, such as funding sources. In addition, the ICF provides a framework and vocabulary useful for occupational therapy clinical practice, research, and education (Pettersson et al., 2012).

OCCUPATIONAL THERAPY PRACTICE FRAMEWORK: DOMAIN & PROCESS, 3RD EDITION

Although the ICF is a useful tool for occupational therapists in thinking about health and disability, that classification system alone is not sufficient as the language of the profession (Mahaffey & Colaianni, 2012; Pettersson et al., 2012). Several decades ago, leaders in the profession recognized the need for a system of uniform terminology. The original document, *Occupational Therapy Product Output Reporting System and Uniform Terminology for Reporting Occupational Therapy Services*, was developed in response to a change in public laws targeted at reducing fraud and abuse of the Medicare and Medicaid systems (AOTA, 1989).

That original document has been revised multiple times and ultimately resulted in the development of the *Occupational Therapy Practice Framework: Domain & Process, 3rd Edition*, hereafter referred to as *OTPF-III* (AOTA, 2014a). The *OTPF-III* is the document that defines and guides professional practice of all occupational therapists and occupational therapy assistants. More specifically, the *OTPF-III* was developed "to articulate occupational therapy's distinct perspective and contribution to promoting the health and participation of persons, groups, and populations through engagement in occupation" (AOTA, 2014a, p. S2). The *OTPF-III* "serves as a reference for questions about practice, guides documentation, and articulates information about occupational therapy to external audiences, including other health care professionals, third-party payers, and consumers" (AOTA, 2014a, p. 139). The *OTPF-III* is divided into two major sections:

1. *Domain*: This section of the document outlines the purview of occupational therapy practice and identifies the areas in which occupational therapy practitioners have knowledge and expertise.

2. *Process*: This section focuses on the delivery of occupational therapy services, with a focus on occupation-centered and client-centered practices.

Domain of Occupational Therapy

The aspects of occupational therapy's domain are viewed as having a dynamic interrelationship that affects "the client's occupational identity, health, well-being and participation in life" (AOTA, 2014a, p. S4). The ultimate goal of occupational therapy is to support a client's engagement in meaningful occupation, and all aspects of the domain are viewed as having equal value. The expertise of an occupational therapy practitioner is required to understand and document the relationship among all aspects and the resulting impact on a client's engagement in areas of occupation. The various aspects of the domain of occupational therapy are summarized as follows:

- *Occupations*: Occupations are "the daily life activities in which people engage" and include activities of daily living, instrumental activities of daily living, rest and sleep, education, work, play, leisure, and social participation (AOTA, 2014a, p. S4-S6).

- *Client Factors*: Client factors "are specific capacities, characteristics, or beliefs that reside within the person and that influence performance in occupations" and include values, beliefs, and spirituality; body function; and body structures (AOTA, 2014a, p. S4-S6).

- *Performance Skills*: Performance skills are "goal-directed actions that are observable as small units of engagement in daily life occupations" and include motor skills, process skills, and social interaction skills.

- *Performance Patterns*: "Performance patterns are the habits, routines, roles, and rituals used in the process of engaging in occupations" (AOTA, 2014a, p. S8).

- *Contexts and Environments*: This aspect includes the physical environment and social environment in which occupations occur as well as elements of the cultural, personal, temporal, and virtual contexts that influence occupational performance (AOTA, 2014a, p. S8-S9).

Process of Occupational Therapy Service Delivery

The process of service delivery in occupational therapy is composed of evaluation, intervention, and targeting of outcomes (AOTA, 2014a). The *OTPF-III* explains that the process of service delivery does not occur in a linear fashion. Rather, it is a dynamic and fluid process that allows occupational therapy practitioners to focus on identified outcomes while continually reflecting on and accommodating new developments and insights throughout the service delivery process. Accurate and effective clinical documentation during all phases of service delivery is essential to communicate the necessity and benefit of occupational therapy to all involved parties. The process of occupational therapy service delivery is summarized as follows (AOTA, 2014a, p. S10):

- **Evaluation**
  - *Occupational Profile*: The occupational therapist gathers information about the client's occupational history, experiences, daily living patterns, interests, values, needs, priorities, and reasons for seeking services.
  - *Analysis of Occupational Performance*: After obtaining a thorough occupational profile, the occupational therapist identifies the client's strengths, problems, and potential problems through observation and assessment of the client's performance.
- **Intervention**
  - *Intervention Plan*: The occupational therapist uses relevant frames of reference and evidence to develop an action plan in collaboration with the client.
  - *Intervention Implementation*: The occupational therapist carries out the action plan and monitors the client's response.
  - *Intervention Review*: The occupational therapist reviews the intervention plan and progress toward targeted outcomes.
- **Targeting of Outcomes**: The occupational therapist uses outcomes assessment information to plan future interactions with the client and to complete program evaluation.

OTHER PUBLICATIONS OF THE AMERICAN OCCUPATIONAL THERAPY ASSOCIATION

The content of this manual reflects the domain and process of contemporary occupational therapy practice as described in the *OTPF-III*. The *OTPF-III* is just one of many *Official Documents* published by the AOTA that influences occupational therapy practice and therefore documentation. *Official Documents* can be divided into the following types (AOTA, 2014b):

- *Guidelines*: Provide descriptions, examples, or recommendations of procedures pertaining to occupational therapy practice and education.
- *Position Papers*: Present the official stance of AOTA on a particular issue or subject.
- *Standards*: Include a general description of a topic relevant to occupational therapy practice and define the minimum requirements for performance and quality.
- *Statements*: Describe and clarify an aspect or issue related to education or practice. Although they do not present an official stance of AOTA, statements are linked to fundamental concepts of occupational therapy.

Each AOTA official document undergoes a standard 5-year document review process by the AOTA Commission on Practice (AOTA, 2015b). This documentation manual incorporates concepts and guidelines from the most recent versions of AOTA *Official Documents* relevant to documentation. However, practitioners should remain informed about *Official Document* revisions that affect practice and documentation. Newly revised *Official Documents* are published each year in *The American Journal of Occupational Therapy*. In addition, all AOTA *Official Documents* are available on the organization's website (http://www.aota.org).

The Accreditation Council for Occupational Therapy Education (ACOTE) publishes accreditation standards for educational programs at the levels of associate degree for the occupational therapy assistant, and master's and doctoral degrees for the occupational therapist. This manual will provide you with a tool for becoming competent in the documentation skills specified in the accreditation standards. Although standards vary according to the requirements of each educational level, the standards for documentation are consistent across all three levels:

- Standard B.1.8. "Demonstrate an understanding of the use of technology to support performance, participation, health and well-being. This technology may include, but is not limited to, electronic documentation systems, distance communication, virtual environments, and telehealth technology" (ACOTE, 2014, p. 19).
- Standard B.4.10. "Document occupational therapy services to ensure accountability of service provision and to meet standards for reimbursement of services, adhering to the requirements of applicable facility, local, state, federal, and reimbursement agencies. Documentation must effectively communicate the need and rationale for occupational therapy services" (ACOTE, 2014, p. 22)

- Standard B.5.32. "Document occupational therapy services to ensure accountability of service provision and to meet standards for reimbursement of services. Documentation must effectively communicate the need and rationale for occupational therapy services and must be appropriate to the context in which the service is delivered" (ACOTE, 2014, p. 28)
- Standard B.7.4. Demonstrate knowledge of various reimbursement systems (e.g., federal, state, third party, private payer), appeals mechanisms, and documentation requirements that affect society and the practice of occupational therapy" (ACOTE, 2014, p. 29)

In summary, there are numerous documents and publications that affect the occupational therapy profession as a whole and clinical documentation in particular. It is the responsibility of each occupational therapy practitioner to be familiar with current literature, standards, and state and federal regulations that affect documentation. Leaders in the profession are continually researching and publishing both revised and novel works that affect occupational therapy practice. Staying current with all professional publications allows occupational therapy practitioners to engage in evidence-based practice, and this must be reflected in clinical documentation.

OVERVIEW

The information in this manual has been arranged in the order that it is most easily learned, with foundational concepts presented first. More complex concepts build on these as clinical reasoning is developed. Chapter 2 provides an introduction to the medical (health) record, including its function, uses, and history. Chapter 3 expands on some of the issues introduced in the previous chapter and provides a general foundation of information to guide documentation in occupational therapy practices. Chapter 4 presents the rules and mechanics of documentation.

Chapter 5 discusses the process of developing functional problem statements that can be positively affected by occupational therapy intervention. Chapter 6 introduces the COAST format for writing goals and objectives. This format was introduced in the previous edition of this textbook and has since been endorsed at the AOTA Specialty Conference on Effective Documentation (Amini, 2014). Worksheets are provided for practice and several examples of problems and goal statements are provided for your reference.

Chapters 7 through 10 teach the four sections of the SOAP format (Subjective, Objective, Assessment, and Plan), which are introduced and explained in Chapters 1 and 2. Multiple examples are presented for each section, and worksheets are provided for practice. Chapter 11 reviews the skills presented in the previous six chapters and provides multiple worksheets to refine those skills. Chapter 12 introduces the intervention planning process that follows an evaluation and provides worksheets to practice this skill.

The last four chapters of this manual serve as a reference as you learn how to document occupational therapy practice. Chapter 13 presents information from *Guidelines for Documentation of Occupational Therapy* (AOTA, 2013) and provides examples of documentation from the different stages of the occupational therapy process. Chapter 14 discusses requirements specific to various settings and funding sources and provides several examples. Chapter 15 introduces some of the common features of electronic documentation software. Chapter 16 provides an array of examples from various stages of the occupational therapy process and numerous practice settings and patient populations.

An appendix with suggestions for completing the worksheets is also provided. It is important to remember that there are multiple "correct" ways to document. As you work through this manual, we recommend that you complete the worksheets on your own before looking at the suggested answers in the appendix.

NEW IN THIS EDITION

The fourth edition of *Documentation Manual for Occupational Therapy: Writing SOAP Notes* is based on the *Occupational Therapy Practice Framework: Domain & Process, 3rd Edition* (AOTA, 2014a) and on the *Guidelines for Documentation of Occupational Therapy* (AOTA, 2013). The fourth edition presents an increased focus on occupation in all areas of documentation, and numerous references have been added throughout the text in an effort to present contemporary evidence-based information.

Chapter 3 expands considerably on information regarding reimbursement that was covered only briefly in the previous edition, with specific attention to Medicare guidelines, CPT codes, and G-Codes. Chapter 15 is also an expansion of information on electronic documentation from the previous edition. Several new examples and screenshots have been included to highlight the features of different electronic documentation software options. Several examples have been updated and added throughout the book to reflect current practice in early intervention, mental health, seating and mobility, driver rehabilitation, work hardening, assistive technology, community practice, and primary care.

All worksheets presented in this manual will be available on a website. This will give students the option of using either the perforated worksheets in the book or accessing them in an electronic version.

In addition to the changes listed previously, this edition also comes with an instructor's manual that will be helpful to occupational therapy instructors teaching courses that involve documentation or fieldwork. The instructor's manual includes recommendations for use of this textbook and the worksheets as learning tools. Additional suggestions and examples of quizzes and assignments are provided. Grading rubrics are provided for evaluating student performance in writing functional problem statements, goals, intervention plans, and SOAP notes. The instructor's manual also includes instructor access to several new videos that may be used for developing documentation skills. A case history and sample documentation accompany each video.

REFERENCES

Accreditation Council for Occupational Therapy Education. (2014). 2011 Accreditation Council for Occupational Therapy Education standards and interpretive guide: December 2014 interpretive guide version. Retrieved from http://www.aota.org.

American Occupational Therapy Association. (1989). Uniform terminology for occupational therapy (2nd ed.). *American Journal of Occupational Therapy, 43*(12), 808-815.

American Occupational Therapy Association. (2013). Guidelines for documentation of occupational therapy. *American Journal of Occupational Therapy, 67*(6), S32-S38. doi: 10.5014/ajot.2013.67S32.

American Occupational Therapy Association. (2014a). *Occupational therapy practice framework: Domain & process* (3rd ed.). Bethesda, MD: AOTA Press.

American Occupational Therapy Association. (2014b). Types of official documents. Retrieved from http://www.aota.org/Practice/Manage/Official/Official-Docs.aspx.

American Occupational Therapy Association. (2015a). About AOTA. Retrieved from http://www.aota.org/AboutAOTA.aspx.

American Occupational Therapy Association. (2015b). AOTA's Commission on Practice (COP). Retrieved from http://www.aota.org/AboutAOTA/Get-Involved/RA/COP.aspx.

American Occupational Therapy Association. (2016). Welcome ceremony. Presentation at the American Occupational Therapy Association 2016 Annual Conference & Expo, Chicago, IL.

Amini, D. (2014). Documentation for occupation-based practice. Presentation at the 2014 AOTA Specialty Conference, Alexandria, VA.

Boyt Schell, B. A., Scaffa, M. E., Gillen, G., & Cohn, E. S. (2014). Contemporary occupational therapy practice. In B.A. Boyt Schell, Gillen, & Scaffa (Eds.), *Willard & Spackman's occupational therapy* (12th ed., pp. 47-58.) Philadelphia, PA: Lippincott Williams & Wilkins.

Mahaffey, L., & Colaianni, D. (2012). Understanding ICF's connection to occupational therapy services. *OT Practice, 17*(7), 7-8.

Pettersson, I., Pettersson, V., & Frisk, M. (2012). ICF from an occupational therapy perspective in adult care: An integrative literature review. *Scandinavian Journal of Occupational Therapy, 19*, 260–273. doi: 10.3109/11038128.2011.557087.

Rexe, K., Lammi, B. M., & von Zweck, C. (2013). Occupational therapy: Cost-effective solutions for changing health system needs. *Healthcare Quarterly, 16*(1), 69-75.

World Health Organization. (2002). *Towards a common language for functioning, disability, and health: ICF.* Geneva, Switzerland: Author. Retrieved from http://www.who.int/classifications/icf/training/icfbeginnersguide.pdf.

The Health Record

The health record, often called the *medical record*, is a compilation of data that includes the client's past and present health information. The purpose of the health record is to serve as the medical and legal document of a client's history, his or her current condition and status, the intervention provided, and the client's response to intervention (Gillum, 2013; Scott, 2013). Like many aspects of health care, the health record is continuously undergoing changes. Before moving on to the specific processes involved in documenting occupational therapy practice, it is important to understand the history of health records in general and the implications for occupational therapy documentation. This chapter will provide a brief history of health records in general, a history and overview of SOAP notes, and a discussion of the many audiences and functions of the health record.

HISTORY OF HEALTH RECORDS

The recording of patient information can be traced back through antiquity from the cave paintings and stone carvings of prehistoric times to Egyptian surgical case reports documented on papyrus (Abdelhak, Grostick, & Hanken, 2012; Gillum, 2013). As civilizations developed, people transitioned to pen and paper for recording events. In the 1700s, ledgers were used to record information for various businesses in the United States including banks, stores, and eventually hospitals. Benjamin Franklin, secretary of one of the first incorporated hospitals in Pennsylvania in the mid-1700s, kept records of clients' names, addresses, disorders, and dates of admission and discharge (Gensel, 2005; University of Pennsylvania, 2015). More formal medical records developed as major teaching hospitals were established across the United States (Gillum, 2013). As medicine has advanced, so has the complexity and detail of the record. A profession, now called *Health Information Management*, was created to oversee the collection, classification, storage, retrieval, and dissemination of health records (American Health Information Management Association [AHIMA], 2015a).

The use of computers to support health records management can be traced back to the late 1960s (Gillum, 2013). Over the last several decades, the use of electronic health records (EHRs) or electronic medical records has transitioned from the exception to the rule in many health care settings (Gillum, 2013; Scott, 2013; Tripathi, 2012). The use of EHRs has the potential to streamline and improve the overall quality of client care, increase efficiency of health practitioners, and reduce health care costs (Gillum, 2013; Scott, 2013).

HISTORY OF THE SOAP NOTE

EHRs allow members of a client's health care team to access information with a few simple clicks of the mouse. While many health care organizations have moved fully or partially to EHRs, printed health records are still in use in many settings and are the default back-up plan when EHRs experience technological glitches. Printed health records are typically organized in one of the following methods (Clark, 2004):

Gateley CA, Borcherding S. *Documentation Manual for Occupational Therapy: Writing SOAP Notes, Fourth Edition (pp 7-13).*
© 2017 SLACK Incorporated

- *Source-oriented*: Documents are grouped together by the source from which they came (e.g., laboratory results, radiology results, physician notes, nursing notes, therapy notes, etc.).
- *Integrated*: Documents from various sources are entered in chronological or reverse chronological order.
- *Problem-oriented*: Documents are organized according to the client's problem list.

Each of these formats has its advantages and disadvantages. However, it is the problem-oriented medical record (POMR) that is the basis for the SOAP note format presented in this manual. The POMR was introduced by Dr. Lawrence Weed in the late 1960s to standardize physician and nursing documentation (Jacobs, 2009). Weed believed that the POMR format offered a more client-centered approach by focusing on the client's problems and the progress made toward solving those problems. As part of the more client-centered approach to documentation, Weed recommended that the progress note be organized into four sections, including the client's own perception of the situation, which previously had been considered irrelevant. He used the acronym SOAP to define the four sections (Martinez, 2013):

1. *"S" (Subjective)*: This section includes the client's report of his or her problems, limitations, and needs as well as the client's perception of treatment and progress. Typically, the subjective section of the progress note is brief. However, in an initial evaluation report, the "S" might be longer since it will include the information obtained in the initial interview.

2. *"O" (Objective)*: This section contains the health professional's observation of the client's performance and the treatment provided. In an initial evaluation note, this section also includes all of the measurable, quantifiable, and observable data that were collected.

3. *"A" (Assessment)*: This section is the health professional's analysis and interpretation of the events reported in the subjective and objective sections. This section shows the practitioner's clinical reasoning. An initial evaluation contains the functional problem list and the client's rehabilitation potential. Subsequent progress notes will focus on one or more problems from that list as well as the progress made and rehabilitation potential.

4. *"P" (Plan)*: This section is the health professional's plan of what to do next, and it includes the anticipated frequency and duration of services. An initial evaluation includes a detailed intervention plan. Subsequent progress notes specify the planned focus for future sessions with the client. This section may also include plans to refer the client to other disciplines when appropriate.

SOAP notes helped standardize documentation among physicians as well as nurses, pharmacists, psychologists, therapists, and many other health care professionals (Barnett, Gallimore, Kopacek, & Porter, 2014; Martinez, 2013; Scott, 2013). In fact, SOAP notes have been described as "the most common method of documentation used by providers to input notes into patients' medical records" (Martinez, 2013, para. 2). Many EHRs are built around the SOAP note concept and contain options for data entry in a SOAP note format.

It is important to remember that SOAP is just a format—an outline for organizing information. Any note can be written in this format, although some work better than others. An initial assessment can be quite lengthy when written in SOAP format because it will contain an occupational profile, prior level of functioning, a summary of functional problems, and the detailed intervention plan including long- and short-term goals. For this reason, many practice settings do not use the SOAP format for the initial evaluation report, but the facility may use the SOAP format for treatment and progress notes.

The SOAP format is an alternative to narrative notes, which tend to be disorganized and subjective. It forces the writer to look at all four aspects of the therapy session and to present the information in an orderly fashion. Learning the SOAP format is an excellent way for students and practitioners to develop the clinical reasoning process that underlies therapeutic intervention. Practitioners who learn to use the SOAP format will be able to adapt their documentation skills to nearly any practice setting as well as to EHRs. A more detailed explanation of each section of the SOAP note is provided in Chapters 7 through 10.

HEALTH INSURANCE PORTABILITY AND ACCOUNTABILITY ACT

In 1996, Congress passed the Health Insurance Portability and Accountability Act (HIPAA) to ensure that employees could maintain health benefits when changing jobs (Scott, 2013). Another major provision of HIPAA was the establishment of federal standards for the security, use, and disclosure of a client's protected health information (PHI). The HIPAA Privacy Rule, effective since 2003, prevents unauthorized disclosure of a client's PHI. Clients are also accorded several rights under HIPAA (U.S. Department of Health & Human Services [HHS], 2015b). These include the following:

- The right to view and obtain a copy of the health record
- The right to request revision or omission of information in the health record that is incorrect
- The right to know how health information is used and shared with others
- The right to decide if PHI can be used for purposes of marketing and research
- The right to authorize the release of health information to selected individuals
- The right to file a complaint if it is believed that health information has been used in a way that violates the law

HIPAA has several implications for occupational therapy practitioners, particularly as many health care settings have transitioned to EHRs. In 2013, the HIPAA Security Rule implemented new requirements to address technological advances (Collmer, 2015). The new rule "not only strengthened privacy and security safeguards for PHI, but it also created steeper civil and criminal penalties for violation" (Collmer, 2015, p. 13). In any practice setting, you should have a clear understanding of your employer's strategies for HIPAA compliance and your role in maintaining client confidentiality. Although not all-inclusive, the following is a list of strategies that will help maintain compliance with HIPAA guidelines (Collmer, 2015):

- Do not discuss client PHI with anyone who does not have a need to know the information.
- Do not discuss client PHI in an area where it may be overheard by others.
- Do not leave paper charts out on a desk for easy access by unauthorized users.
- Do not leave client records open on a computer screen or other electronic device.
- Always log off of electronic devices containing health records.
- When working on electronic devices, position yourself and the device in a manner to prevent others from viewing the screen.
- Make sure electronic devices containing PHI are locked up to prevent physical access by unauthorized users.
- Make sure that you are using encrypted emails or encrypted cloud-based software programs to share electronic PHI with other authorized users.
- Avoid documenting in public areas with unsecured wireless access.

"Compliance with the HIPAA Security Rule means more than following the law. Occupational therapy practitioners who comply with the requirements protect their organization and themselves from hefty penalties and reputational damage" (Collmer, 2015, p. 16). Furthermore, occupational therapy practitioners must follow the American Occupational Therapy Association (AOTA; 2015) *Code of Ethics*. Principle 3 of the *Code of Ethics* states "occupational therapy personnel shall respect the right of the individual to self-determination, privacy, confidentiality, and consent" (AOTA, 2015, p. 4). The related standard of conduct specifies that "occupational therapy personnel shall maintain the confidentiality of all verbal, written, electronic, augmentative, and nonverbal communications, in compliance with applicable laws, including all aspects of privacy laws and exceptions thereto" (e.g., HIPAA, Family Educational Rights and Privacy Act [FERPA]).

In summary, you should also have a clear understanding of the privacy safeguards that exist at your place of employment and your role in ensuring compliance with HIPAA laws. For example, what procedure should you follow if a client asks for a copy of the health record? Is there a form that must be signed in order for you to discuss health information with a client's relative or friend? What should your response be if another client innocently asks, "What's wrong with that person over there?"

FAMILY EDUCATIONAL RIGHTS AND PRIVACY ACT

Congress enacted FERPA in 1974 "to guarantee parental access to student records and to permit access only to person with legitimate reasons to view the records" (Barboza, Epps, Byington, & Keene, 2008, p. 2). FERPA applies to educational institutions that receive government funding through the U.S. Department of Education. School occupational therapy practitioners have access to student educational records and must comply with FERPA regulations. In some instances, school practitioners may also be subject to HIPAA guidelines. For example, if a practitioner is providing occupational therapy services as outlined in the child's Individualized Education Program but Medicaid is billed for the services, the billing procedures must comply with HIPAA guidelines while the documentation for the services becomes part of the educational record and therefore falls under FERPA guidelines (Barboza et al., 2008). When in doubt about whether you can share information about school-based occupational therapy services, you should consult with school administrators and your employer if you are providing contract services and are employed by another entity.

PURPOSES OF CLIENT CARE DOCUMENTATION

The primary and obvious purpose of the health record is to document a client's health information for future reference. It is important to consider the many potential audiences and functions of the health record whenever you make an entry into a client's record. Scott (2013) explained that, with the exception of national defense, no other business endeavor in the United States is as costly or requires the level of comprehensive accurate documentation of services provided as does the health care industry.

CLIENT CARE MANAGEMENT

The health record is one of the ways the treatment team communicates with each other about the day-to-day aspects of the client's care. Other occupational therapy practitioners and members of the interdisciplinary treatment team will read your notes to coordinate care. In your note, you share the results of your evaluation, report the client's progress toward established goals, and advise other members of the team of your plan for continuing care, all of which are important to the treatment team. Good documentation is particularly important in ensuring continuity of care within and between settings as a single client may encounter multiple occupational therapy practitioners during the intervention process.

REIMBURSEMENT

The health record is the source for what services were provided and what services may be billed. Third-party payers such as Medicare, Medicaid, and private insurance companies may review documentation, not only for frequency and duration, but also to determine if the services provided to the client are worth paying for. Documentation in the health record is the primary means of justifying reimbursement for intervention (Scott, 2013). In all settings, but particularly outpatient settings where services are billed on a fee-per-service model, occupational therapy practitioners must ensure that their documentation about the treatment session justifies the billing codes that were used for the client's visit (Valdes, 2014).

UTILIZATION REVIEW AND UTILIZATION MANAGEMENT

The health record may be used for determining whether services provided to a client are appropriate, medically necessary, and efficient according to the policies and procedures established by federal and state regulatory agencies. Freedman (2006) explained the distinction between *utilization review* and *utilization management*, two terms that often are used interchangeably but have different meanings. Utilization review is a review of the health record that occurs after services have been provided to a client. Utilization management involves the proactive processes that take place before and during a client's provision of health services. These processes may include discharge planning from an acute care hospital setting or precertification for an acute care or rehabilitation unit stay. The goals of both utilization review and utilization management are to ensure compliance of health care providers and organizations to regulatory standards and to use a client's funds for health care in the most cost-effective manner. In either situation, documentation of occupational therapy services may help determine whether a client's admission and continued treatment are necessary and appropriate.

THE LEGAL SYSTEM

The health record is a legal document that substantiates what occurred during a client's illness and treatment. Any entries made in the health record, whether in print or electronic format, become a part of that legal document and may be subpoenaed (Scott, 2013). If you as an occupational therapy practitioner have to appear in court to testify, it will be helpful if your documentation is clear, accurate, and thorough. Court cases often occur years after the event or intervention that is being contested. You may not even remember the event or the client. What you have written in the health record will provide you with the information you need to testify. However, Scott (2013) explained that "despite its broad range of variegated uses as a legal instrument, healthcare recordkeeping...should not be carried out with a defensive legal focus. Rather, the creation of patient care records should be guided primarily by patient welfare-oriented healthcare principles" (p. 94).

QUALITY MANAGEMENT

Once referred to as *quality assurance*, the more global concept of quality management changes the emphasis "away from the impossible task of 'assuring' quality to continuously striving to improve the quality of health care delivery" (Scott, 2013, p. 162). Depending on your practice setting, this process may be referred to as *quality improvement, quality assessment and improvement, total quality management, performance improvement,* or other similar terms. Many facilities have a quality management committee that is in charge of identifying and addressing problems in client care. The health record is one of the primary sources of information used in the quality management process. An example of a quality management process is the review of occupational therapy documentation to determine whether practitioners were consistently documenting a client's pain level according to hospital policy, followed by the implementation of measures to increase the compliance with the hospital policy. Another example of a quality management process is the review of client care records to determine whether specific standardized assessments were performed for particular populations according to departmental or facility policy.

ACCREDITATION

Health care settings that bill Medicare and/or Medicaid for services must be accredited by a state survey agency or a national accreditation organization approved by the Centers for Medicare and Medicaid Services (CMS) to ensure compliance with applicable laws and regulations (CMS, 2015). Some health care facilities voluntarily seek accreditation from private entities to improve their professional reputation as a provider of quality health care. For example, the Joint Commission, the oldest and largest health care accreditation entity in the United States, accredits approximately 21,000 health care organizations and programs (Joint Commission, 2015a). The Joint Commission accredits hospitals, nursing care centers, home health agencies, ambulatory health care clinics, and behavioral health care programs (Joint Commission, 2015b). The Joint Commission mission is "to continuously improve health care for the public, in collaboration with other stakeholders, by evaluating health care organizations and inspiring them to excel in providing safe and effective care of the highest quality and value" (Joint Commission, 2015a, para. 2). The Commission on Accreditation of Rehabilitation Facilities (CARF) is another accrediting agency that occupational therapy practitioners may encounter. Founded in 1966 in the United States, CARF International now accredits more than 50,000 programs and services worldwide in the areas of aging services, behavioral health, child and youth services, employment and community services, and medical rehabilitation (CARF International, 2015). Accreditation surveyors always rely heavily on the review of client health records during the accreditation survey of a facility.

EDUCATION AND RESEARCH

The health record may be used as a teaching tool. Students in various health care professions use the health record to gain information about a client's medical history and current clinical condition. An occupational therapy student may review the health record to learn about quality occupational therapy intervention or to gain a better understanding of the roles and interventions of other members of the client's health care team.

The health record may also be used to provide data for research by a variety of individuals. Public health entities may use the health record to identify and document the incidence of certain medical conditions. In recent decades, there has been a demand for evidence-based practice in all health care professions, including occupational therapy, to improve patient outcomes and reduce health care costs (Baker & Tickle-Degnen, 2014). For example, researchers may collect and analyze data from the health record to improve methods of disease and injury prevention or to analyze client outcomes to determine efficacy of specific therapeutic interventions. Good documentation practices help ensure that credible and valid data are available to clinical researchers (Bargaje, 2011; Glasse, n.d.).

BUSINESS DEVELOPMENT AND MANAGEMENT

Management teams use the information contained in the health record to plan and market services provided by a facility. For example, are there enough referrals for outpatient occupational therapy driving evaluations to warrant the cost of purchasing expensive assessment equipment and providing specialized training for staff? Does the number of referrals for inpatient occupational therapy following total joint replacement signify the need for additional occupational therapy staffing on the orthopedic unit?

Health care records can also provide a productivity measure of occupational therapy practitioner workload and performance. Productivity is a measure of the amount of billable time in a practitioner's workday. Although many practitioners cringe at the mention of productivity standards, "workload expectations and productivity measurement are legitimate management tools utilized to ensure appropriate staffing resources for service delivery as well as to maximize reimbursement with the goal of achieving economic sustainability" (AOTA Ethics Commission, 2014).

CLIENT ACCESS

Another significant user of the health record is the client. When you are documenting in the health record, always remember that the client owns the information and may choose to exercise his or her right "to inspect, review, and receive a copy" of his or her health record (HHS, 2015b, para. 1). As health care has evolved to a more client-centered, collaborative approach, encouraging and increasing client access to health records can improve the client's sense of control and foster engagement in the health care process (Giardina, Menon, Parrish, Sittig, & Singh, 2014).

A recent trend in the United States is encouraging clients to use a Personal Health Record (PHR), which is a way to organize and manage health information that may be scattered across various health care facilities and providers (HHS, 2015a). Unlike EHRs, PHRs are maintained and controlled by the client rather than the provider and may be kept in either written or electronic form (AHIMA, 2015b). While providers still maintain a health record on each client, the PHR allows the individual to keep health information in an organized fashion for personal reference and for ease of communication with health care providers. A client may choose to include information in his or her PHR about occupational therapy services you have provided.

REFERENCES

Abdelhak, M., Grostick, S., & Hanken, M. A. (2012). *Health information: Management of a strategic resource* (4th ed.). St. Louis, MO: Elsevier.

American Health Information Management Association. (2015a). Get to know AHIMA: Our history. Retrieved from http://www.ahima.org/about/aboutahima.

American Health Information Management Association. (2015b). What is a personal health record (PHR)? Retrieved from http://www.myphr.com/StartaPHR/what_is_a_phr.aspx.

American Occupational Therapy Association. (2015). Occupational therapy Code of Ethics. Retrieved from http://www.aota.org/-/media/corporate/files/practice/ethics/code-of-ethics.pdf

American Occupational Therapy Association Ethics Commission. (2014). Ethical considerations for productivity, billing, and reimbursement. Retrieved from http://www.aota.org/-/media/Corporate/Files/Practice/Ethics/Advisory/reimbursement-productivity.PDF.

Baker, N., & Tickle-Degnen, L. (2014). Evidence-based practice: Integrating evidence to inform practice. In B. A. Boyt Schell, G. Gillen, & M. E. Scaffa (Eds.) *Willard & Spackman's occupational therapy* (12th ed., pp. 398-412). Philadelphia, PA: Lippincott Williams & Wilkins.

Barboza, S., Epps, S., Byington, R., & Keene, S. (2008). HIPAA goes to school: Clarifying privacy laws in the education environment. *The Internet Journal of Law, Healthcare and Ethics, 6*(2), 1-5.

Bargaje, C. (2011). Good documentation practice in clinical research. *Perspectives in Clinical Research, 2*(2), 59-63. doi: 10.4103/2229-3485.80368.

Barnett, S. G., Gallimore, C., Kopacek, K. J., & Porter, A. L. (2014). Evaluation of electronic SOAP note grading and feedback. *Currents in Pharmacy Teaching and Learning, 6*(4), 516-526. doi: 10.1016/j.cptl.2014.04.010.

Centers for Medicare & Medicaid Services. (2015). Accreditation. Retrieved from https://www.cms.gov/Medicare/Provider-Enrollment-and-Certification/SurveyCertificationGenInfo/Accreditation.html.

Clark, J. (2004). *Documentation for acute care*. Chicago, IL: American Health Information Management Association.

Collmer, V. (2015). Navigating the HIPAA security rule: Practical strategies for the occupational therapy practitioner. *OT Practice, 20*(14), 13-16.

Commission on Accreditation of Rehabilitation Facilities International. (2015). Who we are. Retrieved from http://www.carf.org/About/WhoWeAre/.

Freedman, S. (2006). Understand the nuances of utilization review and utilization management. *Managed Healthcare Executive.* Retrieved from http://managedhealthcareexecutive.modernmedicine.com/mhe/article/articleDetail.jsp?id=282713.

Gensel, L. (2005). The medical world of Benjamin Franklin. *Journal of the Royal Society of Medicine, 98*(12), 534-583. doi: 10.1258/jsrm.98.12.534.

Giardina, T. D., Menon S., Parrish D. E., Sittig D. F., & Singh H. (2014). Patient access to medical records and healthcare outcomes: A systematic review. *Journal of the American Medical Informatics Association, 21*(4), 737-741. doi: 10.1136/amia-jnl-2013-002239.

Gillum, R. F. (2013). From papyrus to the electronic tablet: A brief history of the clinical medical record with lessons for the digital age. *The American Journal of Medicine, 126*(10), 853-857. doi: 10.1016/j.amjmed.2013.03.024.

Glasse, A. (n.d.). Good documentation practices: Clinical research operations & regulatory support. Retrieved from http://miami-ictsi.org/documents/Documentation_Practices_in_Clinical_Research.pdf.

Jacobs, L. (2009). Interview with Lawrence Weed, MD: The father of the problem-oriented medical record looks ahead. *The Permanente Journal, 13*(3), 84-89.

Joint Commission. (2015a). About the Joint Commission. Retrieved from http://www.jointcommission.org/about_us/about_the_joint_commission_main.aspx.

Joint Commission. (2015b). What is accreditation? Retrieved from http://www.jointcommission.org/accreditation/accreditation_main.aspx.

Martinez, X. E. (2013). How SOAP notes paved the way for modern medical documentation. Retrieved from http://www.powery-ourpractice.com/electronic-health-records/how-soap-notes-paved-the-way-for-modern-medical-documentation/.

Scott, R. W. (2013). *Legal, ethical, and practical aspects of patient care documentation: A guide for rehabilitation professionals* (4th ed.). Burlington, MA: Jones & Bartlett Learning.

Tripathi, M. (2012). EHR evolution: Policy and legislation forces changing the EHR. *Journal of AHIMA, 83*(10). 24-29.

University of Pennsylvania. (2015). History of Pennsylvania Hospital. Retrieved from http://www.uphs.upenn.edu/paharc/timeline/1751/

U.S. Department of Health & Human Services. (2015a). Personal health records and the HIPAA privacy rule. Retrieved from http://www.hhs.gov/ocr/privacy/hipaa/understanding/special/healthit/phrs.pdf

U.S. Department of Health & Human Services. (2015b). Understanding health information privacy. Retrieved from http://www.hhs.gov/ocr/privacy/hipaa/understanding/index.html

Valdes, K. (2014). How to comply with Medicare documentation requirements for Part B therapy services. Presented at a Summit on Professional Education seminar, Columbia, MO.

3

Reimbursement, Legal, and Ethical Considerations

The previous chapter provided an overview of the various purposes and uses of the health record and the potential impacts on the documentation of occupational therapy practitioners. Some of those issues warrant further explanation and discussion. Because documentation is the primary means of justifying reimbursement for services (Scott, 2013), it is important for occupational therapy practitioners to understand various reimbursement systems and pertinent terminology. Practitioners must be aware of federal and state laws and regulations that affect reimbursement and documentation. It is also necessary to understand the impact of *Official Documents* of the American Occupational Therapy Association (AOTA) on documentation. In addition, it is important to consider the ethical implications that practitioners may encounter regarding the documentation of occupational therapy services. Reimbursement, legal, and ethical issues vary considerably between practice settings, and occupational therapists practice in diverse health care settings (AOTA, 2015a). This chapter will provide a general foundation of information to guide documentation, but practitioners will need to stay up-to-date on federal, state, and organizational policy changes that affect occupational therapy documentation and practice. As Lohman (2014) explained:

> It is important for all therapists, no matter where they work, to understand payment systems that affect practice and to be proactive by being aware of changes that may affect practice. Why? Because obtaining payment is the "bread and butter" of most practices, and therapists should be involved in obtaining optimal payment. This knowledge helps to support clients in their ability to access occupational therapy services. (p. 1052)

PATIENT PROTECTION AND AFFORDABLE CARE ACT

The Patient Protection and Affordable Care Act (PPACA), introduced and implemented during President Barack Obama's time in office, represents "the strongest attempt to date to change our health care system in both the public and private health markets" (Lohman, 2014, p. 1065). The PPACA was developed in response to large numbers of uninsured and underinsured Americans, the rising proportion of health care expenditures by state and federal governments, and health care market inefficiencies. Although the PPACA remains mired in controversy at the time of this writing and uncertainties exist with presidential and congressional changes, many of the concepts introduced in the PPACA will continue to affect occupational therapy practice well into the future.

SOURCES OF REIMBURSEMENT

The following sections will provide a very brief overview of information related to reimbursement from some of the most common sources for occupational therapy payment. Funding sources are continuously revising regulations

Gateley CA, Borcherding S. *Documentation Manual for*
Occupational Therapy: Writing SOAP Notes, Fourth Edition (pp 15-28).
© 2017 SLACK Incorporated

and guidelines. Your fieldwork educator or employer will be an important resource in helping you understand documentation expectations related to reimbursement. Many employers have separate departments to handle billing issues, but you must understand your role in the reimbursement process.

MEDICARE

Medicare is a federal health insurance program managed by the Centers for Medicare & Medicaid Services (CMS, 2015i; Lohman, 2014). Medicare helps pay the health care costs of people over age 65 years, people under age 65 years with certain disabilities, and people with end-stage renal disease. Medicare benefits are divided into four parts (CMS, 2015i):

1. *Part A*: Covers inpatient care in hospitals and critical access hospitals, skilled nursing facilities (SNFs), home health care, and hospice
2. *Part B*: Covers physicians' services and outpatient care, including occupational therapy; also covers services in long-term care facilities when the client does not qualify for coverage under Part A
3. *Part C*: Private insurance companies contract with Medicare to provide individuals with their Part A and Part B benefits through Medicare Advantage Plans.
4. *Part D*: Covers prescription drug costs

People who are eligible for Medicare have a variety of options to consider when selecting their Medicare coverage. Each individual you treat may have different benefits, co-pays, and deductibles depending on the coverage options they have selected. Occupational therapy services may be billed through Medicare Parts A, B, and C. Occupational therapy services covered under Medicare must be medically necessary and skilled (Bogenrief, 2014). *Medically necessary* means that services are consistent with accepted standards of practice for the client's condition. *Skilled* means that the services provided require the decision making and highly complex competencies of an occupational therapist or occupational therapy assistant with a knowledge base of human functioning and occupational performance. Nonskilled services are those that are routine or maintenance-types of therapy, both of which could be carried out by nonprofessional personnel or caregivers. Furthermore, occupational therapy services should result in documentable improvements within a reasonable and predictable period of time based on contemporary practice standards. Because Medicare regulations and guidelines are constantly changing, it is important that you stay abreast of current issues related to Medicare reimbursement for occupational therapy services. Several online resources are available to help you understand Medicare reimbursement:

- CMS website: https://www.cms.gov/
- Medicare website: https://www.medicare.gov/
- AOTA website: http://www.aota.org/

Medicare Part A

Like many other aspects of health care, Medicare underwent significant changes as a result of the PPACA as government officials attempted to reduce rising health care expenditures. Multiple reimbursement systems exist for Medicare Part A recipients (CMS, 2015a, 2015f, 2015k; Lohman, 2014):

- *Fee-For-Service*: In this reimbursement model, health care providers are paid separately for each service provided.
- *Prospective Payment Systems*: Under a Prospective Payment Systems model of reimbursement, Medicare payments are based on a predetermined fixed amount according to a patient's diagnosis-related group.
- *Bundled Payments*: As part of the PPACA, CMS created the Innovation Center "to test innovative payment and service delivery models that have the potential to reduce…expenditures while preserving or enhancing the quality of care for beneficiaries" (CMS, 2015a, para. 3). The Bundled Payments for Care Improvement initiative was introduced to link payments for the multiple services that a Medicare beneficiary receives during an episode of care. "Under the initiative, organizations enter into payment arrangements that include financial and performance accountability for episodes of care. These models may lead to higher quality and more coordinated care at a lower cost to Medicare" (CMS, 2015a, para. 1). At the time of this writing, four different models of reimbursement were being tested in inpatient hospitals, SNFs, inpatient rehabilitation facilities (IRFs), long-term acute care hospitals (LTACs), and home health agencies.

By now you have probably realized that Medicare has a lot of acronyms to describe various aspects health care delivery, documentation, and reimbursement. The following are a few other terms and acronyms that you may encounter if you work with Medicare Part A beneficiaries:

- *Inpatient Rehabilitation Facility—Patient Assessment Instrument (IRF-PAI)*: "The IRF-PAI contains patient clinical, demographic, and other information and classifies the patient into distinct groups based on clinical characteristics and expected resource needs. Separate payments are calculated for each group, including the application of case and facility-level adjustments" (CMS, 2014a).
- *Functional Independence Measure (FIM) Instrument*: Included in the IRF-PAI, the FIM is a seven-level scale to rate a patient's performance in 18 functional activities during their rehabilitation stay (CMS, 2014a, 2014c). Occupational therapists play an important role in documenting a client's performance in activities of daily living and other functional activities. This information is used to help determine the client's scores on the FIM instrument of the IRF-PAI.
- *Long-Term Care Minimum Data Set (MDS)*: SNFs use an assessment tool called the *MDS* to report data about the client's diagnosis, functional status, and time spent in therapy. Since payment is based partly on the amount of time spent in therapy, complete and accurate documentation by the occupational therapist is essential for appropriate reimbursement (CMS, 2015g).
- *Outcome and Assessment Information Set (OASIS)*: This tool is used to collect information about Medicare beneficiaries receiving home health services. "OASIS data are used for multiple purposes including calculating several types of quality reports which are provided to home health agencies to help guide quality and performance improvement efforts" (CMS, 2015d, para. 3). Although typically completed by nursing or other disciplines, in some situations, occupational therapists may be responsible for completing the OASIS at the beginning of a client's home health care services.

Medicare Part B

Medicare Part B covers occupational therapy services in outpatient and long-term care settings. Clients typically have a monthly premium for this supplemental medical coverage, as well as a deductible and a 20% copayment based on the Medicare-approved amount for the service (CMS, 2015f). In addition, CMS establishes therapy caps, or therapy cap limits, on therapy services. Physical therapy and speech-language therapy have a combined yearly cap. Occupational therapy has its own yearly cap. There are exceptions to the cap limit. If the occupational therapy practitioner documents that services above the therapy cap limit were medically reasonable and necessary, clients may qualify for additional services beyond the therapy cap, up to a designated threshold amount. Occupational therapy practitioners must attach a "KX modifier" to claims to request an exception to the cap. "By using the KX modifier, you are attesting that the services above the therapy cap are reasonable and necessary, and that there is documentation of medical necessity for these services in the medical record" (Sandhu, 2014, p. 6). Any services provided above the threshold amount will automatically be reviewed by a Medicare contractor.

If future services are not reasonable and necessary, or if the client is not expected to demonstrate significant functional improvement within a reasonable amount of time, the occupational therapist must provide the Medicare beneficiary with an Advance Beneficiary Notice of Noncoverage (ABN). The ABN informs clients that services are not likely to be paid by Medicare so they can make decisions about whether they want to receive those services and pay for them out of pocket. Valdes (2014) explained that many clients think that, just because a physician has ordered occupational therapy, Medicare will automatically cover those services. However, the responsibility lies with the occupational therapy practitioner to document the functional status and improvement of the client to prove medical necessity.

Medicare Part C

Medicare Part C plans, also known as *Medicare Advantage Plans*, are offered by private Medicare-approved insurance companies, which administer the client's Part A and Part B benefits (CMS, 2015e, 2015f, 2015i). Although these private insurance companies must follow general rules set by Medicare, they may establish their own rules about how clients access various health care services, including occupational therapy. For example, a Medicare Advantage plan can limit which facilities and providers are covered under the plan. Furthermore, insurance companies administering Medicare Advantage plans can set their own out-of-pocket costs such as deductibles and copayments.

MEDICAID AND CHILDREN'S HEALTH INSURANCE PLAN

Medicaid is a health insurance program jointly funded by the federal government and each individual state (CMS, 2015h, 2015j; Lohman, 2014). It covers individuals who have limited income and meet certain eligibility requirements. Medicaid is administered by each individual state. While all states must follow general federal guidelines, there is considerable variance between states in terms of which individuals are eligible for Medicaid and what services are covered. There may also be differences within a single state between services that are covered by Medicaid for adults versus children. The Children's Health Insurance Plan (CHIP) is another program jointly funded by federal and state government that provides health insurance coverage to children in families who earn too much to qualify for Medicaid. Like Medicaid, CHIP coverage and benefits vary by state. Occupational therapists must become familiar with documentation and reimbursement guidelines for the state in which they are practicing.

PRIVATE INSURANCE

An individual may have private health insurance through his or her employer or through the employer of his or her spouse or parent. The cost of such plans is often subsidized by the employer. In an effort to reduce the number of uninsured individuals in the United States, the PPACA required the establishment of health insurance marketplaces that allow individuals and small business to purchase private health insurance (AOTA, 2015b). There are many different private insurance plans with varying coverage, and there may be specific requirements that must be followed for the insurance company to pay for health care services. These requirements may include seeking health care from only particular providers considered "in network," getting "preauthorization" or prior approval before seeing a health care provider, and limiting the number of visits per year to a particular type of provider (CMS, 2015b). Many health care settings have individuals whose role is to deal with these insurance issues, but occupational therapists may have more direct involvement in the process in some settings. Documentation must meet the requirements of the individual practice setting, and there may be additional documentation required for a client's specific insurance plan.

WORKER'S COMPENSATION

Worker's compensation is a type of business insurance that covers the medical expenses and wages of employees who are injured on the job. Each state has different requirements for its worker's compensation program (AOTA, 2015k). Occupational therapy may be a service covered under the medical expenses of the program. When a client has worker's compensation as the funding source, therapeutic interventions and documentation should focus on improving the individual's capacity to return to work. In some cases, occupational therapists may be called upon to conduct ergonomic assessments to determine if a client's injury, disease, or condition is work related or the result of a pre-existing or concurrent medical condition (Zuccarello, 2010).

SCHOOLS

Part B of the Individuals with Disabilities Education Act (IDEA) of 2004 requires schools to provide students with disabilities a free appropriate public education in the least restrictive environment. The law applies to students aged 3 through 21 years (Mulligan, 2014). Section 504 of the Rehabilitation Act of 1973 and Title II of the Americans with Disabilities Act of 1990 prohibit schools from excluding a student with a disability from participating in educational activities (AOTA, 2011). Occupational therapists may be asked to provide direct services to help a child meet his or her educational goals. They may also be asked to provide consultative services to help the school determine necessary modifications and accommodations. Schools use an Individualized Education Program to document the student's educational needs, goals, and services (Mulligan, 2014). Documentation requirements vary from school to school, but the services provided must be relevant to the educational setting (AOTA, 2011; Mulligan, 2014). In some cases, school-based services may be covered by Medicaid. In such cases, services must meet requirements of both educational relevance and medical necessity (AOTA, 2011, p. S47).

EARLY INTERVENTION PROGRAMS

The Early Intervention Program for Infants and Toddlers with Disabilities (Part C of IDEA) is a federal grant program that assists states in operating a program of early intervention services for infants and toddlers from birth through 2 years of age, along with their families. The program targets children who have a diagnosis associated with developmental delay and children who are deemed at risk for developmental delay. A major provision of Part C is that services are to be provided in a child's natural environment. These include the child's home and community settings that are typical for children without disabilities, such as preschools, daycare centers, and other community settings. Eligibility requirements vary between states based on each state's definition of developmental delays, established risks (e.g., specific diagnoses known to be associated with delays), and potential risk factors for developmental problems (Mulligan, 2014). Just as some school-based services are covered by Medicaid, occupational therapy services provided through early intervention programs may also be covered by Medicaid (AOTA, 2011). Each child served in an early intervention program will have an Individualized Family Service Plan (IFSP) that includes the family's strengths, concerns, and priorities for the child (Mulligan, 2014). Occupational therapy is one of the many services that may be provided as part of the IFSP, and documentation requirements vary across states.

Billing Codes

Occupational therapy practitioners will encounter multiple coding systems as part of their documentation and billing processes. These coding systems are intended to provide a standard language between health care providers and reimbursement sources for describing a client's diagnosis and the services provided (U.S. Department of Health & Human Services [HHS], 2015b). It should be noted that the coding systems described in this section are updated frequently, and practitioners must keep track of changes that may affect their documentation.

ICD-10 Codes

The World Health Organization developed the *International Classification of Diseases* (ICD) in the 1970s as a coding system for signs, symptoms, injuries, diseases, and conditions (Mullin, 1999). The current ICD-10 classification system consists of two parts (HHS, 2015a, 2015b):

1. *ICD-10-CM (Clinical Modification)*: These are diagnosis codes consisting of three to seven alpha and numeric digits. These codes allow a high degree of specificity about a client's condition.
   - Example: I69.351—Sequelae of cerebral infarction, hemiplegia, and hemiparesis affecting right dominant side
2. *ICD-10-PCS (Procedure Classification System)*: These are the codes used to bill for services in inpatient hospital settings only. Like the diagnosis codes, the procedure codes allow for a high degree of specificity.
   - Example: F0FZ1FZ—Caregiver training in dressing using assistive, adaptive, supportive, or protective equipment (Alkaline Software, 2015)

In most hospital and clinic settings, there are individuals or entire departments whose responsibility it is to review documentation and ensure that applicable codes were included in a client's health record and related billing documentation. However, those individuals rely on the detailed documentation of health professionals, including occupational therapy practitioners, to assign the appropriate codes.

Current Procedural Terminology Codes

Current Procedural Terminology (CPT) codes are owned and copyrighted by the American Medical Association (AMA, 2015). The codes are a standardized listing of descriptive and identifying terms for reporting medical services and procedures. CMS adopted the use of CPT codes in 1983 as the mandatory system of coding services under Medicare Part B. CPT codes, also known as *HCPCS Level I codes*, comprise one of the subsystems of the Healthcare Common Procedure Coding System used by Medicare and other health insurance programs to process health care claims. Most managed care and private insurance companies also base their reimbursements on the CPT values established by CMS. CPT codes are continuously reviewed, and new and revised CPT codes are published yearly. Some codes may be deleted and others added. Furthermore, the AMA collaborates with AOTA and other organizations to recommend values per code based on "the mental effort and judgment, technical skill, and psychological stress in providing the service" (AOTA, 2015j, para. 4). It is the responsibility of each occupational therapy practitioner and employer to understand the current codes that may be assigned for services provided. Each year, AOTA provides members with a list of CPT codes from AMA of the most frequently used codes by occupational therapy practitioners to classify and bill for services. The following are just a few of those common codes. Please note that this list is not all-inclusive (AMA, 2013):

- 97003   Occupational therapy evaluation
- 97004   Occupational therapy re-evaluation
- 97110   Therapeutic procedure (therapeutic exercises)
- 97112   Neuromuscular re-education
- 97530   Therapeutic activities

- ◆ 97532   Development of cognitive skills
- ◆ 97533   Sensory integrative techniques
- ◆ 97535   Self-care/home management training
- ◆ 97537   Community/work reintegration
- ◆ 97542   Wheelchair management (assessment, fitting, training)
- ◆ 97545   Work hardening/conditioning
- ◆ 97760   Orthotic management/training
- ◆ 97761   Prosthetic management/training

Besides determining which code to assign for services provided, occupational therapy practitioners must also have a clear understanding of the guidelines for using each code. For example, many codes can be billed in 15-minute units, while other codes can only be billed once regardless of time spent providing the service. There are also restrictions regarding codes that can be billed within the same therapy session to prevent funding sources from paying for overlapping services. CMS provides a National Correct Coding Initiative (NCCI) list of codes that may overlap. However, occupational therapists may bill for two codes on the NCCI list by adding an additional billing modifier to the claim:

> Modifier 59 is used by occupational therapists to indicate that two codes from the NCCI list are actually distinct procedural services. Documentation should support the modifier by documenting: (1) a different session, (2) a different procedure, (3) a different site or organ system, (4) service not ordinarily performed by the same occupational therapist on the same day. (AOTA, 2015c, para. 3)

HCPCS LEVEL II CODES

Whereas CPT codes identify *services and procedures* provided by health care professionals, including occupational therapists, HCPCS Level II codes identify *products and supplies* such as durable medical equipment, orthotics, and prosthetics (CMS, 2015c). Similar to the use of CPT codes, occupational therapy practitioners may encounter certain limitations from payer sources and state regulatory agencies for particular HCPCS Level II codes. Furthermore, you should be aware that not all codes are accepted by Medicare and other payers. Providing a product and bill does not guarantee that the client's funding source will pay for that product. "Always review state rules, the official HCPCS book, and request information from specific insurers concerning use of codes and payment policy" (AOTA, 2015f, para. 1). Here are two examples of HCPCS Level II codes that occupational therapy practitioners may use in various settings:

1. L3650—Shoulder Orthosis, figure of eight design abduction restrainer, prefabricated, off-the-shelf
2. L3906—Wrist-Hand Orthosis, without joints, custom fabricated, includes fitting and adjustment

G-CODES

Occupational therapists billing Medicare Part B for outpatient therapy services must report functional data for clients on their claims to be reimbursed for services. These codes may also be used in hospital settings when a patient's length of stay does not cross two midnights, thus making it an outpatient or observation stay. "Functional data reporting takes the form of new G-codes, which identify the primary issue being addressed by therapy, and modifiers that reflect the patient's impairment, limitation, or restriction" (AOTA, 2015e, para. 1). Medicare uses these data to track achievement of patient goals over time. CMS will reject submitted claims that do not have the required G-codes and modifiers. See Tables 3-1 and 3-2 for a list of G-code categories and modifiers. G-codes are not discipline specific, and occupational therapists "should select the G-code set for the functional limitation that most closely relates to the primary functional limitation being treated" (AOTA, 2013a, para. 5). Although some codes are typically reported by specific disciplines, AOTA encourages practitioners to use codes that reflect the full scope of occupational therapy practice, including memory, attention, and swallowing. It is also important to be familiar with all of the codes to better understand a client's functional status as reported in the documentation of your rehabilitation colleagues in outpatient settings.

Table 3-1

G-Code Categories of Functional Limitations

G-Code Category	Current Status	Goal Status	Discharge Status
Mobility: Walking and Moving Around	G8978	G8979	G8980
Changing and Maintaining Body Position	G8981	G8982	G8983
Carrying, Moving, and Handling Objects	G8984	G8985	G8986
Self-Care	G8987	G8988	G8989
Other PT/OT Primary	G8990	G8991	G8992
Other PT/OT Subsequent	G8993	G8994	G8995
Swallowing	G8996	G8997	G8998
Motor Speech	G8999	G9186	G9158
Spoken Language Comprehension	G9159	G9160	G9161
Spoken Language Expression	G9162	G9163	G9164
Attention	G9165	G9166	G9167
Memory	G9168	G9169	G9170
Voice	G9171	G9172	G9173
Other SLP	G9174	G9175	G9176

Abbreviations: OT, occupational therapy; PT, physical therapy; SLP, speech-language pathology.

Adapted from *Quick Reference Chart: Short & Long Descriptors for Therapy Functional Reporting G-codes.* (CMS, 2012).

Table 3-2

G-Code Modifiers to Indicate Level of Functional Limitation

Severity/Complexity Modifier for G-Code Functional Limitation	Client's Percentage of Functional Impairment, Limitation, or Restriction
CH	0%
CI	1% to 19%
CJ	20% to 39%
CK	40% to 59%
CL	60% to 79%
CM	80% to 99%
CN	100%

Adapted from *Quick Reference Chart: Short & Long Descriptors for Therapy Functional Reporting G-codes.* (CMS, 2012).

AOTA (2015g) published *Selected Tools for Occupational Therapy Reporting of Outpatient Functional Data (G-Codes and Modifiers) to the Medicare Program.* This document lists several standardized assessment tools that can be used to assess client functional status for the G-code categories used most frequently by occupational therapists. However, AOTA reiterated that:

> Occupational therapists are not required by CMS to use a specific functional outcome assessment tool in the selection of a G-code or a modifier, and AOTA is not recommending the use of any one tool or instrument. When selecting a G-code, a therapist is to rely on his/her clinical and professional judgment. (AOTA, 2015g, p. 3)

CMS sets the guidelines for functional reporting, and these may change from year to year. Occupational therapy practitioners must remain informed about current CMS guidelines. AOTA also provides a summary of the guidelines for when G-codes and modifiers must be reported (AOTA, 2013a):

- On the initial date of service for a new therapy episode of care
- At least once every 10 treatment days
- When an evaluation procedure is provided and billed (CPT codes 97003 and 97004)
- When the client is discharged from a therapy episode of care
- When a particular functional limitation has ended, but more therapy is necessary
- When a new functional limitation is being reported

LEGAL, REGULATORY, AND ETHICAL GUIDELINES

Occupational therapy practitioners must be aware of legal, regulatory, and ethical standards that affect documentation. The AOTA publishes several *Official Documents* that guide occupational therapy practice and have direct implications on documentation. In addition, each state has a practice act that further regulates occupational therapy practice. This section will highlight the key points of several documents that affect the documentation of occupational therapy practitioners. Keep in mind that AOTA *Official Documents* are revised approximately every 5 years, and state practice acts may be updated annually. Occupational therapy practitioners must be familiar with the most current documents available.

SCOPE OF PRACTICE

This document delineates the domain and process of occupational therapy practice and describes the educational and certification requirements for occupational therapy practitioners. Occupational therapy is defined as "the therapeutic use of everyday life activities (occupations) with individuals or groups for the purpose of enhancing or enabling participation in roles, habits, and routines in home, school, workplace, community, and other settings" (AOTA, 2014c, p. S35). Documentation should demonstrate that the services provided to a client fall within the scope of practice for the occupational therapy profession. Furthermore, practitioners must abide by state laws for licensure, continuing education, and supervision. Such laws may affect the credentials included in a practitioner's signature on documentation and the type of documentation required to reflect that appropriate supervision has been provided to occupational therapy assistants during the delivery of services.

STANDARDS OF PRACTICE FOR OCCUPATIONAL THERAPY

This document defines the standards that must be met to practice as an occupational therapist or occupational therapy assistant (AOTA, 2015h). It outlines the education, examination, and licensure requirements for occupational therapy practitioners. The document goes on to clarify professional roles during the process of service delivery and states that documentation must meet the "time frames, formats, and standards established by practice settings, federal and state law, other regulatory and payer requirements, external accreditation programs, and AOTA documents" (AOTA, 2015h, p. 4).

GUIDELINES FOR SUPERVISION, ROLES, AND RESPONSIBILITIES DURING THE DELIVERY OF OCCUPATIONAL THERAPY SERVICES

This document outlines the roles, responsibilities, and supervision requirements of occupational therapists, occupational therapy assistants, and occupational therapy aides in the provision of occupational therapy services, including documentation practice (AOTA, 2014a).

Occupational Therapists

Occupational therapists are considered autonomous practitioners, meaning they are independent of all aspects of service delivery, including documentation of the evaluation, intervention plan, intervention implementation, and outcomes. Occupational therapists initiate and direct the evaluation, interpret the data, develop and direct the intervention plan, modify or discontinue the intervention plan when appropriate, and interpret outcomes of a client's occupational performance. They collaborate with occupational therapy assistants by delegating selected assessments and interventions and exchanging information throughout the evaluation and intervention process. Documentation should reflect an occupational therapist's involvement throughout the delivery of occupational therapy services.

Occupational Therapy Assistants

Occupational therapy assistants must deliver services under the supervision of an occupational therapist. The amount of supervision that must be provided will vary depending on the state of practice and funding source. Occupational therapy assistants may contribute to the evaluation process by implementing assessments that have been delegated by the occupational therapist and providing verbal and written reports of the client's performance to the occupational therapist. They may collaborate with the occupational therapist during the development of the intervention plan. They are responsible for knowing the client's occupational therapy goals and targeted outcomes, and provide written documentation and verbal reports to the occupational therapist about the client's progress toward those goals and outcomes. Finally, in collaboration with the supervising occupational therapist, occupational therapy assistants select, implement, and modify "occupational therapy interventions, including, but not limited to, occupations and activities, preparatory methods and tasks, client education and training, and group interventions consistent with demonstrated competency levels, client goals, and the requirements of the practice setting" (AOTA, 2014a, p. S20). Their accompanying documentation should reflect that all guidelines have been followed throughout the delivery of occupational therapy services.

Occupational Therapy Aides

Occupational therapy aides provide supportive non-skilled services specifically delegated by the occupational therapist or occupational therapy assistant. Ultimately, the occupational therapist is responsible for the use and actions of the aide, but aides may be supervised by the occupational therapy assistant. Aides may provide non–client-related tasks such as clerical, maintenance, and work area or equipment preparation. They may also perform routine client-related tasks under stable, predictable circumstances if they have previously demonstrated competence in the task. Occupational therapy practitioners must adhere to state and payer regulations when using aides and documenting the services provided by an aide.

Occupational Therapy Students and Occupational Therapy Assistant Students

Although not addressed in an *Official Document*, AOTA has issued clarification of the supervision requirements for students when occupational therapy services are billed under Medicare. State laws and facility guidelines may be even more restrictive. The supervision requirements summarized by AOTA (2013b) are as follows:

- *Medicare Part A—Hospital and Inpatient Rehabilitation*: No specific CMS rules; state laws should be followed.
- *Medicare Part A—SNF*: Services of an occupational therapy student and/or occupational therapy assistant student may be recorded on the MDS as minutes of therapy received by the client. CMS no longer requires that services be provided within the line-of-sight of an occupational therapist. "Supervising therapists and therapy assistants…must determine whether or not a student is ready to treat patients without line-of-sight supervision. The supervising therapist/assistant may not be engaged in any other activity or treatment, with the exception of documenting" (AOTA, 2013b, p. 2). Supervising therapists and therapy assistants should be physically present in the facility and immediately available for guidance as needed by the student.

- *Medicare Part A—Hospice*: No specific CMS rules; state laws should be followed. AOTA recommends that the approach for Part A inpatient settings be followed.
- *Medicare Part A—Home Health*: CMS regulations define "qualified personnel" who may provide and bill for home health services. Students are not included in the definition of qualified personnel. AOTA offered the following clarification: "CMS has not issued specific restrictions regarding students providing services in conjunction with a qualified OT or OTA. Services can be provided (as allowed by state law) as part of a home health visit, when the student is supervised by an OT or OTA in the home" (AOTA, 2013b, p 3).
- *Medicare Part B—Outpatient/SNF/Home Health Part B*: There are very specific rules regarding the use of occupational therapy students in the provision of services under Part B reimbursement. "Services performed by a student are not reimbursed under Medicare Part B," regardless of whether the services were provided under direct or line-of-sight supervision (CMS, 2001, p. 1). However, the presence of an occupational therapy student in the room does not make the services unbillable. AOTA has further explained that students can assist a qualified practitioner in the provision of occupational therapy services. "Students can participate in the delivery of services when the qualified practitioner (OT) is directing the service, making the skilled judgment, responsible for the assessment and treatment in the same room as the student, and not simultaneously treating another patient. The qualified practitioner is solely responsible and must sign all documentation" (AOTA, 2013b, p. 2).

GUIDELINES FOR DOCUMENTATION OF OCCUPATIONAL THERAPY

This document articulates the purposes of documentation, explains different types of documentation, and lists the fundamental elements that should be present in all occupational therapy documentation. There should be documentation any time occupational therapy services are provided to a client. The term *client* may be used to describe an individual, group, or population as defined in the *OTPF-III* (AOTA, 2014b). According to the *Guidelines for Documentation of Occupational Therapy*, "the purpose of documentation is to:

- Communicate information about the client from the occupational therapy perspective;
- Articulate the rationale for provision of occupational therapy services and the relationship of those service to client outcomes, reflecting the occupational therapy practitioner's clinical reasoning and professional judgment; and
- Create a chronological record of client status, occupational therapy services provided to the client, client response to occupational therapy intervention, and outcomes" (AOTA, 2013c, p. S32).

There are several different types of documentation that occur throughout the occupational therapy process of screening, evaluation, intervention, and outcomes. They include the following:

- Screening report
- Evaluation report
- Re-evaluation report
- Intervention plan
- Contact report
- Progress report
- Transition plan
- Discharge or discontinuation report (AOTA, 2013c)

The different types of documentation will be explained in more detail in Chapter 13. Regardless of the type of documentation, there are several essential elements that must be present in all documentation:

- Client's full name and case number (if applicable)
- Date and type of occupational therapy contact
- Type of documentation; name of agency and department
- Signature immediately after the documentation with practitioner's name and professional credentials
- Cosignature of documentation by students in accordance with payer policy, state laws, and facility standards
- Terminology and abbreviations acceptable to the setting
- All errors noted and signed
- Adherence to professional standards regarding technology used for purposes of documentation
- Compliance with confidentiality standards
- Compliance with legal and agency requirements for storage and disposal of records

◆ "Documentation should reflect professional clinical reasoning and expertise of an occupational therapy practitioner and the nature of occupational therapy services delivered in a safe and effective manner. The client's diagnosis or prognosis should not be the sole rationale for occupational therapy services" (AOTA, 2013c, p. S37).

OCCUPATIONAL THERAPY CODE OF ETHICS AND ETHICS STANDARDS

This document is based on the core values of the occupational therapy profession and outlines the principles intended to promote and maintain high professional standards of conduct. It is intended to guide decision making when ethical issues arise. In simple terms, practitioners must always consider the implications of their decisions and actions on occupational therapy clients. The six principles and standards of conduct are summarized as follows (AOTA 2015d):

1. *Beneficence*: Practitioners will demonstrate concern for the safety and well-being of their clients.
2. *Nonmaleficence*: Practitioners will not harm or impose risks of harm for their clients.
3. *Autonomy*: Practitioners will collaborate with clients to determine goals, obtain informed consent for services, respect the client's right to refuse services, and protect all confidential information.
4. *Justice*: Practitioners will provide fair, unbiased, and equitable services to their clients.
5. *Veracity*: Practitioners will provide objective, accurate information in all forms of communication and avoid communication that is false, fraudulent, or deceptive.
6. *Fidelity*: Practitioners will demonstrate respect, fairness, discretion, and integrity in all professional relationships.

These ethical principles have many direct implications for documentation of occupational therapy services. An individualized evaluation and plan of care should be documented for each client, and the collaborative process between practitioner and client must be well documented. Documentation and accompanying billing must accurately reflect the services that were provided and must be in compliance with applicable laws, guidelines, and regulations. Documentation must include accurate credentials of the practitioner providing service and a description of appropriate levels of supervision during service delivery when applicable to comply with legal and facility guidelines. Documentation should not contain false information or fabricated data, and practitioners must keep documentation confidential at all times.

PRACTICE ACTS

Each state regulates the practice of occupational therapy. State practice acts address issues such as scope of occupational therapy practice, qualifications and licensure requirements, continuing competence, supervision of students and occupational therapy personnel, and referral requirements (AOTA, 2015i). Each of these issues may have either direct or indirect implications on a practitioner's documentation, and it is the responsibility of each practitioner to know and abide by statutes that govern occupational therapy practice.

REIMBURSEMENT, LEGAL, AND ETHICAL ISSUES

When practitioners do not abide by all of the guidelines presented in this chapter that affect practice and documentation, they may encounter unfortunate reimbursement, legal, and ethical situations. In some cases, even those practitioners who consistently meet all guidelines still find themselves in unfortunate situations. Some of the common situations involving occupational therapy documentation will be discussed in this section.

REIMBURSEMENT DENIALS

Medicare and other reimbursement sources look at health care documentation with increasing scrutiny when determining whether billed services will be reimbursed. Appealing a reimbursement denial requires valuable time and resources. Denials can often be avoided by consistently providing thorough documentation that meets all necessary requirements. Valdes (2014), Scott (2013), and Brennan (2015) listed several reasons for reimbursement denials by Medicare and other payers related to occupational therapy documentation:

◆ Use of abbreviations unknown to the claim reviewer
◆ Illegible documentation
◆ Incomplete documentation (patient name, signatures, dates, minutes of treatment)

- Missing physician order or signed plan of care
- Lack of support for billing codes
- Failure to document progress within reasonable time frame
- Skilled care not justified
- Lack of support for medical necessity
- Standardized scores reported without interpretation of functional impact for client
- Repetitive documentation between sessions with no evidence of significant improvement
- Excessive duration of sessions and/or duration of care
- Excessive use of KX modifiers to override therapy caps
- Lack of required co-signatures for students and/or therapy assistants
- Lack of thorough explanation of client's comorbidities and prior/current functional status
- Failure to document rationale for changing intervention plan or frequency/duration of treatment
- Too much emphasis on client factors (e.g., strength, range of motion) without relation to function
- Documentation suggests duplication of service with another discipline

BILLING FRAUD AND ABUSE

Scott (2013) defined fraud as "a false misrepresentation of a material fact, made with the intent to deceive, which causes another person to take some action detrimental to his or her own (or the public's) interest" (p. 210). Examples of billing practices that may constitute fraud include knowingly filing claims for services that were not rendered and knowingly billing for services at a higher complexity level than what was provided, such as billing for individual occupational therapy services when multiple clients were treated simultaneously. CMS (2014b) cautioned that "committing Medicare fraud exposes individuals and entities to potential criminal and civil remedies, including imprisonment, fines, and penalties....Providers and health care organizations that commit health care fraud risk exclusion from participation in Federal health care programs and the loss of their professional licenses" (p. 3).

CMS described abuse as "practices that, either directly or indirectly, result in unnecessary costs to the Medicare Program" (CMS, 2014b, p. 3). Examples include billing for services that were not medically necessary, charging excessively for services or supplies, and misuse of codes to maximize reimbursement. Occupational therapy practitioners must be diligent in documenting and billing for their services appropriately to avoid claims of fraud and abuse.

MALPRACTICE AND OTHER LEGAL CLAIMS

Health care malpractice claims may result from professional negligence, breach of client-professional contractual promise, liability for defective equipment or abnormally dangerous care-related activities that cause injury, or intentional misconduct. From a legal perspective, the documentation that appears in a client's health record is often considered the best evidence of what transpired between the client and health care provider. It is essential that occupational therapy practitioners document client interactions accurately and completely. If an occupational therapy practitioner is found guilty of malpractice, he or she may face serious consequences, including monetary loss, loss of reputation, and state and/or federal punitive action including loss of license to practice (Scott, 2013).

ETHICAL DILEMMAS

Many occupational therapy practitioners will encounter ethical dilemmas involving their documentation at some point in their careers. For example, suppose it is time to provide a progress note to a client's insurance company to request authorization for additional outpatient visits. In your opinion, the client has made great progress and really does not need any additional services, but the client tells you that she hopes she can keep seeing you for a few more weeks so she can get even stronger. While you always have the client's best interests in mind, you should never falsify or withhold information about a client's performance in your documentation.

The issue of productivity expectations can also lead to ethical dilemmas. Productivity is measured by comparing the number of units or minutes billed to the number of hours worked (Yamkovenko, 2014). Many settings have stringent productivity targets with the expectation that clients will be treated concurrently or in groups. While treating multiple clients simultaneously is not unethical, the services must be documented and billed appropriately. Occupational therapy practitioners may find themselves torn between meeting the productivity expectations of their employer and providing quality, individualized care to their clients. In 2014, AOTA, along with the professional associations for physical therapy and speech-language therapy, drafted the Consensus Statement on Clinical Judgment in Health Care Settings. This document reiterated the importance of clinical judgment and expertise in providing optimal client care. "Overriding or ignoring clinical judgment through administrative mandates, employer pressure to meet quotas, or inappropriate productivity standards may be a violation of payer rules, may be in conflict with state licensure laws, and may even constitute fraud" (AOTA, American Physical Therapy Association, & American Speech-Language-Hearing Association, 2014, p. 1). Examples of ethical issues related to occupational therapy practice and documentation include the following:

- Placing or keeping clients on caseload who do not need skilled services or meet payer coverage criteria
- Administrative mandates regarding treatment frequency, duration, or intensity
- Providing treatment without client consent
- Counting non-billable time as treatment time
- Inappropriate coding or changes to coding without approval of the treating therapist
- Falsifying or changing documentation to misrepresent services delivered or time spent with client

The Consensus Statement listed the following suggestions for therapy practitioners who find themselves faced with ethical dilemmas such as those listed previously:

- Stop the questionable practice
- Contact an administrator or corporate compliance officer for the facility
- Contact state and national professional associations for guidance (i.e., AOTA)
- Consider seeking legal counsel
- If appropriate, consider reporting information to CMS or the Office of the Inspector General for the HHS

REFERENCES

Alkaline Software. (2015). ICD-10-PCS: Physical rehabilitation and diagnostic audiology. Retrieved from http://www.icd10data. com.

American Medical Association. (2013). 2015 CPT codes for occupational therapy. Retrieved from http://www.aota.org.

American Medical Association. (2015). CPT – Current Procedural Terminology. Retrieved from http://www.ama-assn.org.

American Occupational Therapy Association. (2011). Occupational therapy services in early childhood and school-based settings. *American Journal of Occupational Therapy, 65*(Suppl.), S46-S54.

American Occupational Therapy Association. (2013a). Functional data collection requirements for outpatient therapy. Retrieved from http://www.aota.org.

American Occupational Therapy Association. (2013b). OT/OTA student supervision & Medicare requirements. Retrieved from http://www.aota.org.

American Occupational Therapy Association. (2013c). Guidelines for documentation of occupational therapy. *American Journal of Occupational Therapy, 67*(Suppl.), S32-S38. doi: 10.5014/ajot.2013.67S32.

American Occupational Therapy Association. (2014a). Guidelines for supervision, roles, and responsibilities during the delivery of occupational therapy services. *American Journal of Occupational Therapy, 68*(Suppl.), S16-S22. doi: 10.5014/ajot.2014.686S03.

American Occupational Therapy Association. (2014b). *Occupational therapy practice framework: Domain & process* (3rd ed.). Bethesda, MD: AOTA Press.

American Occupational Therapy Association. (2014c). Scope of practice. *American Journal of Occupational Therapy, 68*(Suppl.), S34-S40. doi: 10.5014/ajot.2014.686S04.

American Occupational Therapy Association. (2015a). 2015 American Occupational Therapy Association salary & workforce survey: Executive summary. Retrieved from http:/www.aota.org.

American Occupational Therapy Association. (2015b). Health insurance marketplaces/exchanges. Retrieved from http://www. aota.org.

American Occupational Therapy Association. (2015c). Occupational therapists should continue Modifier 59 use. Retrieved from http://www.aota.org.

American Occupational Therapy Association. (2015d). Occupational therapy code of ethics. *American Journal of Occupational Therapy, 69*(Suppl. 3), 691341003, 1-8. doi:10.5014/ajot.2015.696S03.

American Occupational Therapy Association. (2015e). Resources for G-Code functional data reporting. Retrieved from http:// www.aota.org.

American Occupational Therapy Association. (2015f). Selected 2015 HCPCS Level II codes. Retrieved from http://www.aota.org.

American Occupational Therapy Association. (2015g). Selected assessment tools for occupational therapy reporting of outpatient functional data (G-codes and modifiers) to the Medicare program. Retrieved from http://www.aota.org.

American Occupational Therapy Association. (2015h). Standards of practice for occupational therapy. *American Journal of Occupational Therapy, 69*(Suppl.), 6913410057, 1-6. doi: 10.5014/ajot.2015.696S06.

American Occupational Therapy Association. (2015i). State OT statutes and regulations. Retrieved from http://www.aota.org.

American Occupational Therapy Association. (2015j). Survey on evaluation and re-evaluation Current Procedural Terminology codes. Retrieved from http://www.aota.org.

American Occupational Therapy Association. (2015k). Worker's compensation. Retrieved from http://www.aota.org.

American Occupational Therapy Association, American Physical Therapy Association, and American Speech-Language-Hearing Association. (2014). Consensus statement on clinical judgment in healthcare settings. Retrieved from http://www.aota.org.

Bogenrief, J. B. (2014, September). Medicare Part A update. Presentation at AOTA Specialty Conference on Effective Documentation, Alexandria, VA. Retrieved from http://www.aota.org.

Brennan, C. (2015). The do's & don'ts of documentation. *OT Practice, 20*(15), 8-11.

Centers for Medicare & Medicaid Services. (2001). Program memorandum: Questions and answers regarding payment for the services of therapy students under Part B of Medicare. Retrieved from https://www.cms.gov.

Centers for Medicare & Medicaid Services. (2012). Quick reference chart: Short & long descriptors for therapy functional reporting G-codes. Retrieved from https://www.cms.gov.

Centers for Medicare & Medicaid Services. (2014a). IRF-PAI training manual. Retrieved from https://www.cms.gov.

Center for Medicare & Medicaid Services. (2014b). Medicare fraud & abuse: Prevention, detection, and reporting. Retrieved from https://www.cms.gov.

Centers for Medicare & Medicaid Services. (2014c). Payment system fact sheet series: Inpatient Rehabilitation Facility Prospective Payment System. Retrieved from https://www.cms.gov.

Centers for Medicare & Medicaid Services. (2015a). Bundled Payments for Care Improvement (BPCI) initiative: General information. Retrieved from http://innovation.cms.gov.

Centers for Medicare & Medicaid Services. (2015b). Glossary. Retrieved from https://www.healthcare.gov.

Centers for Medicare & Medicaid Services. (2015c). HCPCS: General information. Retrieved from https://www.cms.gov.

Centers for Medicare & Medicaid Services. (2015d). Home health quality initiative. Retrieved from https://www.cms.gov.

Centers for Medicare & Medicaid Services. (2015e). How do Medicare Advantage plans work? Retrieved from https://www.medicare.gov.

Centers for Medicare & Medicaid Services. (2015f). How plans work. Retrieved from https://www.medicare.gov.

Centers for Medicare & Medicaid Services. (2015g). MDS 3.0 for nursing homes and swing bed providers. Retrieved from http://cms.gov.

Centers for Medicare & Medicaid Services. (2015h). Medicaid eligibility. Retrieved from http://www.medicaid.gov.

Centers for Medicare & Medicaid Services. (2015i). Medicare program: General information. Retrieved from https://www.cms.gov.

Centers for Medicare & Medicaid Services. (2015j). The Children's Health Insurance Program (CHIP). Retrieved from https://www.healthcare.gov.

Centers for Medicare & Medicaid Services. (2015k). Your Medicare coverage: Physical therapy / occupational therapy/speech-language pathology services. Retrieved from https://www.medicare.gov.

Lohman, H. (2014). Payment for service in the United States. In B. A. Boyt Schell, G. Gillen, & M. E. Scaffa (Eds.) *Willard & Spackman's occupational therapy* (12th ed., pp. 1051-1067). Philadelphia, PA: Lippincott Williams & Wilkins.

Mulligan, S. (2014). *Occupational therapy evaluation for children: A pocket guide* (2nd ed.). Philadelphia, PA: Lippincott Williams & Wilkins.

Mullin, R. (1999). A brief history of ICD-10-PCS. *Journal of AHIMA, 70*(9), 97-98.

Sandhu, S. (2014). What will Medicare Part B changes mean for you in 2015? *OT Practice, 19*(22),6.

Scott, R. W. (2013). *Legal, ethical, and practical aspects of patient care documentation: A guide for rehabilitation professionals* (4th ed.). Burlington, MA: Jones & Bartlett Learning.

U.S. Department of Health & Human Services. (2015a). Basic introduction to ICD-10-CM. Retrieved from https://www.cms.gov.

U.S. Department of Health & Human Services. (2015b). ICD-10-CM/CPS: The next generation of coding. Retrieved from https://www.cms.gov

Valdes, K. (2014). How to comply with Medicare documentation requirements for part B therapy services. Presented at the Summit on Professional Education seminar, Columbia, MO.

Yamkovenko, S. (2014). How are you dealing with productivity? Retrieved from http://otconnections.aota.org/aota_blogs.

Zuccarello, V. (2010). The use of ergonomic analysis in medical causation cases to support or debunk compensability claims for musculoskeletal disorders. *Special Interest Section Quarterly: Work & Industry, 24*(3), 1-4.

General Guidelines for Documentation

The first three chapters of this book have detailed the importance of good documentation skills. The health record is a communication tool while the client is receiving services, but it is also the source for financial, legal, and clinical accountability. Occupational therapy documentation should always contain the following:

- What services were provided and when they were provided
- What was said and what happened
- How the client responded to the service provided
- Why the skill of an occupational therapy practitioner was required rather than the services of an aide, a family member, or another professional

Before you write anything in the record, make these assumptions:

- Someone else will have to read and understand what I write because I may be sick or out of town the next time this client needs to be treated.
- This entry I am about to make will be scrutinized by a third-party payer. If I were a Medicare reviewer, would I want to pay for the services I am about to record?
- My client will exercise his or her right to read this record.

As discussed in Chapter 3, it is critical to know your payment sources when documenting. Some payers are looking for different outcomes than others. With a Medicare client, you will discuss activities of daily living (ADLs) and instrumental activities of daily living (IADLs), and write goals for self-care and home management. With a workers' compensation client, you will write goals that are oriented toward returning to work. In home health care, you may need to document that your client is unable to leave home to receive services or that education on safety issues was provided to the caregiver. With a child, you will need to focus on educationally relevant services identified in the Individualized Education Program (IEP).

It is essential to remember that your documentation is a reflection of your professional identity and abilities. It is also a reflection of your academic institution, your department, and occupational therapy as a profession. Unless they have witnessed you treating a client, your documentation may be the primary way that others form an impression about your skills and professionalism. This chapter will review general rules for documenting in the health record, guidelines for documenting special situations, considerations in electronic documentation, abbreviations and symbols for documentation, and common documentation errors.

General Rules for Documenting in the Health Record

There are several rules that should always be followed when documenting in the health record (Brennan, 2015; Sames, 2014; Scott, 2013):

Gateley CA, Borcherding S. *Documentation Manual for*
Occupational Therapy: Writing SOAP Notes, Fourth Edition (pp 29-44).
© 2017 SLACK Incorporated

- *Always use waterproof, nonerasable black ink*: This prevents smearing, erasing, or otherwise changing the health record.
- *Correct errors*: Never use correction fluid or correction tape! It is considered an illegal alteration of the record. If you make an error in a written health record, draw a single line through it, write your correction, and initial the change:

CG
Pt. able to dress lower body with ~~verbal cues~~ min Ⓐ using a reacher.

  - If you inadvertently write your note in the wrong client's chart, draw a single line through the entire entry and write "wrong chart" beside it with your signature.
  - If you need to add something after you have written and signed your note, write an addendum with the current date and time.

- *Be sure all required data are present*: The *Guidelines for Documentation in Occupational Therapy* (American Occupational Therapy Association [AOTA], 2013) specify the content for each type of note you may be writing. This information will be covered in Chapter 13.
- *Be as concise as possible without leaving out pertinent data*: You will have limited time for documentation under today's productivity standards, and other busy professionals appreciate being able to read what you have written in the shortest time possible.
- *Sign and date every entry*: Some facilities and funding sources also require you to document the time of day or number of minutes that the client received services. The standard format is first name, middle initial, last name, and credentials. Required credentials may vary by state. In written health records, if your signature is not legible, be sure to print your name below your signature. In electronic health records (EHRs), you will be able to sign your name electronically with your electronic user identification and password. Notes by students must be co-signed by a supervising therapist, and in some settings, notes by occupational therapy assistants must be co-signed by the supervising occupational therapist.
  - Signature Example for Students: *Crystal A. Gateley, OTS*
  - Signature Example for Therapists: *Crystal A. Gateley, PhD, OTR/L*
- *Identify the client on every page of documentation*: In a written health record, every page must include the client's full name and other identifying information as required by the facility in indelible ink or in the form of a stamp.
- *Document in a timely manner*: It is best to document as soon after a session as possible. This allows for the best communication between team members. It also ensures that your recollection of events will be accurate. As many facilities move toward the use of EHRs, occupational therapy practitioners are being asked to complete point-of-service documentation, in which the therapist electronically documents the occupational therapy session during the session (Waite, 2012).
  - If you encounter a situation in which you need to document a session that occurred on another date, you should document "Late entry for (date)" at the beginning of the note.
- *Use appropriate terminology for the recipient of services*: When referring to the persons who receive occupational therapy services, the terms *client, patient, consumer, resident, veteran, participant, individual, student, teacher, child, caregiver, employer,* or *family* may be used. Use the term that is considered most respectful for your practice setting.
- *Be prudent in using abbreviations*: Use only the abbreviations that are approved by your facility. This will be discussed in further detail later in this chapter.
- *Focus on the client's experience and leave yourself out*: Unless it is absolutely relevant, do not mention yourself in the note. It is not necessary to say, "Therapist provided caregiver with skilled instruction in assisting client with self-care." Simply say, "Caregiver received skilled instruction in assisting client with self-care." In the rare cases when it is necessary to mention yourself in the note, refer to yourself in the third person. Do not use "I" or "me." Instead, use "the therapist," "the clinician," or "the occupational therapist." For example: "Client cursed and pushed therapist's hand away when physical assistance was provided for grooming task." Chapter 8 will provide additional examples about how to write from the client's point of view while simultaneously showing the skilled therapy that was provided.
- *Always adhere to legal and ethical guidelines*: Be familiar with laws, regulatory guidelines, facility policies, and AOTA *Official Documents* that affect documentation.
- *Write legibly*: Others must be able to read and understand what you have written.

- *Always be accurate and objective*: Report what was actually observed and avoid judging or interpreting the observations other than in the assessment portion of your note.
- *In terms of fiscal and legal accountability, "If it's not documented, it didn't happen"*: No activity or contact is ever considered a service that has been provided until a clinical entry has been made in the health record. In the current era of health care reimbursement scrutiny, you should also think to yourself, "If it's not documented well, my company might not get reimbursed."
- *Avoid spelling, grammar, and punctuation errors*: As previously stated, your documentation is a reflection of your skills and professionalism. Errors in documentation can also present safety concerns for your client if another professional misinterprets your documentation due to such errors. Although some software programs for EHRs offer a spell-check option, many do not.
- *Be aware of "red-flag" words*: Words such as *continued* and *maintained* suggest that progress is not occurring and funding sources may not reimburse for those services. However, the U.S. Supreme Court ruling in the *Jimmo v Sebelius* case "clarified that improvement is not required to obtain services in Medicare" (AOTA, 2015, para. 2). Rather, occupational therapy may be provided when skilled care is "required in order to prevent or slow deterioration and maintain a beneficiary at the maximum practicable level of function" (Centers for Medicare & Medicaid Services, 2015, p. 1). In such cases, be very clear in your documentation that the skills of an occupational therapy practitioner were required due to the nature of the client's condition or the complexity of the intervention.

Documenting Special Situations

Change in Client Status

Any unusual situations regarding the client should be documented. In many cases, therapy personnel may be the first to recognize a change in patient status indicative of a significant underlying medical issue (Szanzer, 2014). For example, suppose during your morning ADL session with a client that you observe pain and swelling of the lower leg (symptoms of a blood clot) or a decrease in cognition from previous sessions. Those symptoms should be documented in the health record. It is also important to communicate any status change to the client's nurse and/or physician and to document that you have passed the information on to the appropriate person. Example:

> *During lower body dressing, client observed to have redness, pitting edema, and pain in lower Ⓛ LE. Skin also noted to be warm to touch. Discontinued ADL session. Notified nurse and physician of patient status.*

In another example, suppose you are working with a toddler diagnosed with hydrocephalus. When you arrive to the child's home for a scheduled early intervention session, you note that the child is more irritable and lethargic than you have observed in previous sessions, and the parent reports that the child has been hitting her head repeatedly, all of which are signs of shunt malfunction (Cincinnati Children's Hospital Medical Center, 2015). You should document your follow up actions. Example:

> *Upon arrival to child's home for occupational therapy session, Chloe noted to be significantly more irritable and lethargic than previous sessions. Parent reports Chloe has been crying and hitting right side of her head all morning. Redness noted at shunt site. Recommended parent seek immediate medical attention for Chloe to rule out shunt malfunction. Family transported Chloe to emergency department at Children's Hospital. Notified Chloe's pediatrician and Early Intervention case manager. No other occupational therapy intervention provided this date.*

Missed Visits

Any scheduled or attempted visits that are missed should be documented with an explanation for the missed visit and any other pertinent information regarding follow-up:

- *Client cancelled scheduled outpatient visit due to inclement weather. Confirmed next appointment on 12-1-2017.*
- *Attempted twice this date to see pt. for initial OT eval. Pt. off unit to diagnostic testing (TEE) in am, then on bed rest this pm following sedation from test. Will reattempt tomorrow.*
- *Resident declined participation in therapeutic exercise this am, citing fatigue. Rescheduled for this pm.*
- *Child missed two scheduled OT sessions on 11/1 & 11/3 due to being absent from school 11/1–11/4/2017 with illness. Will resume 30-minute sessions 2x/wk next week.*
- *Attempted scheduled home visit for early intervention. Child and family not home at scheduled time/date. Attempted twice to contact by phone, no answer, left message on voicemail. Notified service coordinator of situation.*

LACK OF COMPLIANCE

A client's lack of compliance with medical and therapy recommendations is another situation that should be documented. For example, if a client is not following safety recommendations, such as hip precautions or the use of an assistive device for ambulation during ADLs, it is important to document these observations along with any reasons that the client may provide for choosing not to follow the recommendations. It is, however, necessary to distinguish between voluntary lack of compliance and cognitive deficits that limit the client's ability to remember to comply with recommendations. Examples:

- *Client does not consistently adhere to postsurgical hip precautions during ADL performance. Reviewed hip precautions. Client able to articulate 3 of 3 precautions but reports difficulty remembering to follow them during functional activities.*
- *During home health visit, client reported she had not been using shower chair for bathing as recommended to reduce fall risk. "I just don't like having all that stuff cluttering up my bathroom."*
- *Child has missed 4 of 8 scheduled therapy visits this month. Caregiver reports difficulty balancing therapy schedule with numerous other medical and school-related appointments. After discussion with caregiver, frequency of sessions reduced to 1x/wk with a plan for increased emphasis on home program activities. Insurance case manager notified.*

INCIDENT REPORTS

Another special situation that requires documentation is an incident report. An incident report should be completed for events such as client falls, skin tears, inadvertent removal of IV or catheter, and other unplanned events that led to injury or had the potential to lead to the injury of a client, visitor, or staff person. Scott (2013) reiterated that the incident report should not be contained in the health record, as it contains administrative information about follow-up of the incident. The health record should contain only the objective clinical information related to the event, and no mention of the incident report. Example:

> *Client experienced ½-inch skin tear to dorsal aspect of Ⓛ hand when reaching into kitchen cabinet during cooking activity. Pressure and gauze bandage applied; nursing notified. Client stated, "I'm fine" and continued with cooking activity.*

Health care settings have special forms and procedures for documenting incident reports, which serve the following purposes:

- Ensuring that optimal care was provided to the injured party
- Protecting the staff member and facility from unwarranted liability exposure
- Identifying the need for further staff training to prevent similar incidents

Each facility will have a particular form (written or electronic) for documenting adverse incidents. The following information is typically included in an incident report (Scott, 2013):

- Administrative data such as name, address, date of birth, and incident date and location
- Patient diagnosis and summary of care received following the incident
- Type of incident (e.g., fall, skin tear, modality-related, equipment malfunction, etc.)
- Condition of person affected by incident
- Course of action
- Witnesses, if appropriate
- Concise yet thorough explanation of event in objective terms, without speculation of cause

An incident involving injury to you will require additional documentation because it is considered a workers' compensation issue. Examples include injuring your back while transferring a client, slipping on a wet floor in a client's room, or being struck or bitten by a client. When any event occurs that would require an incident report, it is essential that you notify your supervisor immediately so that appropriate responses can be carried out and documented.

PEOPLE FIRST LANGUAGE

Snow (2013) suggested that professionals should always make an intentional effort to refer to the individual first rather than the diagnosis. "People first language puts the person before the disability, and describes what the person *has*, not who the person *is*" (Snow, 2013, p. 3). For example, rather than "the Down baby," we should say "the infant with Down syndrome." Rather than "the stroke in Room 203," we should say "the patient in Room 203 who had a stroke."

This concept of people first language fits well within our profession. One of the guiding principles for the occupational therapy profession is client-centered practice (Boyt Schell, Scaffa, Gillen, & Cohn, 2014). One way to demonstrate client-centered practice is by using people first language not just in our verbal interactions, but also in our documentation. We should write our notes in terms of what the client needs rather than stating that the client is a particular assist level. Our clients are much more than their assist levels.

Please say: "*Veteran needs max assist...*" or "*Veteran requires max assist...*"

Rather than "*Veteran is max assist...*"

CONSIDERATIONS IN ELECTRONIC DOCUMENTATION

While EHRs provide many advantages in terms of efficiency, connectivity, and legibility, they also present unique concerns, particularly in regard to confidentiality. The HIPAA Security Rule established federal standards for the security of EHRs. All employees who have access to EHRs must take precautions to prevent unauthorized access, alteration, or disclosure of a client's health information (Scott, 2013). Occupational therapy practitioners who have access to EHRs will generally have a username and/or password to access client records and to sign documentation that has been entered about occupational therapy services. The following precautions should be taken to adhere to the HIPAA Security Rule (Collmer, 2015):

- Do not share your username or password with anyone.
- Logout when you are leaving an electronic workstation.
- Do not access any EHRs that you do not have a direct need to see. This includes your own EHR or those of family, friends, etc. Access to unauthorized EHRs can be traced back to your username and may be grounds for disciplinary action, termination of employment, and legal action.
- Be aware of your surroundings and make sure that unauthorized individuals cannot read the screen. Electronic workstations are often located in high traffic areas such as nurses' stations, patient rooms, hallways, therapy gyms, and shared offices.
- Be familiar and compliant with your employer's EHR safeguards, including the transmission of personal health information via facsimile or electronic mail.

While EHRs increase legibility of documentation, they do not eliminate the potential for errors. Many programs have a spell check feature to reduce spelling errors, but such programs may not catch typographical errors such as the reversal of letters resulting in a different, correctly spelled word. Occupational therapy practitioners should carefully review what they have entered into an EHR prior to providing an electronic signature.

AVOIDING COMMON DOCUMENTATION ERRORS

As previously stated, your documentation is a reflection of you and the profession of occupational therapy. Mistakes in spelling, grammar, and punctuation may give others a negative impression of your knowledge, skills, and professionalism (Moore, 2015; Scott, 2013). Such errors can also lead to serious consequences for you or your client. This section will review several rules to help you avoid common documentation errors:

- Use quotation marks when documenting the exact words that a client or another person said.
    - Incorrect: *Client stated I can't feel my right arm.*
    - Correct: *Client stated, "I can't feel my right arm."*
- Do not use quotation marks when paraphrasing what a client or another person said.
    - Incorrect: *Client reports she "can't feel her right arm."*
    - Correct: *Client reports she cannot feel her right arm.*
- Be consistent in the use of verb tense.
    - Incorrect: *Client demonstrated upper body dressing with min Ⓐ. Client threads Ⓡ UE into sleeve first. Client transfers to toilet with SBA. Client completed grooming tasks independently.*
    - Correct: *Client demonstrated upper body dressing with min Ⓐ. Client threaded Ⓡ UE into sleeve first. Client transferred to toilet with SBA. Client completed grooming tasks independently.*

- Indicate plurals by adding an "s" to the end of a word without an apostrophe.
  - Incorrect: *The client's participated in a group discussion about time management and ADL's. The OT's then provided additional suggestion's.*
  - Correct: *The clients participated in a group discussion about time management and ADLs. The OTs then provided additional suggestions.*
- Indicate possession of a single person or object by using an apostrophe before the "s."
  - Incorrect: *The clients' spouse was present during the session.*
  - Correct: *The client's spouse was present during the session.*
- Indicate possession of more than one person or object by using and apostrophe after the "s."
  - Incorrect: *The three clients group discussion focused on coping skills.*
  - Correct: *The three clients' group discussion focused on coping skills.*
- Use a singular pronoun to refer to one person.
  - Incorrect: *The client has difficulty putting on their shirt.*
  - Correct: *The client has difficulty putting on his shirt.*
- Use a plural pronoun to refer to more than one person.
  - Incorrect: *They blame themself for the situation.*
  - Correct: *They blame themselves for the situation.*
- Follow the general rules for capitalization (Table 4-1).
- Know the appropriate spelling of commonly misspelled words (Table 4-2).

Table 4-1

General Rules for Capitalization

CAPITALIZE	DO NOT CAPITALIZE
Proper names in medical terminology • e.g., Alzheimer's disease	Common nouns in medical terminology • e.g., virus, appendectomy, scapula
Trade names of products and medications • e.g., Jobst stocking, Advil	Generic drugs and products • e.g., compression glove, pain reliever
Specific organizations • e.g., Joint Commission	Generic organizations • e.g., accrediting agency
Academic degrees and professional designations after the person's name • e.g., Crystal Gateley, PhD, OTR/L	General degrees or generic professional designations • e.g., an associate's degree, an occupational therapist
Exact test titles • e.g., Peabody Developmental Motor Scales	Generic test • e.g., sensory test, cognitive test
Specific department proper names • e.g., Midwest Hospital Occupational Therapy Department	Generic department names • e.g., an occupational therapy department, the rehab department
Official titles as part of a name • e.g., Dr. Wolf, Father O'Malley	Generic or descriptive titles • e.g., the doctor, the clergyman

Information compiled from Moore (2015) and Villemaire & Villemaire (2005).

Table 4-2

Commonly Misspelled Words

Words That Sound Alike	"I" Before "E" Except After "C" Words	Miscellaneous Words
• accept (*She wouldn't accept it.*) • except (*all except that one*) • affect (*He had a flat affect. That didn't affect his participation.*) • effect (*That has no effect on me.*) • aid (verb—*to help*; noun—*a helping device, such as a "visual aid"*) • aide (*person, such as the occupational therapy aide*) • aloud (*She said it aloud.*) • allowed (*Children aren't allowed in there.*) • brake (*Lock the wheelchair brake.*) • break (*Take a break. He will break his arm.*) • gait (*ambulation*) • gate (*an entrance*) • lay (*Lay it on the desk.*) • lie (*He wants to lie on the bed.*) • loose (*not tight*) • lose (*I want to lose weight.*) • patience (*Have some patience!*) • patients (*The patients were in their rooms.*) • peace (*I want some peace and quiet.*) • piece (*piece of the puzzle*) • principal (*the school principal*) • principle (*principles of NDT*) • stationary (*not moving*) • stationery (*writing paper*) • than (*I have more than you.*) • then (*Then he went to bed.*) • their (*It was their house.*) • there (*Put it there.*) • they're (*they are*) • wait (*Wait here.*) • weight (*Her weight has declined.*) • you're (*you are*) • your (*It's your turn.*)	• achieve (after "ch" is still "ie") • believe • brief • hygiene • piece • receive • relieve • retrieve	• activity • Alzheimer's • asymmetry • catheterization • clavicle • current • deferred • definitely • developmentally • dining • doctor • doff • doffed • doffing • dominant • don • donned • equilibrium • exercise • immobilize • independent • input • intention • interest • judgment • paraffin • perform • putty • recommendations • remember • rotator cuff • schizophrenia • stabilization • strength • symmetry • technique • toilet • tolerate • transferring • writing

Information compiled from Merriam-Webster (2015).

ABBREVIATIONS AND SYMBOLS

Using abbreviations and symbols when documenting in the client's health record saves valuable time, but these should be used with discretion (Scott, 2013). Remember that your notes may be read by someone who knows little about occupational therapy, and that individual may determine whether to pay for your services. You should be sure that the individual will be able to understand the information you are trying to convey. Health care settings typically have a list of approved abbreviations. You should be familiar with that list and use only abbreviations that are approved for your setting. Do not make up abbreviations. Many people commonly use acronyms or shorthand when chatting online or texting, but those abbreviations are not appropriate for the health record. Also remember that while it is permissible to use abbreviations, it is not required. You may write out any word instead of shortening it. In this manual, you will find that some notes use more abbreviations and symbols than others. Table 4-3 lists commonly used abbreviations. Please note that this list is not all inclusive. The Joint Commission, which accredits many hospitals and other health care facilities, does not maintain a list of acceptable abbreviations and symbols for use in documentation. However, the Joint Commission has published an *Official "Do Not Use" List of Abbreviations* (Joint Commission, 2015). The list contains abbreviations and symbols prohibited on all orders, along with handwritten, pre-printed, and electronic forms regarding medications. A few examples of prohibited abbreviations are qd (every day) and qod (every other day) because they can be mistaken for each other. While occupational therapy practitioners would rarely have involvement with documentation regarding medications, some facilities prohibit the use of the abbreviations and symbols on the *"Do Not Use" List* by any health care provider in any type of documentation. You must be familiar with the list of acceptable and prohibited abbreviations and symbols for your facility.

Table 4-3

Abbreviations and Symbols

ABBREVIATIONS FOR DIAGNOSES, PROCEDURES, AND BODY PARTS					
AAA	abdominal aortic aneurysm	A/P	anterior/posterior	CAT	computerized axial tomography
Ⓐ	assistance	ARF	acute renal failure	cath.	catheter; catheterization
A&Ox4	alert and oriented to person, place, time, situation	ASCVD	atherosclerotic cardio-vascular disease	CBC	complete blood count
		ASHD	arterial sclerotic heart disease	c-diff	*C. difficile* (bacteria)
ā	before			CF	cystic fibrosis
abd	abduction	ASIS	anterior superior iliac spine	chemo	chemotherapy
ABG	arterial blood gas	Ⓑ	bilateral	CHF	congestive heart failure
add	adduction			CHI	closed head injury
ADD	attention deficit disorder	BE	below elbow	CMC	carpometacarpal
ADHD	attention deficit hyper-activity disorder	Bi-PAP	bi-level positive airway pressure	CNS	central nervous system
		BK	below knee	C/O	complains of
AE	above elbow	BKA	below knee amputation	CO$_2$	carbon dioxide
AIDS	acquired immunodefi-ciency syndrome	BM	bowel movement	COPD	chronic obstructive pul-monary disease
		BP	blood pressure		
AK	above knee	BRP	bathroom privileges	CP	cerebral palsy
AKA	above knee amputation	c̄	with	CPAP	continuous positive air-way pressure
ALS	amyotrophic lateral sclerosis	CA	cancer; carcinoma	CPM	continuous passive motion (machine)
		CABG	coronary artery bypass graft		
AMA	against medical advice			CPR	cardiopulmonary resuscitation
ant.	anterior	CAD	coronary artery disease		
appt.	appointment				

(continued)

Table 4-3 (continued)

Abbreviations and Symbols

ABBREVIATIONS FOR DIAGNOSES, PROCEDURES, AND BODY PARTS					
CRF	chronic renal failure	HR	heart rate	PCA	personal care attendant
CSF	cerebrospinal fluid	HTN	hypertension	PDD	pervasive developmental disorder
CT	computed tomography	hx	history		
CTR	carpal tunnel release	I&D	incision and drainage	PEG	percutaneous endoscopic gastrostomy
CVA	cerebrovascular accident	IM	intramuscular		
CXR	chest x-ray	I&O	intake and output	peri.	perineal
DDD	degenerative disk disease	IV	intravenous	PET	positron emission tomography
DIP	distal interphalangeal joint	Ⓛ	left		
		LLQ	left lower quadrant	PIP	proximal interphalangeal joint
DJD	degenerative joint disease	LMN	lower motor neuron		
		LOC	loss of consciousness	PMH	previous medical history
DM	diabetes mellitus	LP	lumbar puncture	PNS	peripheral nervous system
DNR	do not resuscitate	LUQ	left upper quadrant		
DOB	date of birth	MCP	metacarpalphalangeal	PO	by mouth; orally
DTR	deep tendon reflex	MD	muscular dystrophy; medical doctor	postop	postoperatively
DVT	deep vein thrombosis			preop	preoperatively
dx	diagnosis	meds.	medications	PSIS	posterior superior iliac spine
ECG	electrocardiogram	mets.	metastases		
ECHO	echocardiogram	MI	myocardial infarction	PVD	peripheral vascular disease
EEG	electroencephalogram	MRA	magnetic resonance angiogram		
EKG	electrocardiogram			Ⓡ	right
EMG	electromyogram	MRI	magnetic resonance imaging	RA	rheumatoid arthritis
ENT	ear, nose, throat			RBC	red blood cell count
EOM	extraocular movement	MRSA	Methicillin-resistant *Staphylococcus aureus* (bacteria)	RLQ	right lower quadrant
ESRD	end stage renal disease			R/O	rule out
EtOH	ethanol (alcohol use/ abuse)			RSD	reflex sympathetic dystrophy
		MS	multiple sclerosis		
FBS	fasting blood sugar	MVA	motor vehicle accident	RTC	return to clinic
FTT	failure to thrive	NC	nasal cannula	RTO	return to office
F/U	follow-up	NG	nasogastric (tube)	RUQ	right upper quadrant
fx	fracture	NKA	no known allergies	Rx	prescription
GB	gallbladder	NKDA	no known drug allergies	s̄	without
GERD	gastroesophageal reflux disease	NOS	not otherwise specified	SCI	spinal cord injury
		NPO	nothing by mouth	SDH	subdural hematoma
GI	gastrointestinal	N/V	nausea and vomiting	SLE	systemic lupus erythematosus
GSW	gunshot wound	O$_2$	oxygen		
H/A	headache	OA	osteoarthritis	SOB	shortness of breath
HEENT	head, eyes, ears, nose, throat	ORIF	open reduction internal fixation	S/P	status post
				S/S	signs and symptoms
HIV	human immunodeficiency virus	p̄	after	sx	symptoms
		PCA	patient controlled analgesia	Sz	seizure
H&P	history and physical			TB	tuberculosis

(continued)

Table 4-3 (continued)

Abbreviations and Symbols

ABBREVIATIONS FOR DIAGNOSES, PROCEDURES, AND BODY PARTS					
TBI	traumatic brain injury	TKR	total knee replacement	US	ultrasound
TEDS	thromboembolic disease stockings	tPA	tissue plasminogen activator	UTI	urinary tract infection
				VC	vital capacity
TEE	transesophageal echocardiogram	TPN	total parenteral nutrition	VRE	Vancomycin-resistant *enterococci* (bacteria)
		tx	treatment		
THA	total hip arthroplasty	UA	urinalysis	WBC	white blood cell count
THR	total hip replacement	UMN	upper motor neuron	wt.	weight
TIA	transient ischemic attack	URI	upper respiratory infection	y.o.	year old
TKA	total knee arthroplasty			yr.	year

ABBREVIATIONS FOR FREQUENCY AND TIME					
ad lib	as desired	PTA	prior to admission	1x/wk	once a week
AM/am	morning	qd	every day	2x/wk	twice a week
ASAP	as soon as possible	qid	four times a day	3x/wk	three times a week
bid	twice a day	qod	every other day	1x/mo	once a month
noc	night or bedtime	STAT	immediately	2x/mo	twice a month
PM/pm	afternoon	tid	three times a day	3x/mo	three times a month
prn	as needed				

ABBREVIATIONS FOR LOCATION AND SETTINGS					
CCU	coronary (cardiac) care unit	LTAC	long-term acute care	PACU	post-anesthesia care unit
		LTC	long-term care	PICU	pediatric intensive care unit
ECF	extended care facility	MICU	medical intensive care unit		
ED	emergency department			RCF	residential care facility
ER	emergency room	NICU	neonatal intensive care unit	SICU	surgical intensive care unit
HH	home health				
ICU	intensive care unit	OP	outpatient	SNF	skilled nursing facility
IP	inpatient	OR	operating room	SNU	skilled nursing unit

ABBREVIATIONS FOR LEVELS OF ASSISTANCE					
Ⓘ	independent	Min Ⓐ	minimal assistance	Ⓓ	dependent assistance
Mod Ⓘ	modified independent	Mod Ⓐ	moderate assistance	x1	assistance of 1 person
SBA	stand by assistance	Max Ⓐ	maximal assistance	x2	assistance of 2 people
CGA	contact guard assistance				

MISCELLANEOUS COMMON THERAPY ABBREVIATIONS					
AAROM	active assistive range of motion	ATNR	asymmetrical tonic neck reflex	COTA	certified occupational therapy assistant
ADLs	activities of daily living	BADLs	basic activities of daily living	COTA/L	certified occupational therapy assistant/ licensed
AFO	ankle foot orthosis				
amb.	ambulation; ambulated	CHT	certified hand therapist		
AROM	active range of motion			CST	craniosacral therapist
				D/C	discontinue; discharge

(continued)

Table 4-3 (continued)
Abbreviations and Symbols

MISCELLANEOUS COMMON THERAPY ABBREVIATIONS					
DME	durable medical equipment	LOS	length of stay	pt.	patient
ELOS	estimated length of stay	MMT	manual muscle testing	PTA	physical therapist assistant
EOB	edge of bed or explanation of benefits	N	normal (muscle grade)	PWB	partial weightbearing
e-stim	electrical stimulation	NDT	neurodevelopmental treatment	rehab	rehabilitation
eval.	evaluation	NMES	neuromuscular electrical stimulation	SI	sensory integration
ext.	extension	NWB	non-weightbearing	SLP	speech language pathologist
F	fair (muscle grade)	OOB	out of bed	SOAP	subjective, objective, assessment, plan
FIM	Functional Independence Measure	OT	occupational therapist; occupational therapy	SOC	start of care
flex.	flexion	OTR	occupational therapist, registered	STG	short-term goal
ft.	foot; feet			STM	short-term memory
FWB	full weightbearing	OTR/L	occupational therapist, registered/licensed	STNR	symmetrical tonic neck reflex
G	good (muscle grade)	OTS	occupational therapy student	TDWB	touch down weightbearing
HEP	home exercise program			TENS	transcutaneous electrical nerve stimulation
HOB	head of bed	P	poor (muscle grade)		
HOH	hand over hand, or hard of hearing	PAM	physical agent modality	TTWB	toe touch weightbearing
IADLs	instrumental activities of daily living	PLOF	prior level of function	UE	upper extremity
		PNF	proprioceptive neuromuscular facilitation	WBAT	weightbearing as tolerated
IEP	Individualized Education Program	POC	plan of care	w/c	wheelchair
KAFO	knee ankle foot orthosis	PT	physical therapist; physical therapy	WFL	within functional limits
LE	lower extremity			WNL	within normal limits

MISCELLANEOUS SYMBOLS					
♀	female	'	feet	~	approximately
♂	male	°	degree	%	percent
↓	decrease	+	plus, positive	&	and
↑	increase	–	minus, negative	@	at
c̄	with	#	number (#1); pounds	↔	to and from
s̄	without	/	per	→	to; progressing toward
ā	before	<	less than	1°	primary
p̄	after	>	greater than	2°	secondary; due to
"	inches	=	equals		

Information compiled from Marks (2015) and Unbound Medicine (2015).

REFERENCES

American Occupational Therapy Association. (2013). Guidelines for documentation of occupational therapy. *American Journal of Occupational Therapy, 67*(Suppl.), S32-S38. doi: 10.5014/ajot.2013.67S32.

American Occupational Therapy Association. (2015). Jimmo: The court case that promotes skilled therapy. Retrieved from http://www.aota.org.

Boyt Schell, B. A., Scaffa, M. E., Gillen, G., & Cohn, E. S. (2014). Contemporary occupational therapy practice. In B.A. Boyt Schell, Gillen, & Scaffa (Eds.) *Willard & Spackman's occupational therapy* (12th ed., pp. 47-58.) Philadelphia, PA: Lippincott Williams & Wilkins.

Brennan, C. (2015). The do's & don'ts of documentation. *OT Practice, 20*(15), 8-11.

Centers for Medicare & Medicaid Services. (2015). Jimmo v. Sebelius settlement agreement fact sheet. Retrieved from https://www.cms.gov.

Cincinnati Children's Hospital Medical Center. (2015). Shunt malfunction signs. Retrieved from http://www.cincinnatichildrens.org.

Collmer, V. (2015). Navigating the HIPAA security rule: Practical strategies for the occupational therapy practitioner. *OT Practice, 20*(14), 13-16.

Joint Commission. (2015). Facts about the Official "Do Not Use' list of abbreviations. Retrieved from whttp://www.jointcomission.org.

Marks, J. W. (Ed.). (2015). List of common medical abbreviations and terminology. Retrieved from http://www.medicinenet.com.

Merriam-Webster. (2015). Merriam-Webster's online dictionary. Retrieved from http://dictionary.reference.com.

Moore, B. (2015). Medical records and documentation. Retrieved from http://www.infusionceus.com.

Sames, K. M. (2014). Documentation in practice. In B. A. Boyt Schell, G. Gillen, & M. E. Scaffa (Eds.) *Willard & Spackman's occupational therapy* (12th ed., pp. 466-475). Philadelphia, PA: Lippincott Williams & Wilkins.

Scott, R. W. (2013). *Legal, ethical, and practical aspects of patient care documentation: A guide for rehabilitation professionals* (4th ed.). Burlington, MA: Jones & Bartlett Learning.

Snow, K. (2013). People first language. Retrieved from http://www.disabilityisnatural.com.

Szanzer, F. M. (2014). Deep vein thrombosis: The silent killer. *Advance for Physical Therapy & Rehab Medicine.* Retrieved from http://physical-therapy.advanceweb.com.

Unbound Medicine. (2015). Medical abbreviations. *Taber's online medical dictionary.* Retrieved from http://www.tabers.com.

Villemaire, D., & Villemaire, L. (2005) *Grammar & writing skills for the health professional* (2nd ed.). Clifton Park, NY: Thomson Delmar Learning.

Waite, A. (2012). Point-of-service documentation strategies help practitioners beat the time crunch. *OT Practice, 17*(1), 9-12.

WORKSHEET 4-1

Avoiding Common Documentation Errors

Identify and correct the errors in the following statements.

1. Pt. stated my head really hurts this morning.

2. Resident reported "her right hand is working better today."

3. Student used right hand to cut with scissors. Student then switches to left hand for coloring tasks. Student did not demonstrate consistent hand preference.

4. The client's expressed excitement about the upcoming visit to the mall.

5. An occupational therapy referral was recieved from the childs' teacher.

6. The child was unable to button their coat.

7. The resident's were all in the dinning room weighting for there meal.

8. Client demonstrated appropriate social interaction by responding your welcome to another group member.

9. Pt. required moderate assistance to use dominate right hand in hygeine tasks.

10. Client does not demonstrate awareness of the affect of his mood on other member's of the group.

11. Pt. expressed intrest in getting dressed. Pt. required verbal cues when doning pullover shirt to utilize adaptive teckniques due to right rotary cup injury.

WORKSHEET 4-1 (CONTINUED)

Avoiding Common Documentation Errors

Identify and correct the errors in the following statements.

12.   The ot noticed assymetry in the childs sitting posture. Parents reports that the client is unable to sit independantly.

13.   The OTR preformed a Cognitive Test on the client.

14.   The Doctor called to check on the Patients status.

15.   Client demonstrated poor judgement by attempting to stand up without their walker.

16.   Pt. had right arm imobilized due to a clavical fracture.

17.   Client required several breif rest brakes during ADL's.

18.   The clinic employs three otr's and two ota's.

19.   The students principle stated Jimmy is disruptive at school.

20.   A child at this age should be able to dress themselves.

21.   The childrens' mother has difficulty keeping all they're appointment's.

22.   Client needed a visual aide to help them learn how to preform self-catherization.

WORKSHEET 4-2

Using Abbreviations

Translate each sentence written with abbreviations into full English phrases or sentences.

1. Client C/O pain in Ⓡ MCP joint p̄ ~15 min PROM.

2. Pt. A&Ox4.

3. Client transferred w/c → mat c̄ sliding board & max Ⓐ x2.

4. 1° dx Ⓛ BKA, 2° dx COPD, CHF, DM, & PVD.

5. Pt. is S/P Ⓡ THR. Orders received for OT 2x/day for ADLs & IADLs, TTWB Ⓡ LE.

Shorten these sentences using only the standard abbreviations in this chapter.

6. Client has thirty degrees of passive range of motion in the left distal interphalangeal joint, which is within functional limits.

7. Client is able to put on her socks with standby assistance, but requires moderate assistance with putting on and taking off left shoe.

8. The client requires contact guard assistance for balance during her morning dressing, which she performs while sitting on the edge of her bed.

WORKSHEET 4-2 (CONTINUED)

Using Abbreviations

Shorten these notes using only the standard abbreviations in this chapter.

9.   The patient participated in a bedside evaluation of activities of daily living. She was able to perform bed mobility with moderate assistance, but she needed maximum assistance to put on her adult undergarment. She was able to go from a supine position to a sitting position with minimum assistance and from a sitting position to a standing position with moderate assistance.

10.   The resident came to the occupational therapy clinic via wheelchair escort. The resident was observed to lean toward his left. The resident needed verbal cues and minimum assistance in positioning his body in the wheelchair to maintain midline orientation and symmetrical posture. The resident transferred from his wheelchair to the toilet with moderate assistance of one person to help him keep his balance using a standing pivot transfer. He needed verbal cues and visual feedback from a mirror to maintain upright posture.

11.   The veteran participated in an evaluation in his room to determine relevant client factors. The veteran's short-term memory was three out of three for immediate recall, one out of three after 1 minute, and zero out of three with verbal cues after 5 minutes. The left upper extremity shoulder flexion was a grade of 4, shoulder extension was a grade of 4, elbow flexion was a grade of 4, elbow extension was a grade of 4, wrist flexion was a grade of 4 minus, wrist extension was a grade of 4 minus, and grip strength was 8 pounds. The left upper extremity light touch was intact. The right upper extremity muscle grades and sensation were within functional limits.

5

Writing Occupation-Based Problem Statements

As a part of the initial assessment, the occupational therapist develops a "problem list" identifying the major areas of occupation that have been affected by the client's condition. The contributing factors that affect the client's occupational performance are also identified. Priorities are then set with the client and caregivers so the problems that are most important to them will be addressed. Some clients may need clarification of occupational therapy's role to identify problem areas that fall within the scope of occupational therapy practice. Educating the client about the purpose and potential benefits of occupational therapy is an important part of establishing a therapeutic relationship (DeCleene, 2013). For example, when you ask a client in the hospital what his or her goal is, a common response is, "I want to walk." However, ambulation alone is a physical therapy goal. You can probe deeper by asking, "What things do you need to walk for?" Ask about activities such as meal preparation, gathering clothes to wear, and carrying items from place to place at home, school, or work. Clients that take an active role in goal setting often have improved functional outcomes and report greater satisfaction with the rehabilitation process (Tripicchio, Bykerk, Wegner, & Wegner, 2009; VanPuymbrouck, 2014).

There are two parts to a functional problem statement: the area of occupation that is a concern and the contributing factors that are interfering with the client's engagement in that area of occupation. Let's take a closer look at information that was presented in Chapter 1 about occupational therapy's domain.

AREAS OF OCCUPATION

Occupational therapy practitioners provide interventions for people who have difficulty engaging in an area of occupation. The focus on ability to engage in occupation is what distinguishes the occupational therapy profession from other health care disciplines. The *OTPF-III* (American Occupational Therapy Association [AOTA], 2014) categorizes the areas of occupation (Table 5-1) that may be addressed by occupational therapy practitioners.

It is essential to remember that the entities and agencies that provide reimbursement for occupational therapy services have different priorities. You should have a good understanding of the funding source regulations, and your documentation should target areas of occupation that the funding source considers necessary and reimbursable (Amini, 2014; Brennan, 2014). For example, Medicare is likely to be most concerned with problems and goals that target ADLs and IADLs to help get the client back to living as independently as possible (Valdes, 2014). In worker's compensation cases, problem statements and goals should focus on work (King & Olson, 2014). In school-based therapy, education is the area of occupation that should be addressed in problems and goals (Swinth, 2014).

Gateley CA, Borcherding S. *Documentation Manual for Occupational Therapy: Writing SOAP Notes, Fourth Edition (pp 45-55).*
© 2017 SLACK Incorporated

Table 5-1

Areas of Occupation

Area of Occupation	Description	Examples
ADLs	Activities necessary for care of one's own body and personal independence. May also be referred to as *basic activities of daily living* (BADLs) or *personal activities of daily living* (PADLs)	◆ Bathing/showering ◆ Dressing ◆ Feeding ◆ Functional mobility (during performance of functional activities) ◆ Personal device care ◆ Personal hygiene and grooming ◆ Sexual activity ◆ Toileting and toilet hygiene (including care of bowel and bladder management and menstrual needs)
IADLs	Activities involving participation in the home or community that often require more complex problem-solving and social skills than ADLs	◆ Care of others ◆ Care of pets ◆ Child rearing ◆ Communication management ◆ Community mobility and driving ◆ Financial management ◆ Health management and maintenance ◆ Home establishment and management ◆ Meal preparation and clean up ◆ Religious and spiritual activities ◆ Safety and emergency maintenance ◆ Shopping
Rest and sleep	Activities related to obtaining the rest and sleep necessary for successful engagement in other areas of occupation	◆ Rest ◆ Sleep participation ◆ Sleep preparation
Education	Includes activities necessary for learning and participating in an educational environment	◆ Formal education participation ◆ Informal personal educational needs or interests exploration ◆ Informal personal education participation
Work	Includes seeking and carrying out paid employment or volunteer activities	◆ Employment interests and pursuits ◆ Employment seeking and acquisition ◆ Job performance ◆ Retirement preparation and adjustment ◆ Volunteer exploration ◆ Volunteer participation
Play	Activities that provide enjoyment or entertainment; may be spontaneous or organized	◆ Play exploration ◆ Play participation
Leisure	Intrinsically rewarding activities that are engaged in when an individual is not obligated to perform other occupations	◆ Leisure exploration ◆ Leisure participation
Social participation	Interaction with others that is within expected contextual norms	◆ Community ◆ Family ◆ Peer, friend

Information compiled from American Occupational Therapy Association. (2014). *Occupational therapy practice framework: Domain & process* (3rd ed.). Bethesda, MD: AOTA Press.

Table 5-2

Potential Contributing Factors

POTENTIAL CONTRIBUTING FACTORS	DESCRIPTION	EXAMPLES
Client factors	"…specific capacities, characteristics, or beliefs that reside within the person…" (AOTA, 2014, p. S7)	◆ Values, beliefs, and spirituality ◆ Body functions ▪ *Mental*: Attention, memory, perception, sequencing, emotions, personality traits ▪ *Sensory*: Vision, hearing, vestibular, tactile, pain, proprioceptive ▪ *Neuromusculoskeletal*: Joint mobility and stability, muscle tone, strength, range of motion, voluntary movement ▪ *Cardiovascular, hematological, immunological, and respiratory*: Blood pressure, heart rate, physical endurance ◆ Body structures
Performance skills	"goal-directed actions that are observable as small units of engagement in daily life occupations (AOTA, 2014, p. S7)	◆ *Motor skills*: Bending, reaching, gripping, coordinating, maintaining balance, manipulating ◆ *Process skills*: Attending, choosing, handling, sequencing, initiating ◆ *Social interaction skills*: Initiating interactions, expressing emotions, transitioning, taking turns
Performance patterns	Patterns of behavior related to the activities of an individual, organization, or population	◆ *Habits*: Repetitive rocking in response to stress ◆ *Routines*: Morning routine for dressing and grooming ◆ *Rituals*: Holiday meal preparation ◆ *Roles*: Caregiver, worker, student
Contexts and environments	"…a variety of inter-related conditions that are within and surrounding the client…" (AOTA, 2014, p. S28)	◆ *Cultural*: Customs, beliefs, behavioral expectations ◆ *Personal*: Age, gender, socioeconomic status, educational status, group membership ◆ *Temporal*: Stage of life, time of day, time of year, duration, history ◆ *Virtual*: Communication via audio and electronic devices ◆ Physical: ▪ *Natural environment*: Terrain, plants and animals, sensory qualities ▪ *Built environment*: Buildings, objects, tools, devices ◆ *Social*: Presence, relationships and expectations of others

Information compiled from American Occupational Therapy Association. (2014). *Occupational therapy practice framework: Domain & process* (3rd ed.). Bethesda, MD: AOTA Press.

CONTRIBUTING FACTORS

The second part of the problem statement identifies the contributing factors that limit engagement in the desired occupation. Table 5-2, although not all inclusive, lists several potential contributing factors. The *OTPF-III* (AOTA, 2014) is an excellent resource for identifying contributing factors relevant to occupational performance. The various aspects that comprise occupational therapy's domain are all viewed as having equal value and "together they interact to affect the client's occupational identity, health, well-being, and participation in life" (AOTA, 2014, p. S4). While there may be multiple contributing factors to a limitation in occupational performance, your documentation should focus on those factors that can be addressed through occupational therapy intervention.

WRITING PROBLEM STATEMENTS

Note: In this manual, the terms *client, patient, student, child, infant, consumer, resident, individual, veteran,* and first names have been used to reflect the terms used in various practice settings. Names have been fabricated to protect the confidentiality of those people who receive our services. If a note says, "Mr. P was seen in his home..." please understand that he is being called "Mr. P" for purposes of confidentiality. In your documentation, please use the term or format that is considered most respectful in your setting.

As occupational therapy practitioners, we recognize that a client's sense of well-being depends partly on the ability to participate in the life roles desired at home, at work, at school, and in the community. To gather information about the client, we develop an occupational profile of the client and conduct an analysis of occupational performance (AOTA, 2014). Through these various evaluation procedures, we identify the areas of occupation affected by a client's condition and the factors contributing to the functional limitation. Whenever possible, we also specify the extent to which occupational performance is limited. It is important to note that the client's diagnosis is not the problem. The contributing factors may be the result of the diagnosis, but it is our responsibility to identify those specific factors that contribute to functional limitation. To summarize, you need to identify the following:

- An area of occupation
    - If possible, a measurement of the functional limitation
- A contributing factor to be addressed in occupational therapy
    - If possible, a measurement for the contributing factor
    - Optional: The diagnoses causing this factor

Let's take a look at an example of a functional problem statement:

    Client is <u>unable to dress self Ⓘ</u> due to ↓ AROM in Ⓑ UE.

          Area of Occupation   Contributing Factor

This statement has the essential elements of the area of occupation and a contributing factor, but more specific measurable information would be helpful in documenting progress toward goals. Based on the problem statement listed previously, you will not be able to show any increase in function until the client demonstrates full active range of motion (AROM) and is independent in dressing. Rather than saying that the client is **unable to perform** a given activity independently, it is better to state the assist level needed. It is also helpful to provide the **amount** of AROM that is limited.

For example:

    Client requires max Ⓐ to dress self due to ½ AROM in Ⓑ UE.

With this reworded problem statement, you now will be able to document progress when the client demonstrates an increase in AROM or when the client is able to complete dressing with mod Ⓐ. It may also be helpful to add the diagnosis.

For example:

    Client requires max Ⓐ to dress self due to ½ AROM in Ⓑ UE 2° to infection of the spinal cord.

It is not mandatory to list the diagnosis in the problem statement since it will be documented in other parts of your initial evaluation. In some cases, however, it is helpful to document the diagnosis since there may be a difference in the interventions that will be provided based on the diagnosis.

For ease of writing, you can use the following formula to write a functional problem statement:

Client requires _____ in _____ due to _____.

          assist level   performing what occupational task   contributing factor

A few more examples:

- *Child requires mod Ⓐ to hold scissors to complete art activities in school due to high tone in Ⓡ UE.*
- *Veteran requires min Ⓐ in completing toilet transfer due to trunk instability resulting from Ⓡ CVA.*
- *Consumer requires maximal verbal cues to complete 3-step lunch preparation due to decreased sequencing and problem-solving skills.*

If a client is unable to perform an activity independently, the assist level will be specified. However, sometimes the activity is one that the client either **can** or **cannot** do, with no assist levels in question. In that case, you can use the following format:

Client unable to _____ due to _____.

                engage in what occupational task   what contributing factor

For example:

- *Consumer is unable to sustain employment more than 2 weeks due to absence of stress management skills.*
- *Client is unable to grasp a writing instrument for more than 3 minutes due to pain level of >5/10 with finger flexion of Ⓡ hand.*
- *Child is unable to do jumping jacks to participate in gym class due to motor planning deficits.*

In the last example, the child cannot do the task with any level of assistance. It is a "can" or "cannot" activity. The child is not dependent in jumping jacks; she just cannot do them.

It is not mandatory that these formats be used. These are useful ways of wording functional problem statements, but there are others. Sometimes a slightly different format is more useful:

_____ results in _____.

             Contributing factor   what occupational deficit

For example:

- *Three steps leading to front door limit client's independence in entering house.*
- *Inability to perform simple math calculations results in need for caregiver assistance in IADL tasks such as balancing checkbook.*
- *Pain level >6 at end range shoulder flexion limits ability to don shirt overhead.*
- *Aggressive behavior results in limited opportunities for social participation and repeated involvement with the juvenile justice system.*

Although any of these three formats are acceptable for writing a functional problem statement, students and new practitioners often find that the last format lends itself best to incorporation into the "A" (Assessment) part of a SOAP note, which will be highlighted in Chapter 9.

EXAMPLES OF FUNCTIONAL PROBLEM STATEMENTS

When formulating problem statements, be sure that the problem identified is one that will respond to occupational therapy treatment. There is no need to identify problems that you do not intend to treat. As previously stated, you also need to focus on problems for which treatment is considered necessary and reimbursable by the funding source.

Note: There is a cardstock pullout at the end of this manual that lists the three formulas for writing functional problem statements as well as several examples. Pull it out and carry it with you to use as a quick reference guide.

ACTIVITIES OF DAILY LIVING

- *Poor task initiation and sequencing result in client's need for max verbal cues during dressing activity.*
- *Client requires mod Ⓐ to don pants 2° 3+ UE strength.*
- *Attention span of <3 minutes results in need for mod verbal and tactile cues during grooming tasks.*
- *Client tolerates less than 10 minutes of ADL participation due to severe shortness of breath.*
- *5 out of 10 Ⓡ elbow pain results in veteran needing max Ⓐ to comb hair.*
- *Resident requires hand over hand assist to keep food on fork due to poor motor planning.*
- *Oral tactile defensiveness results in limited variety of food intake.*
- *Patient requires min Ⓐ in dressing activities 2° low vision.*

- *Poor balance and lack of adaptive equipment results in decreased safety while bathing.*
- *Child needs mod Ⓐ in upper body hygiene 2° pronator spasticity, which limits Ⓡ forearm supination by ½ range.*
- *Decreased strength in trunk and UEs results in resident needing max Ⓐ for dressing EOB.*
- *Child unable to feed self due to asymmetrical positioning in w/c.*
- *Client is dependent on caregiver to empty catheter bag due to limited Ⓑ UE function resulting from C5 SCI.*

Instrumental Activities of Daily Living

- *Impaired short-term memory results in safety concerns during meal preparation and child care.*
- *Client unsafe in home management tasks secondary to inability to recognize fatigue when standing.*
- *Client demonstrates ↓ safety in all IADL tasks due to impaired judgment and sequencing.*
- *Focused attention on auditory hallucinations makes consumer unsafe to live alone.*
- *Client requires mod verbal cues for safety during cooking tasks due to impaired Ⓡ UE sensation.*
- *Lifting and bending restrictions due to postsurgical back precautions result in client being unable to complete laundry tasks.*
- *Client unable to write checks for bill paying due to limited grip strength and coordination of dominant Ⓡ hand.*
- *Decreased memory and problem solving result in resident being unable to locate emergency fire exit.*
- *Frequent alcohol use impairs consumer's ability to operate a motor vehicle safely.*
- *Client requires max verbal cues to navigate city bus route to doctor's office due to impaired sequencing and problem solving.*
- *Inability to count money limits client's ability to make independent purchases in the community.*
- *Client is unable to change infant's diaper due to decreased strength and sensation in Ⓑ hands.*

Rest and Sleep

- *Auditory hallucinations result in client obtaining < 3 hours sleep nightly.*
- *Impaired judgment results in resident not calling for assistance when needing to use commode during the night.*
- *Client requires mod Ⓐ to manage bed linens in preparation for sleep due to impaired sensation and strength of Ⓑ hands resulting from multiple sclerosis.*

Education

- *Sierra requires mod Ⓐ to complete art assignment requiring use of a ruler 2° bilateral incoordination.*
- *Sensory-seeking behaviors and decreased attention result in inability to complete classroom assignments in a timely manner.*
- *Slow handwriting speed related to Juvenile Rheumatoid Arthritis results in client's inability to keep up with note-taking during college lectures.*
- *Jose requires step-by-step verbal cues to obtain lunch tray and pay attendant due to impaired sequencing and problem solving.*
- *Tactile defensiveness results in inability to tolerate unexpected touch from peers during circle time.*

Work

- *Preference for youth-culture specific dress limits client's ability to find employment.*
- *Inattention to personal hygiene interferes with consumer's ability to find employment.*
- *Client is unable to perform carpentry work due to grip strength of 3# in Ⓡ hand.*
- *Patient unable to grasp and hold tool with Ⓛ hand due to pain level > 5/10 with flexion of Ⓛ index finger.*
- *< 60° AROM in Ⓡ shoulder abduction limits client's ability to perform work tasks.*
- *Daily cocaine use results in client's inability to hold a job.*
- *Client requires assistance to complete electronic job application due to decreased vision.*
- *Client unable to complete volunteer duties at hospital gift shop due to decreased endurance.*
- *Decreased balance results in inability to lift and carry 20# bucket to feed farm animals.*

PLAY

- *Preoccupation with aligning objects limits child's pretend play interactions with preschool classmates.*
- *Child needs max verbal and tactile cues to transfer toys from one hand to the other due to inattention to Ⓡ side of the body.*
- *Ian is unable to engage in age-appropriate play activities due to sensory processing deficits.*
- *Impulsive behaviors result in teen's need for mod verbal cues for turn taking during group board games.*

LEISURE

- *Resident unable to complete needlework due to impaired coordination of Ⓡ hand.*
- *Impaired problem-solving skills limit consumer's ability to utilize public transportation to attend weekly bowling league.*
- *Decreased fine motor skills result in client's need for mod Ⓐ to manage camera functions when taking pictures.*

SOCIAL PARTICIPATION

- *Belief in government conspiracy limits consumer's willingness to participate in social activities in the community.*
- *Child unable to communicate with peers verbally due to progressive oral motor weakness resulting from muscular dystrophy.*
- *Anxiety in crowds limits client's willingness to leave home for participation in social events.*
- *Individual's aggressive behavior results in social isolation.*
- *Drug-seeking and drug-using behaviors limit client's social participation in non–drug-related activities.*

REFERENCES

American Occupational Therapy Association. (2014). *Occupational therapy practice framework: Domain & process* (3rd ed.). Bethesda, MD: AOTA Press.

Amini, D. (2014). *Documentation for occupation-based practice.* Paper presented at the 2014 AOTA Specialty Conference, Alexandria, VA.

Brennan, C. (2014). *Write it right: What really matters in documentation.* Paper presented at the 2014 AOTA Specialty Conference, Alexandria, VA.

DeCleene, K. E. (2013). Therapists as educators: The importance of client education in occupational therapy. *The Open Journal of Occupational Therapy, 4*(1), 1-21. Retrieved from http://scholarworks.wmich.edu.

King, P. M., & Olson, D. L. (2014). Work. In B.A. Boyt Schell, Gillen, & Scaffa (Eds.) *Willard & Spackman's occupational therapy* (12th ed., pp. 678-696.) Philadelphia, PA: Lippincott Williams & Wilkins.

Swinth, Y. L. (2014). Education. In B.A. Boyt Schell, Gillen, & Scaffa (Eds.) *Willard & Spackman's occupational therapy* (12th ed., pp. 653-677.) Philadelphia, PA: Lippincott Williams & Wilkins.

Tripicchio, B., Bykerk, K., Wegner, C., & Wegner, J. (2009). Increasing patient participation: The effects of training physical and occupational therapists to involve geriatric patients in the concerns-clarification and goal-setting processes. *Journal of Physical Therapy Education, 23*(1), 55-63.

Valdes, K. (2014). *How to comply with Medicare documentation requirements for Part B therapy services.* Summit Professional Education seminar held August 23, 2014 in Columbia, MO.

VanPuymbrouck, L. H. (2014). Promoting client goal ownership in a clinical setting. *The Open Journal of Occupational Therapy, 2*(2), 1-20. Retrieved from http://scholarworks.wmich.edu.

WORKSHEET 5-1

Identifying the Contributing Factors

Complete each of the following functional problem statements with at least three possible contributing factors. (Hint: It may be helpful to refer to Table 5-2 for potential contributing factors.)

1. *Area of Occupation = Work*
   - Consumer is unable to sustain employment longer than 2 weeks due to

   - Consumer is unable to sustain employment longer than 2 weeks due to

   - Consumer is unable to sustain employment longer than 2 weeks due to

2. *Area of Occupation = ADLs*
   - Veteran needs 1½ hours to complete grooming tasks due to

   - Veteran needs 1½ hours to complete grooming tasks due to

   - Veteran needs 1½ hours to complete grooming tasks due to

3. *Area of Occupation = Education*
   - Child is unable to complete grade-appropriate written worksheets due to

   - Child is unable to complete grade-appropriate written worksheets due to

   - Child is unable to complete grade-appropriate written worksheets due to

WORKSHEET 5-2

Writing Occupation-Based Problem Statements

Use the following descriptions to write occupation-based problem statements for each client. Make them specific enough to:
- Show the area of occupation that is a concern
- Show the contributing factor(s) that affect this area of occupation
- Serve as a baseline against which to measure progress

You may use any of the three formats provided in this chapter for writing the functional problem statements.

1. *The client has an acquired injury to his brain. As a result, he is not able to pay attention to task for very long at a time, and he is having trouble completing his morning routine. Usually he can pay attention to what he is doing for about 2 minutes, and needs to be redirected back to the task after that.*

2. *The child is having trouble in school because she has difficulty staying within the lines when she is writing. She habitually grips her pencil in a gross grasp, although with help (someone's hand placed over hers) she can hold it with her thumb and two fingers.*

3. *The resident is not very cognitively aware. About 40% of the time, she has trouble figuring out what to do first if she has to complete a self-care task, and she doesn't remember what she has just been told.*

4. *Mr. J has recently sustained a ⓡ CVA. His ⓛ arm is flaccid and he forgets that it is there. He needs physical and verbal help with ADL tasks about 60% of the time.*

5. *The consumer has had trouble finding a job. His appearance is unkempt and he has a strong body odor, neither of which seem troubling to him.*

6. *The client is unable to transfer safely w/c ↔ toilet without someone to remind him that he needs to follow his total hip precautions.*

Writing Measurable Occupation-Based Goals and Objectives

Goals and objectives used in a treatment plan must be written in occupation-based, measurable, observable, action-oriented terms. They must also be realistic for the client and achievable in a reasonable amount of time within the client's current practice setting. Goals are formulated from the problem list compiled in collaboration with the client. For successful intervention, it is critical to work on goals that are important to the client. Occupational therapy practitioners have a responsibility to include clients in discussions regarding the goals and interventions that will direct their care (American Occupational Therapy Association [AOTA], 2014).

Occupational therapy goals must focus on functional improvements in occupational performance. The client factors that contribute to such progress, such as strength and range of motion, are much less important to a third-party payer than what the client can actually do, even though the gains in those contributing factors may be essential to achieving the functional outcome.

Lamb (2014) emphasized the importance of "demonstrating the distinct value of occupational therapy through documentation" and encouraged practitioners to "approach documentation as an ethical and fiscal responsibility, as a marketing tool, and as a means of obtaining data for current and future research projects" (pp. 1, 5). There is also a movement toward evidence-based practice and communicating that evidence in clinical documentation. Occupational therapy practitioners can combine scientific research evidence with the information that is gathered through interviews and observations of clients (Baker & Tickle-Degnen, 2014). Using these approaches, we can collaborate with our clients to establish outcome measures that demonstrate functional improvements and the ability to participate in meaningful occupation.

GOALS

Goals in an intervention plan are also called *long-term goals* (LTGs) or *outcomes*. These are usually discharge goals—what the client hopes to accomplish by the time of discharge from occupational therapy services in the current setting. For each problem you have identified, you will have at least one LTG, and often more than one.

OBJECTIVES

Objectives are also called *short-term goals* (STGs). These are goals that are met in smaller increments while progressing toward the discharge goals.

For example, if your LTG is:

Client will complete 3-step stove top meal preparation with modified independence using walker within 1 week.

then one of your STGs might be:

Client will retrieve and transport items from refrigerator to stove using walker and wheeled cart with CGA within 3 days.

Gateley CA, Borcherding S. *Documentation Manual for Occupational Therapy: Writing SOAP Notes, Fourth Edition (pp 57-72).* © 2017 SLACK Incorporated

If your LTG is:

Client will move 35# objects needed for work from table to counter without ↑ in pain by discharge in 2 weeks.

then one of your STGs might be:

Client will be able to lift 10# objects needed for work without ↑ in pain within 1 week.

You may have several STGs (objectives) for each LTG. For example, suppose you are treating Mr. Hawkins, a 45-year-old executive who sustained a Ⓡ CVA a few days ago and has Ⓛ hemiplegia. On evaluation, you find that he is oriented x 4, verbal, intelligent, and able to learn, and he has a supportive wife. After talking with him about what he would like to achieve in occupational therapy, you and he decide upon a goal of modified independence in upper body dressing. You believe that this is a realistic goal, provided that he receives skilled instruction and the necessary adaptive equipment. You set the following series of STGs:

1. Seated edge of bed, client will reach for clothing items at arm's length with CGA to maintain dynamic sitting by the end of the 3rd treatment session.

2. By the 6th treatment session, client will be able to participate in dressing activities for > 10 minutes without rest break seated edge of bed with CGA.

3. After skilled instruction, client will be able to don shirt sitting EOB using one-handed techniques with min verbal cues by the 8th treatment session.

4. Client will be able to button shirt using a button hook with 2 or fewer verbal cues by 10th treatment session.

5. Client will complete all upper body dressing tasks with modified independence seated EOB by discharge in 2 weeks.

As you can see, each of these STGs is measurable, observable, and action-oriented. The first four STGs are steps to the ultimate LTG (Figure 6-1).

Figure 6-1. Steps to the ultimate LTG.

An intervention plan is always a work in progress. Unexpected events and conditions can affect the progress your client will be able to make toward his or her goals. If you find a goal unrealistic, you are obligated to change it. It is not useful to continue with a plan that is not working. For example, suppose that your client begins to have some motor function return in his involved Ⓛ upper extremity. You now know that he may be able to dress his upper body without adaptive techniques or equipment, and he wants very much to do that. You would need to write a new set of STGs for him.

GOAL WRITING: THE COAST METHOD

There are several formats available for writing goal statements (Sames, 2015). In this manual, we advocate the use of a format that was first introduced in the previous edition of this textbook: the COAST method. This method was designed around the principles put forth by Crepeau, Boyt Schell, and Cohn (2009) that contemporary practice should be client centered and occupation centered. The AOTA recently established an annual specialty conference entitled *Effective Documentation—The Key to Payment & Articulating Our Distinct Value.* The COAST method has been presented at the conference as a way to ensure that occupational therapy practitioners are communicating our inherent focus on occupational performance to third-party payers (Amini, 2014).

Just as the SOAP format is one way of learning to document occupational therapy services, the COAST method is simply one way of learning to write goals. While settings may vary in the format used, learning the COAST method will ensure that you consistently include all necessary information in your goal statements.

- ◆ C—Client   Client will perform
- ◆ O—Occupation   What occupation?
- ◆ A—Assist Level   With what level of assistance/independence?
- ◆ S—Specific Condition   Under what conditions?
- ◆ T—Timeline   By when?

> There has been considerable debate about the concepts of *occupation*, *activity*, and *task*, with definitions varying between conceptual models (Brown, 2014). It is not within the scope of this textbook to engage in that debate. The *OTPF-III* (AOTA, 2014) provides multiple definitions of occupation that include the terms *activity* or *task*. For purposes of this textbook, it can be assumed that the "O" in the COAST acronym encompasses any activity or task that is related to the performance of an area of occupation as defined by the *OTPF-III* (AOTA, 2014).

To write goals and objectives in a way that can be measured, the elements to be included are very specific. Let's take a closer look at each category.

C (CLIENT)

In writing treatment goals, the **client** is the key player. Goals should be written in terms of what the client will do, not what the therapist will do. The therapist's actions are documented later, under intervention strategies. An action verb is also inserted here, such as *perform*, *demonstrate*, or *complete*.

For example:

>   *Client will perform*...

O (OCCUPATION)

This is the specific **occupation** to which this goal pertains and should relate to the problem statements that have been established. Improving an individual's ability to engage in occupation is the core of occupational therapy practice. It is the first thing you think of in writing goals, and it should be the essential focus of the goal statement.

For example:

>   *Client will perform a 3-step cooking process*...

A (ASSIST LEVEL)

This is where you specify the **level of assistance** expected, which ultimately translates into the level of independence that the client is expected to demonstrate. This should include the physical and/or verbal cues that will be required in order for the client to complete the activity.

For example:

>   *Client will perform a 3-step cooking process with 2 or fewer verbal cues for sequencing and safety*...

> Note: The method used to describe the level of assistance will vary between settings and funding sources. For example, settings in which Medicare is a primary funding source, such as inpatient rehabilitation centers and long-term care facilities, often use the Functional Independence Measure instrument as a common measure of client outcomes (Centers for Medicare & Medicaid Services, 2015). You need to be aware of the common terminology used in your setting and incorporate it into your goal writing.

Be careful not to mix levels of assistance. This is a common mistake made by students when first learning to write goals.

For example:

>   *Client will perform a 3-step cooking process with modified independence and 2 or fewer verbal cues*....

Inherent in the definition of modified independence is that no verbal cues are required. You cannot use both levels of assistance in the same goal.

S (SPECIFIC CONDITIONS)

This is where you **specify any other conditions** under which the client is expected to perform the desired action such as location, adaptive equipment, or modified technique.

For example:

Client will perform a 3-step cooking process with 2 or fewer verbal cues for sequencing and safety <u>from w/c level in rehab kitchen</u>...

The "A" and "S" together make your goal statement **measurable** and allow you to show your client's progress. Other examples include the following:

- *...by using a dressing stick with 2 or fewer verbal cues*
- *...using walker with CGA*
- *...with mod Ⓐ using sliding board*
- *...3 out of 4 attempts without verbal cues*
- *...independently from standing position*
- *...using medication organizer with weekly supervision for set-up*
- *...3 out of 5 attempts during evening meal*
- *...with modified independence using tub bench and hand-held shower hose*
- *...during group sessions without use of profanity*
- *...seated EOB with CGA for balance*

In rare cases, it is acceptable to omit either the "A" or the "S," **but never both**. You may write a goal for a task that either can or cannot be done, and assistance would not be applicable. For example, suppose you have a client who presents with pain in her Ⓡ CMC joint. She is able to complete most IADL tasks independently, but reports pain during tasks such as opening doorknobs. Your LTG may look like this:

Client will open doorknobs using Ⓡ hand without report of wrist pain within 2 weeks.

In this example, no assist level is mentioned, but "without report of wrist pain" makes this goal measurable. Another example:

Client will complete all dressing tasks Ⓘ by discharge.

In this example, the assistance level (or in this case the lack of assistance level) is stated, but there are no other specific conditions that are necessary for this goal.

T (TIMELINE)

This is the time frame within which the goal is expected to be accomplished. For an LTG, this may be the anticipated discharge date. Please note that in many of the examples throughout this book, when specific dates are used, the examples provide only a month and day. However, if you use this method in your practice setting, you should also provide the year, such as *by 3-20-18*.

For example:

- *Client will perform a 3-step cooking process with 2 or fewer verbal cues for sequencing and safety from w/c level in rehab kitchen <u>by March 20th</u>.*
- *Client will perform a 3-step cooking process with 2 or fewer verbal cues for sequencing and safety from w/c level in rehab kitchen <u>within 2 weeks</u>.*

Depending on your setting, the timeline for your STGs may be daily, weekly, or by number of sessions. For example:

- *Client will prepare a sandwich with 2 or fewer verbal cues for sequencing and safety from w/c level in rehab kitchen <u>by March 16th</u>.*
- *Client will prepare a sandwich with 2 or fewer verbal cues for sequencing and safety from w/c level in rehab kitchen <u>within 1 week</u>.*
- *Client will prepare a sandwich with 2 or fewer verbal cues for sequencing and safety from w/c level in rehab kitchen <u>by 5th treatment session</u>.*

It is important to remember that the time frame for the client's LTG must be realistic to the setting in which you are working. For example, if you work in an acute care hospital setting where the average length of stay is only a few days, it does not make sense to write a goal about what the client will do in 3 weeks. By that time, the client may be working with a home health or outpatient occupational therapist. You have to estimate what you will be able to accomplish in the time frame that is typical for your setting. This sounds challenging, but it does get easier with experience. The following is a rough guideline of maximum time frames for common occupational therapy practice settings:

- *Inpatient acute care*: Often just a few days. As soon as the patient is medically stable, he or she likely will be discharged to a different setting such as inpatient rehabilitation, home with home health therapy services, or home with outpatient therapy services.
- *Inpatient rehabilitation facility*: A few to several weeks depending on setting and severity of impairments.
- *Outpatient clinic*: A few to several weeks. Funding sources may require updates every 30 days, so 4 weeks is a good time frame for a LTG.
- *Skilled nursing facility*: A few to several weeks. Updates to the physician and/or funding source may be required at certain intervals.
- *Schools*: Yearly basis. If a child requires special education services and occupational therapy is listed in the child's plan as a related service, LTGs are updated annually.
- *Early intervention*: A few to several months. Each state sets its own guidelines regarding documentation requirements.
- *Community-based practice*: Varies greatly depending on the type of setting and client population.

It is also important to note that the time frames listed previously are general guidelines for the maximum length of time for an LTG. This does not mean that every client's condition will justify that length of time. Your time frames should be driven by your best estimate of how long it will take the client to achieve maximum function in your setting. Consistently setting the same time frame on goals for every client you see can be a red flag to claim reviewers for third-party payers (Valdes, 2014).

EXAMPLES OF GOAL STATEMENTS

The COAST method is useful as you are learning to write, although the order may need to be changed slightly in order for your sentence to make sense. As long as all of the required elements are present, it does not matter with which element you begin your sentence. Let's take a look at a few examples:

C: *Client will*
O: *feed self 50% of meal*
A: *with min physical Ⓐ to scoop*
S: *using built-up spoon*
T: *within 3 tx sessions.*

The elements of this goal statement can be rearranged without changing the meaning of the goal:

- *Within 3 tx sessions, client will feed self 50% of meal using built-up spoon with min physical Ⓐ to scoop.*
- *Using built-up spoon, client will feed self 50% of meal with min physical Ⓐ to scoop within 3 sessions.*

Here is another example:

C: *Client will perform*
O: *bed-making activity*
A: *with min verbal cues*
S: *while adhering to postsurgical back precautions*
T: *by discharge in 3 days.*

The elements of this goal statement can be rearranged without changing the meaning of the goal:

With min verbal cues, client will perform bed-making activity while adhering to postsurgical back precautions by discharge in 3 days.

While acceptable to rearrange some elements of the COAST goal, the "C" and the "O" should always be kept together to help keep the focus on the occupation.

Incorrect example: *Client will use adaptive equipment with modified independence to complete lower body dressing within 3 days.*

Correct example: *Client will complete lower body dressing using adaptive equipment with modified independence within 3 days.*

In the first example, the focus is on the adaptive equipment rather than the occupation of lower body dressing. Make it easy for the insurance reviewer to discern the most important part of your goal. The client will do what? The client will complete lower body dressing.

ACTIVITIES OF DAILY LIVING

- *Brittney will don coat using over-the-head method with mod Ⓘ within 1 month.*
- *Client will fasten 3 buttons in 2 minutes using button hook with min verbal cues by May 2nd.*
- *Within 3 treatment sessions, Mr. S will complete toileting using raised toilet seat with min Ⓐ for balance during clothing adjustment.*
- *Pt. will complete bathing tasks seated on tub bench using long-handled sponge with SBA within 1 week.*
- *Child will feed self 50% of meal using adaptive spoon with mod Ⓐ within 3 weeks.*
- *Pt. will empty catheter leg-bag with min verbal cues for technique within 1 week.*
- *Client will demonstrate safe clothing retrieval and transport from closet using walker with CGA by November 30th.*
- *Caregiver will demonstrate correct application of client's postsurgical back corset during upper body dressing tasks without verbal cues by end of 2nd treatment session.*
- *Within 1 week, resident will complete grooming tasks from w/c level with min tactile cues to attend to left side.*
- *Caitlyn will demo ability to doff coat and place on coat hook with min Ⓐ by end of school year.*

INSTRUMENTAL ACTIVITIES OF DAILY LIVING

- *By June 23rd, client will transfer 10 laundry items from washer to dryer with 3 or fewer verbal cues to adhere to postsurgical back precautions.*
- *Client will demonstrate ability to change infant's diaper using adaptive one-handed methods with 2 or fewer verbal cues within 2 weeks.*
- *Rachel will analyze bill statement and write check for correct amount 3 of 4 attempts with min verbal cues by August 19th.*
- *Within 3 days, client will demonstrate safe transfer in/out of car with supervision while adhering to postsurgical hip precautions.*
- *Resident will identify and navigate safe route from bedroom to exit of residential care facility with modified independence using 4-wheeled walker by July 5th.*
- *Client will locate phone numbers of emergency services in the telephone directory without physical or verbal cues by end of 3rd treatment session.*
- *Brian will navigate public bus system from home to doctor's office with supervision during next treatment session.*
- *Within 2 weeks, Mrs. S will make bed with modified independence while incorporating energy conservation techniques.*

REST AND SLEEP

- *Using visual checklist as memory aid, Taylor will remember to lock doors before bedtime on 5 consecutive nights by September 21st.*
- *Consumer will go to bed before midnight at least 75% of weeknights within 2 weeks to obtain adequate sleep for effective participation at job.*
- *Within 1 month, teen will complete 3-step bedtime routine using visual schedule with 2 or fewer verbal cues.*

EDUCATION

Note: Therapists working in public schools use a slightly different terminology. In education, goals for one school year are called *objectives* or *behavioral objectives*. Educational goals often are not measured by time, such as *by 5/7/11* or *within 3 weeks*. Since the Individualized Education Program is written annually, the time frame for educational goals is assumed to be annual. Children sometimes exhibit a new behavior inconsistently before it is really established. Therefore, measurement used for children is more likely to reflect whether the behavior is <u>established</u>. For example:

Li Mei will obtain and transport lunch tray to table with mod Ⓘ from w/c level 9 of 10 days.

- *Na'Kyra will cut out circle independently during classroom activities using supinated grasp on scissors with < 2 deviations from line on 75% of attempts.*
- *Child will maintain seated position at desk for 5 minutes with 2 or fewer verbal cues 4 of 5 consecutive days.*
- *Child will print upper case alphabet independently on wide-ruled notebook paper, demonstrating proper letter formation and staying on line, with < 3 errors 75% of attempts.*
- *Student will don/doff coat without physical assistance 90% of the time to be independent with beginning and end-of-day school routine.*
- *Addison will take turns on playground equipment without adult intervention 3 of 4 consecutive days.*
- *Child will copy 10 math problems from whiteboard to paper with < 2 errors and no verbal cues 80% of attempts.*
- *Logan will complete assigned classroom tasks within allotted time with fewer than 3 verbal cues 75% of the time.*
- *Mia will participate in group activities for up to 10 minutes without exhibiting aggressive behaviors toward classmates 4 of 5 consecutive days.*

WORK

- *Without staff support, Malik will request at least one job application from a restaurant within 1 week.*
- *Client will transfer 10# boxes from floor to shelf during simulated work tasks, demonstrating proper body mechanics without verbal cues by October 17th.*
- *By May 4th, client will count correct change from a $20 bill without verbal cues to return to position as volunteer in hospital gift shop.*
- *Alejandro will identify at least 2 opportunities for community volunteer service independently by next group session.*
- *Client will navigate power w/c in work environment without bumping into objects or people within 3 weeks.*
- *Client will demonstrate ability to type 20 words per minute during simulated work tasks using Ⓑ wrist cock-up splints within 2 weeks.*

PLAY

- *Infant will engage in play with parent or sibling by visually tracking a toy 45 degrees past midline in both directions by June 30th.*
- *Within 2 months, Joaquin will stabilize pop-up toy with Ⓛ UE while activating toy with Ⓡ hand with min physical facilitation.*
- *Child will place 3 shapes into puzzle board with no verbal cues in 3 months.*
- *Katrina will engage in pretend play activity with peers for > 3 minutes with minimal adult facilitation by February 28th.*
- *Infant will engage in Ⓑ UE play activity while independently sitting unsupported > 1 minute by December 10th.*
- *Child will catch tennis ball in Ⓑ hands on 8 of 10 attempts when tossed from 10 feet within 3 weeks.*
- *Lauren will stack 6 or more 1" blocks independently using Ⓡ hand to stabilize tower within 1 month.*

SOCIAL PARTICIPATION

- *Consumer will choose and participate in at least one social activity per week independently, 3/3 weeks within 1 month.*
- *With mod verbal cues, consumer will ask roommate to smoke outside the building next time the situation arises.*
- *Matias will make at least 2 verbal contributions to group discussions with min verbal prompts 5/5 days within 1 week.*
- *Within 2 months, Liam will tolerate unexpected touch from peers during circle time without demonstrating aggressive behaviors 80% of the time per daycare provider report.*
- *Using visual schedule and min verbal cues, Myah will transition between home and preschool environment without expressing anxiety or fear at least 50% of the time within 3 months.*

LEISURE

- *Independently, client will identify at least 3 leisure activities that are not associated with drinking by September 8th.*
- *Within 3 weeks, client will demonstrate sufficient coordination to manipulate toothpaste caps, buttons, and knitting needles without dropping.*

> Note: There is a cardstock pullout at the end of this manual that reviews the COAST formula and provides several examples of goal statements. Pull it out and carry it with you to use as a quick-reference guide.

Medical Necessity

As occupational therapists, we view a client holistically, considering the whole person with his or her needs, interests, problems, strengths, and priorities. We know that leisure is an important part of the total picture. When this is the client's priority, we might be inclined to write problem statements and goals focusing on leisure skills and interests, such as:

- Problem: *Client is unable to play softball due to ↓ AROM and ↑ pain in ℝ wrist.*
- LTG: *Client will pitch a softball without wrist pain within 6 weeks.*

However, we know that both Medicare and private insurance are very frugal with our health care dollars and approve expenditures only for medical necessity. Since even adaptive equipment such as a raised toilet seat is not always considered medically necessary, treatment focused on a client's leisure goals is likely to be denied under our current reimbursement system. In consideration of the client's holistic needs and the reimbursement limitations, we may address some of the contributing factors that enable the client to perform a variety of functional tasks in the intervention plan. Documentation would focus on goals and interventions that provide the client with skills for self-care and work, as well as the leisure activities that are so important to the quality of life. Worksheet 6-1 will allow you to practice this documentation skill.

In the example here, we might suspect that the client is also having difficulty with household or work tasks requiring ℝ UE use. It would be more appropriate to write an IADL goal, such as:

> *Client will lift pots and pans during dishwashing without wrist pain in 6 weeks.*

Interventions would be targeted toward the client factors of active range of motion and pain, and improvements in these client factors would result in an increased ability for the client to pursue her leisure interests as well.

> Note: **DO NOT** use participation in treatment as a goal. For example:
>
> *Client will do 20 reps of shoulder ladder with 1# wt. to ↑ endurance to become more ① in IADLs.*
>
> Instead, write a goal that specifies the amount of endurance the client needs to demonstrate during an occupation-based activity. For example:
>
> *Client will complete seated cooking task >5 minutes without rest breaks with SBA within 2 weeks.*

GOALS IN DIFFERENT SETTINGS

The COAST format works well in many occupational therapy settings. This method of goal writing allows you to demonstrate the specific need for occupational therapy services by focusing on areas of occupation affected by the client's condition. In some settings, problem statements and goals are written differently due to the nature of services provided.

MENTAL HEALTH AND SUBSTANCE ABUSE

In mental health and substance abuse practice settings, problem statements and goals are often multidisciplinary and are written to be addressed by the treatment team rather than by one specific discipline.

For example:
- ◆ Problem: *Alcohol use*
- ◆ Behavioral manifestation: *Kyle admits to drinking at least 8 oz. of liquor and 7 to 8 beers nightly, resulting in failing grades and involvement with the law due to physical violence toward peers.*
- ◆ STG: *By next group session, Kyle will identify 2 leisure activities not associated with drinking.*

Another example:
- ◆ Problem: *Noncompliant behavior*
- ◆ Behavioral manifestation: *Amanda is noncompliant with family rules and social norms (attending school, abiding by the law), resulting in assignment to a parole officer and 3 failed foster home placements.*
- ◆ STG: *Amanda will demonstrate willingness to cooperate with family norms by entering into a behavioral contract with her parents within 1 week.*

EARLY INTERVENTION

In recent years, early intervention programs that provide services for children from birth to 3 years of age have moved toward a family-centered, transdisciplinary model of service delivery (Mulligan, 2014; Myers, Case-Smith, & Cason, 2015). One aspect of a family-centered approach is that, rather than the professionals setting the goals for the child, families identify the "outcomes" that they hope their child will achieve. For example, the family may identify outcomes such as the following:

- ◆ *Jayden will use words during playtime and meals to express his needs.*
- ◆ *Jayden will express his emotion in positive ways when he is excited.*
- ◆ *Jayden will show interest in potty training.*
- ◆ *Jayden will walk up and down the stairs at home unassisted.*
- ◆ *Jayden will use a spoon to feed himself at least half of his meal.*

The transdisciplinary aspect of early intervention means that families will interact directly with only one or two individuals of the team on a regular basis, with other disciplines providing services on a consultative basis. Occupational therapists providing early intervention services under a transdisciplinary model may encounter the need for role release, which is "the commitment of professionals to teaching, learning, and providing direct services that may not be traditionally within their discipline-specific roles" (Mulligan, 2014, p. 15). If you work in an early intervention setting, your documentation and interventions should reflect the service delivery model required by the agency.

REFERENCES

American Occupational Therapy Association. (2014). *Occupational therapy practice framework: Domain & process* (3rd ed.). Bethesda, MD: AOTA Press.

Amini, D. (2014). *Documentation for occupation-based practice.* Paper presented at the 2014 AOTA Specialty Conference, Alexandria, VA.

Baker, N., & Tickle-Degnen, L. (2014). Evidence-based practice. In B.A. Boyt Schell, Gillen, & Scaffa (Eds.), *Willard & Spackman's occupational therapy* (12th ed., pp. 398-412.) Philadelphia, PA: Lippincott Williams & Wilkins.

Brown, C. E. (2014). Ecological models in occupational therapy. In B.A. Boyt Schell, Gillen, & Scaffa (Eds.), *Willard & Spackman's occupational therapy* (12th ed., pp. 494-504.) Philadelphia, PA: Lippincott Williams & Wilkins.

Centers for Medicare & Medicaid Services. (2015). IRF Patient Assessment Instrument. Retrieved from https://www.cms.gov.

Crepeau, E., Boyt Schell, B., & Cohn, E. (2009). Contemporary occupational therapy practice in the United States. In E.B Crepeau, E.S. Cohn, & B.A. Boyt Schell (Eds.), *Willard & Spackman's occupational therapy* (11th ed., pp. 216-221). Philadelphia: Lippincott Williams & Wilkins.

Lamb, A. J. (2014). *Documenting the distinct value of occupational therapy through documentation.* Presentation at the 2014 AOTA Specialty Conference – Effective Documentation: The Key to Payment & Articulating Our Distinct Value held September 12-13, 2014 in Alexandria, VA.

Mulligan, S. (2014). *Occupational therapy evaluation for children: A pocket guide* (2nd ed). Philadelphia, PA: Lippincott Williams & Wilkins.

Myers, C. T., Case-Smith, J., & Cason, J. (2015). Early intervention. In J. Case-Smith & J. Clifford O'Brien (Eds.), *Occupational therapy for children and adolescents* (7th ed., pp. 636-663). St. Louis, MO: Elsevier.

Sames, K. M. (2015). *Documenting occupational therapy practice* (3rd ed.). Boston, MA: Pearson.

Valdes, K. (2014). *How to comply with Medicare documentation requirements for Part B therapy services.* Summit Professional Education seminar held August 23, 2014 in Columbia, MO.

WORKSHEET 6-1

Choosing Goals for Medical Necessity

Below is a scenario for a client who has stated a priority for leisure interests. You will have the opportunity to write goals that focus on other areas of occupation while still addressing the same contributing factors that are affecting her performance of leisure activities.

- ♦ Problem: *Client unable to perform sewing due to 2+/5 strength in ® hand musculature.*
  - ▪ LTG: *Client will perform embroidery Ⓘ for 20 minutes within 8 weeks.*
  - ▪ STG: *To ↑ performance of embroidery, client will use needle continuously for 5 minutes within 2 weeks.*

1. What other problems might this woman have due to decreased strength in her ® hand?

2. What LTG might you use that would show medical necessity for increasing ® UE strength?

3. What STG might be used as a step to achieve that LTG?

WORKSHEET 6-2

Evaluating Goal Statements

Refer to the COAST elements to determine which of the following goals has each of the necessary components to be useful in occupational therapy documentation. For each goal that you find to be incomplete or inaccurate in some way, indicate what is missing.

1. *By the time of discharge in 2 weeks, client will dress himself with min Ⓐ for balance using a sock aid and reacher while sitting in w/c.*
   ___ This goal has all of the necessary COAST components.
   ___ This goal lacks:

2. *Client will tolerate 10 minutes of treatment daily.*
   ___ This goal has all of the necessary COAST components.
   ___ This goal lacks:

3. *Client will demonstrate increased coping skills when communicating with her daughter within 2 weeks.*
   ___ This goal has all of the necessary COAST components.
   ___ This goal lacks:

4. *Client will demonstrate 15 minutes of activity tolerance without rest breaks using Ⓑ UEs to complete ADL tasks before breakfast each morning.*
   ___ This goal has all of the necessary COAST components.
   ___ This goal lacks:

5. *OT will teach lower body dressing using a reacher, dressing stick, and sock aid within 3 treatment sessions.*
   ___ This goal has all of the necessary COAST components.
   ___ This goal lacks:

6. *Patient will demonstrate ability to balance his checkbook.*
   ___ This goal has all of the necessary COAST components.
   ___ This goal lacks:

WORKSHEET 6-3

Writing Client-Centered, Occupation-Based, Measurable Goals

Write goals for the scenarios below that are client-centered, occupation-based, and measurable. Please remember that we set goals <u>with</u> the client. Assume for this worksheet that you have already collaborated with the client regarding his or her goals.

1. Ayana is not able to attend to task for more than a few minutes, which makes IADL activities difficult for her. Since she likes to cook and plans to return to cooking after discharge, you have been working with her in the kitchen. You would like to see her able to attend to a task for 10 minutes by the time she is discharged next week. Write a goal that addresses Ayana's attention span during cooking.

   C: _____
   (Client will perform)
   O: _____
   (Occupation)
   A: _____
   (Assist level)
   S: _____
   (Specific conditions)
   T: _____
   (Timeline—by when?)

2. Now write a goal for Ayana to be able to follow directions so that she can read the back of a boxed meal, and eventually a recipe, when she is cooking.

   C: _____
   (Client will perform)
   O: _____
   (Occupation)
   A: _____
   (Assist level)
   S: _____
   (Specific conditions)
   T: _____
   (Timeline—by when?)

3. Scott is having trouble dressing himself after his stroke. You have been teaching him an over-the-head method for putting on his shirt, and have given him a buttonhook to use. Write a dressing goal for Scott.

   C: _____
   (Client will perform)
   O: _____
   (Occupation)
   A: _____
   (Assist level)
   S: _____
   (Specific conditions)
   T: _____
   (Timeline—by when?)

WORKSHEET 6-3 (CONTINUED)

Writing Client-Centered, Occupation-Based, Measurable Goals

Write goals for the scenarios below that are client-centered, occupation-based, and measurable. Please remember that we set goals <u>with</u> the client. Assume for this worksheet that you have already collaborated with the client regarding his or her goals.

4. Nikki is very weak, and she wants to be able to go back to work as a receptionist. She also wants to be able to care for her 4-month-old child. Write a goal that addresses her activity tolerance during an occupation-based activity.

C: _____
(Client will perform)
O: _____
(Occupation)
A: _____
(Assist level)
S: _____
(Specific conditions)
T: _____
(Timeline—by when?)

5. Demarco wants to live independently in the community, but lacks basic money management skills. Write a goal for Demarco to improve his money management skills.

C: _____
(Client will perform)
O: _____
(Occupation)
A: _____
(Assist level)
S: _____
(Specific conditions)
T: _____
(Timeline—by when?)

6. Tiffany has become increasingly more depressed over the past several weeks and was admitted after a suicide attempt. You estimate that you will have her in group for 1 week. You would like to see her mood change in that week. Write an occupation-based goal that will indicate an improved mood.

C: _____
(Client will perform)
O: _____
(Occupation)
A: _____
(Assist level)
S: _____
(Specific conditions)
T: _____
(Timeline—by when?)

Writing the "S"—Subjective

The first section of the SOAP note contains *subjective* information obtained from the client, giving his or her perspective on his or her condition or treatment. Subjective data are information that cannot be verified or measured during the treatment session. In this section, the therapist records the client's report of limitations, concerns, and problems, as well as what the client said was relevant to treatment, such as significant complaints of pain; fatigue; or other expressions of feelings, attitudes, concerns, goals, and plans. When direct quotes are used in the subjective sections of the SOAP note, it is understood that the statement came from the individual receiving therapy unless otherwise stated.

The information obtained from the client will be of greater significance and relevance to your note if it is specific in nature. For instance, if the client tells you, "My shoulder hurts," you may question him further, asking, "Where does it hurt?" or "When does it hurt?" so your note can communicate more detailed information on his condition. You may either use a direct quote or summarize what the client has said, so his description might be written as:

> "My right shoulder hurts when I try to put my shirt on."

or

> Client reports Ⓡ shoulder pain when he tries to put his shirt on.

EXAMPLES OF "S" STATEMENTS

- "I don't need therapy."
- Resident reports pain in Ⓡ shoulder when reaching up to comb hair.
- Patient asked for help when it was needed during the session.
- Client reports, "I keep blowing up at home and yelling at everyone, and I don't know what to do about it."
- "I can't wash the dishes or zip my coat."
- Veteran reports that his fingers "feel kind of dead."
- Pt. reported that he needed to go meet someone and get to work when the session began. When asked questions such as "Can you hear me?" he often responded, "I need to go."
- Resident reports he feels "pretty good" now and his goal is to "get back as independent as I can."
- Consumer reports being fearful of leaving her home.
- Client reports that his doctor has ordered "some home health for a few days to help me learn how to take care of myself."
- Client reported that her shoulder feel better after application of kinesiotape to reduce subluxation. "My short-term goal is to be able to write, and my long-term goal is to return to work."

Gateley CA, Borcherding S. *Documentation Manual for
Occupational Therapy: Writing SOAP Notes, Fourth Edition* (pp 73-79).
© 2017 SLACK Incorporated

- Cindy called the emergency room last night to report a burning sensation in her "gut," which made her afraid she was going to die. Today she reports that she has been worrying about dying and has not showered since the day before yesterday.
- Resident reports being able to bathe and dress self Ⓘ, but does not open dresser drawers and closet doors due to a recent fall from opening a dresser drawer that resulted in a hip fx. She was able to state the correct day and month when asked.
- Pt. commented that she used to use her Ⓛ hand to hold a cup but now is unable to do so. Pt. also complained of soreness in Ⓛ shoulder and inquired about agencies that can help with housekeeping tasks when she returns home.
- Client stated that she has experienced several episodes of bladder incontinence when trying to make it to the bathroom.
- Consumer reports that the hardest feelings for her to deal with are worry and fear about her physical problems, which might go undetected. She reports being unable to function at home (cannot cook, keep house, or do laundry) when she is "sick with depression," but wants to do these things again. Consumer reports that exercise, prayer, and volunteer work are her primary coping strategies, and that she would like to learn more about relaxation techniques.
- Student reports frustration with handwriting tasks, stating, "I'm just no good at it. I hate writing!"

As part of the initial evaluation process, an occupational therapist works toward establishing a collaborative relationship with the client by interviewing the client about his or her concerns and priorities and developing an occupational profile. The occupational profile is "a summary of the client's occupational history and experiences, patterns of daily living, interests, values, and needs" (American Occupational Therapy Association, 2014, p. S13). Additional information for the occupational profile may be gathered from discussions with family or caregivers, and through the review of existing health records. In an evaluation note, the "S" may contain all or part of the client's occupational profile.

For example:

- Client reports that she was admitted after a fall that resulted in confusion and left-sided weakness. Prior to admission, she was living alone in a one-story home and was Ⓘ in all ADLs. She reports that she is a retired librarian, widowed 10 years ago. She says she values her independence and fully intends to return to her own home. She reports that her activities are primarily sedentary, including sewing, reading, and playing cards with friends. She says her daughter lives two blocks away and provides transportation when needed.

Another example:

- The client talked about his current symptoms and the events leading up to his hospitalization. He reports losing his job with a construction company after not reporting to work for 2 weeks due to depression, having an argument with his wife, and taking an overdose. He says that he has always "worked construction" and does not know how to do anything else. He reports concerns that his former employer will not give him "a decent reference." He says he really has no leisure interests except "going out drinking with the guys after work" and sometimes going hunting in the fall.

Sometimes the client is not able to speak or does not make any relevant comments. In such cases, include that information in the "S" section.

For example:

- Client unable to communicate verbally due to expressive aphasia.
- Client did not speak without cueing.
- Using her augmentative communication device, pt. reported that she wanted to be able to take care of herself.
- Resident does not clearly verbalize during treatment, but smiles and nods appropriately when asked questions.
- Client nonverbal throughout most of session but did expression agitation and displeasure with therapy tasks through facial expressions, gestures, and occasional vocalizations of "No, no, no."

Sometimes you will include information that the family or caregiver provided about the client if this is pertinent to the session or the client's progress. This is common when treating infants and very young children.

For example:

- Mother reports difficulty with diapering and dressing the infant, stating, "He just gets all stiff and arches his back."
- Foster parents report that child exhibits excessive energy, constantly running around the house and jumping on furniture. They also report that child is aggressive toward foster siblings and the family pet, and he will not remain seated at mealtimes.

- *Parents report child has difficulty remaining in upright seated position for feeding in standard high chair. "She just keeps falling to the right side."*

Although the "S" is primarily reserved for the client's view, occasionally it is acceptable to report comments from caregivers and other professionals if the comments are directly related to the client's occupational therapy services. This allows you to demonstrate the collaborative efforts of the treatment team.

For example:

- *Pt. tearful throughout session, with very little verbalization. Social worker reports pt.'s family just informed pt. they cannot care for her at home and that she will have to go to a skilled nursing facility.*
- *Classroom teacher reports significant improvement in child's ability to remain seated at desk since implementing use of sensory-cushion in chair to provide additional proprioceptive input. Child states, "I love the bumpy feel of it!"*
- *Physical therapist reports patient should use sliding board for all transfers because she is unable to maintain weightbearing precautions for pivot transfers. Patient states, "I can use that board getting from the wheelchair to the bed, but I'm afraid I'll fall off if I use it to get to the toilet."*
- *Client reports no difficulty with financial management, but spouse reports multiple errors in bill paying and checkbook management in recent months.*

COMMON ERRORS

NOT USING COMMUNICATION TIME WITH THE CLIENT EFFECTIVELY

The most common error that new therapists make in gathering subjective information is in failing to make good use of time when communicating with the client during treatment sessions. Instead of using the time in therapy to talk socially, a good therapist will use the time to listen effectively and to ask questions that will provide pertinent information about the client's attitudes and concerns. This information can be used to ensure effective treatment as well as appropriate documentation. Instead of talking to your client about the weather or Monday Night Football, why not ask him how he thinks he is doing in therapy or what his feelings are related to his upcoming discharge placement? As therapists gain experience, they begin to use the treatment session to gather relevant data regarding occupational history, functional status, prior level of functioning, motivation, priorities, and family support.

Effective communication and interviewing during treatment sessions can seem just like a conversation on the surface. However, as a skilled therapist, you are directing the conversation to topics that are meaningful to client care rather than allowing it to remain superficial. Use this opportunity to expand your occupational profile of the client and to gather data that are vital to providing the very best occupational therapy possible. In having a conversation with your client, guide the discussion to your client's history, problems, needs, strengths, support systems, living situation, and goals for treatment. Without knowing this information from your client's point of view, you will have difficulty planning effective treatment. When a therapist does not listen effectively during treatment, the "S" may read:

- *Client talked about grandchildren visiting.*
- *Patient reports he is reading a good book.*

While these statements are within the scope of the "S," they are not particularly helpful pieces of information to spend the time and space reporting.

NOT WRITING CONCISE, COHERENT STATEMENTS

The second most common error made by new therapists writing the subjective section of the note is simply listing all remarks that the client makes about his or her condition. For example, during one treatment session, the following subjective information was gathered:

- *Client said, "I can't feel anything with my hands."*
- *Client stated, "I'm as wobbly as all get out today."*
- *Client expressed dizziness after bending down to touch the floor while in a seated position.*
- *Client acknowledged improvement in his sitting balance in comparison to the previous week.*

Many of these statements have to do with stability, balance, and safety. Although the quotations are a very objective way of reporting data, and all the statements are relevant to the intervention session, it is more effective to summarize the client's remarks in a concise and coherent manner instead of listing each of these statements separately in the "S" section of the note.

For example:

- *Client expressed lack of sensation in both hands and dizziness in sitting position with dynamic movement (a "wobbly" sensation). He also acknowledged improvement in sitting balance since last week.*

or

- *Client acknowledged improved sitting balance compared to previous week. However, he experienced dizziness after bending down while sitting, and reported feeling "wobbly." Client also reported inability to feel anything with his hands.*

In Worksheet 7-1, you will have the opportunity to combine a client's statements into a coherent and concise "S" statement.

REFERENCE

American Occupational Therapy Association. (2014). *Occupational therapy practice framework: Domain & process* (3rd ed.). Bethesda, MD: AOTA Press.

WORKSHEET 7-1

Writing Concise, Coherent "S" Statements

1. Mrs. P is recovering from a total hip replacement. During a treatment session, she makes the following statements:
   - *"I used that dressing stick and sock aid like you showed me to get dressed without bending down this morning."*
   - *"My hip doesn't hurt when I stand up or sit down, especially with that new toilet seat you got for me."*
   - *"It's getting easier for me to get dressed now."*
   - *"My daughter said they delivered all that bathroom equipment to her house yesterday."*

   Using these statements, write your own concise and organized version for the "S" portion of the SOAP note:

2. Tanner is a 14 year old recently admitted to an inpatient adolescent psychiatric unit following an unsuccessful suicide attempt by overdose with his mother's sleeping pills. During a group session, he makes the following comments:
   - *"I have nothing to live for."*
   - *"I don't have any friends."*
   - *"My family would be better off without me anyway."*
   - *"The teachers at my school all hate me."*
   - *"Maybe next time I should do it right and just use a gun!"*

   Using these statements, write your own concise and organized version for the "S" portion of the SOAP note:

WORSHEET 7-2

Choosing a Subjective Statement

An occupational therapist wrote the following observation after treating Mrs. W, a 62-year-old woman who had a stroke 3 weeks ago:

O: *Client participated in 45-minute OT session in hospital room and rehab gym for UE activities to ↑ AROM in Ⓡ shoulder, activity tolerance, UE strength, and dynamic standing balance, to ↑ independence in ADL tasks.*

ADLs: In room, client was instructed in safety techniques and adaptive equipment use in toileting. Client needs Ⓑ grab bars in bathroom for safe sit → stand transition during toileting. Client attempted to stand by pulling on walker and one grab bar. Client was educated on safety issues and the use of Ⓑ grab bars; she verbalized understanding of recommendations.

Performance Skills: Client required CGA for balance during sit ↔ stand. To address activity tolerance, dynamic standing balance, and ↑ AROM in Ⓡ shoulder, client moved canned goods from counter to cupboard for 5 minutes before needing a 2-minute seated rest break. After resting, she participated in activities to ↑ dynamic standing balance by pouring liquid from a pitcher while standing with CGA for balance. After a 1-minute seated rest, client continued activities to ↑ dynamic standing balance and safety by retrieving objects from floor using reacher while ambulating c̄ wheeled walker and CGA.

Client Factors: Ⓡ shoulder abduction AROM < 90°. Ⓡ shoulder abduction PROM WFL.

The treatment session included all of the following. Which would be best to use as the subjective portion of the SOAP note?

1. *Client was very cooperative and engaged in social conversation throughout the tx session.*
2. *Client remarked that her grandson will be coming to visit later in the week, and that she will be very glad to see him.*
3. *Client reports that she feels "pretty good" today.*
4. *Client says she has difficulty moving Ⓡ UE, although she does not know why it will not move. She reports, "It really doesn't hurt. It's just tight."*
5. *Nursing staff report client is incontinent at night.*

Writing the "O"—Objective

The next part of the note is the *objective* section, where you will record all measurable, quantifiable, and observable data obtained during the treatment session. In this section, you will present a picture of the intervention session you have provided. Once you start looking at things with your professional eyes, they can look quite different. Instead of seeing a child playing with a toy, now you begin to note the child's asymmetrical posture, lack of bilateral hand use, difficulty crossing midline, and immature grasp and pinch patterns. The trick in writing the "O" is knowing what kind of material to include and what to omit. At first your "O" may tend to be longer than that of an experienced therapist, but with time you will learn to write notes that are both complete and concise.

STEPS TO WRITING GOOD OBSERVATIONS

There are four important steps to remember when writing the "O" section of your SOAP note:
1. Begin with a statement about the length, setting, and purpose of the treatment session.
2. Next, provide a brief overview of the key deficits that are affecting the client's performance.
3. Follow the opening statements with a summary of what you observed.
4. Be professional, concise, and specific.
We will look at each of these steps more in depth in the following sections.

STEP 1: BEGIN WITH A STATEMENT ABOUT THE LENGTH, SETTING, AND PURPOSE OF THE TREATMENT SESSION

This opening statement gives the reader an introduction to the remainder of the "O" section. It explains the "where," "what," "how long," and "why" about the client's occupational therapy services. Your documentation is the basis for answering any questions about the services that a client received. In Chapter 3, you learned about Current Procedural Terminology (CPT) codes. Most CPT codes are based on the number of minutes of each specific service the client received. Even though not all settings charge for occupational therapy by the number of minutes provided, it is still in best practice to state the total length of the therapy session in the opening statement of the "O" section.

Sames (2015) suggested that practitioners move away from the passive terminology of the client was "seen" in occupational therapy, and instead state that the client "participated in" the occupational therapy session (p. 15). This distinction is important since funding sources want evidence that the client is actively participating in the habilitation or rehabilitation process.

Gateley CA, Borcherding S. *Documentation Manual for Occupational Therapy: Writing SOAP Notes, Fourth Edition (pp 81-97).*
© 2017 SLACK Incorporated

If you are utilizing occupations or occupation-based activities (American Occupational Therapy Association [AOTA], 2014), use the following format for your opening statement:

Client participated in __ -minute OT session _____ for _____.
    #   in what setting   occupation-based intervention

For example:

- *Client participated in 45-minute OT session in rehab kitchen for meal-preparation activity.*
- *Consumer participated in 2-hour supervised outing involving use of public transportation system for community mobility.*
- *Patient participated in 30-minute OT session in hospital room for completion of morning bathing, dressing, and grooming routine using adaptive equipment.*
- *Patient participated in 30-minute OT session in rehab gym bathroom to practice transfer using tub bench for increased safety and independence during bathing.*

If the session focuses on preparatory methods or tasks (AOTA, 2014), then add a reference to the relevant area of occupation in the opening statement:

Client participated in __ -minute OT session _____ for _____ for _____.
    #   in what setting   intervention   what expected
                                                                                 occupational gain

For example:

- *Child participated in 30-minute OT session in outpatient clinic focusing on improving postural control and Ⓑ UE coordination for increased success in play activities.*
- *Student participated in 30-minute OT session in classroom with focus on improving sensory processing and selective attention needed for engagement in classroom activities.*
- *Client participated in 30-minute OT session in hospital room for skilled instruction in energy conservation during IADLs.*
- *Joe participated in role-playing during 30-minute assertion group in outpatient mental health setting to explore alternative ways to meet his social needs.*
- *Client participated in 30-minute OT session in outpatient hand clinic to address ⓇRhand strengthening and scar desensitization in preparation for return to construction work.*
- *Child participated in 30-minute OT session in therapy room to ↑ strength and tone needed to improve handwriting at school.*

It is essential that you show **the need for your skill as an occupational therapist** in this opening statement. So rather than simply saying, "Client participated in 45-minute OT session at bedside for ADL training," you might instead say:

- *Client participated in 45-minute OT session at bedside for skilled instruction in compensatory dressing techniques.*
- *Resident participated in 45-minute OT session at bedside for skilled instruction in use of adaptive equipment to increase safety during ADL tasks.*
- *Veteran participated in 45-minute OT session at bedside to facilitate attention to Ⓛ side during self-care activities.*

STEP 2: PROVIDE A BRIEF OVERVIEW OF THE CLIENT'S KEY DEFICITS

In an ideal world, other team members and insurance reviewers would read every note that you have written to gain a full understanding of your client's deficits. In reality, a therapist taking over your client might read only your most recent note to get an idea of what to do next. Or, an insurance reviewer might be reviewing certain dates of claims to determine whether payment for your services will be issued. Muir (2015) explained that the best documentation paints a picture of the client. In other words, if there are multiple clients seated in a waiting room or rehabilitation gym, someone reading your documentation should be able to pick out your client based on what you have described. Provide a one to two sentence description of your client's key deficits. For example:

- *Client seated in w/c and presents with dense hemiparesis of Ⓛ UE and Ⓛ LE, edema of Ⓛ hand, and severe Ⓛ neglect.*
- *Client presents with Ⓡ BKA with protective brace in place; Ⓑ shoulder AROM limited to 90° due to severe osteoarthritis.*
- *Client supine in bed upon therapist's arrival; wound VAC in place on nonhealing incision from lumbar discectomy and fusion.*
- *Infant presents with Ⓡ torticollis and positional plagiocephaly with molding helmet in place.*
- *Child exhibited significant sensory seeking behaviors throughout session; also demonstrated escape behaviors when therapist attempted to engage him in functional activities seated at desk.*

STEP 3: FOLLOW THE OPENING STATEMENTS WITH A SUMMARY OF WHAT YOU OBSERVED

After you have established the setting and purpose and provided a very brief overview of the client's deficits, you will discuss the interventions that were completed and the client's response to those interventions. There are different ways that are acceptable in organizing the information of the "O":

- *Chronologically*: Discuss each treatment event in the order it occurred during the treatment session.
- *Categorically*: Organize the information according to categories. The categories you select will vary depending on the client and the purpose of the treatment session. You can refer to the *OTPF-III* (AOTA, 2014) for potential categories. For example, it may be helpful to organize the objective information by areas of occupation, client factors, or performance skills:
  - Areas of occupation (e.g., ADLs, IADLs, work, social participation)
    - Note how each of the performance skills and client factors observed affect performance in the relevant areas of occupation. Include assist levels and set-up required, adaptive equipment or techniques used, types of cueing provided, caregiver education, related positioning and mobility issues, and client's response to the treatment provided. Describe consumer's awareness of others in group, initiation of conversation, and interaction with peers in a group setting.
  - Client factors (e.g., ROM, strength, edema, sensation, attention, reflexes)
    - Provide specific measurements such as girth or volumetric measurements for edema, grip and pinch strength, PROM and AROM, type of sensation that is intact or impaired, length of attention to task, involuntary motor reflexes observed or elicited.
  - Performance skills (e.g., balance, coordination, cognition, behavior)
    - Note whether balance was static or dynamic. Consider whether the client leans in one direction, has rotated posture, or has uneven weight distribution. Describe hand dominance, types of prehension used, purposeful grasp and release, and gross motor versus fine motor ability. Report on orientation, task initiation, ability to stay on task, sequencing, judgment, and ability to follow directions. Document client's agitations, lethargy, affect, compulsivity, anxiety, or demanding behaviors.

Let's take a look at a few examples of the different ways to organize the "O."

Chronologically

One way to organize the "O" section of your SOAP note is to document events in the order in which they happened during the treatment session. Think of this method as giving the reader a "play-by-play" of the session.

For example:

- *Client participated in anger management group for 45 minutes today to improve social interaction skills and ability to maintain employment. Client initially required verbal prompting from nursing staff and security aides to attend group. Client presented with disheveled appearance, kept arms crossed throughout group, and made limited eye contact with other group participants. He displayed displeasure at being asked to attend the group by using profanity. During the group, client related 2 instances in which individuals on the unit consistently bother him, and discussed the way he usually handles the situation. Peer feedback was given on other possible ways he might handle the situation. Client indicated that he would consider these alternatives next time a bothersome situation arises.*
- *Client participated in 30-minute evaluation in OT clinic for assessment of low back pain and instruction in proper body mechanics during IADLs. Client noted to wince in pain when transitioning sit ↔ stand and was*

observed to sit with her weight shifted to her Ⓛ hip. Client demonstrated the way she usually removes items from the refrigerator, washes dishes, cleans the floors, and lifts. She was then instructed in proper body mechanics for completing IADL tasks including using a golfer's lift, squats, stepping toward the item she wished to retrieve, facing the load, and keeping it close to her body. Client demonstrated these techniques with minimal verbal cues and was provided with educational handouts to remind her of correct positioning.

Categorically

Many students and new practitioners initially prefer to arrange the "O" chronologically. However, the resulting "O" can be too lengthy. Alternately, you may choose to organize your information into categories. When categorizing your information, choose categories that make sense for your note. Ask yourself, "What was important about this session?" For example, suppose that today you saw a client in the kitchen for a cooking session in preparation for discharge. She plans to cook when she returns home, but you are not certain of her safety or her ability to perform all the steps of the activity from her wheelchair. You wonder if her strength, activity tolerance, and ability to use her involved hand and arm are sufficient for cooking, and you also want to assess her judgment and ability to problem solve. You therefore choose the following categories, using a combination of client factors and performance skills:

- Functional mobility
- UE range and strength
- Hand function and strength
- Functional endurance
- Cognition

Your note might look like this:

O: *Client participated in 1-hr. OT session in clinic kitchen for skilled instruction in compensatory techniques for safe and independent cooking. Pt. uses w/c for functional mobility due to decreased balance and decreased endurance following MS exacerbation.*

Functional Mobility: Client maneuvered throughout kitchen in w/c with verbal cues to place w/c in appropriate position for reaching objects in kitchen. Client required min Ⓐ in stabilizing items while transporting them in lap and maneuvering w/c simultaneously.

UE ROM and Strength: WFL for reaching items in drawers, opening oven door, and putting dishes in the sink Ⓘ. UE strength adequate for opening refrigerator door and stirring batter Ⓘ. Client required min Ⓐ in opening a plastic storage container.

Hand Function and Strength: Adequate for unscrewing lids, cracking egg, and opening muffin box Ⓘ. Client able to use necessary tools for carrying out task Ⓘ. Client able to set oven dial and put muffins in oven Ⓘ.

Functional Endurance: Client Ⓘ took a 3-minute break after approximately 20 minutes of activity.

Cognition: Client able to respond to verbal instruction and questions with correct response 3/3 times. Client said that she did not think it would be safe for her to take the muffins out of the oven. Client able to problem solve Ⓘ about repositioning her w/c 75% of tx time.

Let's look at another example of a note organized by category. Suppose you work in a school setting and you have a child on your caseload who has been receiving occupational therapy services on a consultative basis one time monthly. During your monthly visit, you consult with the classroom teacher and the child's paraprofessional and observe the child in the classroom. Although the child's handwriting performance and ability to meet classroom expectations without disruptive behaviors appear much improved following previous occupational therapist recommendations, staff report a new concern that the child is displaying aggression toward classmates when going through the lunch line. You then observe the child during lunch and make recommendations to the teacher and paraprofessional. Your note might look like this:

O: *30-minute monthly consultation completed this date including observation of student in classroom and cafeteria, and recommendations to teacher and paraprofessional to help improve child's ability to participate effectively during lunch. Lucas calms to deep pressure sensory input but reacts aggressively to unexpected touch.*

Classroom Observations: Lucas demonstrated ability to remain seated at desk to complete worksheet for 8 minutes while wearing weighted vest for increased proprioception. He is now able to write all letters of the alphabet legibly using adaptive paper with alternating highlighted lines and a rubber pencil grip.

Cafeteria Observations: Lucas exhibited verbal and physical aggression (pushing) toward classmate on two separate occasions when inadvertently bumped in line. Follow-up questioning with Lucas indicates that he perceives unexpected touch as "painful."

Staff Education: Classroom teacher and Lucas' paraprofessional were educated regarding sensory processing deficits related to unexpected touch. Recommendation was made to either allow Lucas to leave classroom a few minutes early to go to cafeteria or to have him stand at the beginning or end of the line to reduce the chances of classmates bumping into him. Staff verbalized understanding and plan to implement suggestions tomorrow.

Students and new practitioners often have difficulty discerning what goes in "S" versus what goes in "O" when occupational therapy sessions are primarily verbal in nature. In mental health settings and cognitive rehabilitation, much of the evaluation and intervention involves talking with the client rather than performing physical tasks. However, it is still important to distinguish what is the *subjective* report of the client and what are the *objective* findings of the session that can be used for future comparison. Categorical organization of the "O" can be very helpful in this process. For example:

S: Client states that she would like to live on her own. However, family expresses concern about teen's residual cognitive deficits from TBI 1 year ago. During challenging tasks presented during evaluation, client stated, "This is stupid. I don't know why my family is making me do this."

O: Client participated in 45-minute evaluation in outpatient setting to assess cognitive abilities in regard to ADL and IADL performance. Throughout session, client had difficulty maintaining attention to task more than 2 minutes and frequently pushed activities away when she was unsuccessful.
Memory: Client able to correctly name all members of immediate family. Client able to repeat 3 of 3 words immediately; able to recall 1 of 3 words after 5-minute delay with other tasks presented during that time.
Problem Solving: Client was presented with a simple recipe and asked to create a grocery list of the necessary items. Client read recipe aloud correctly, but omitted 3 of the 8 items in the recipe when creating written list.
Money Management: Client able to correctly count out given amounts of money involving only one type of coin or bill (e.g., 10 cents, 50 cents, $5.00, $20.00). Client required max verbal cues to count out given amounts of money involving multiple coins and/or bills (e.g., 72 cents, $1.42, $17.87).
Safety Awareness: Client able to identify 4 of 10 home safety hazards from pictures. Client required moderate verbal cues to identify potential solutions to those safety hazards.
Medication Management: Client unable to state name, purpose, or correct dosage of her 3 daily medications. Client required max verbal cueing to fill weekly pill organizer based on directions on medication labels.
Daily Routines: Client required moderate verbal cues to list the steps of her typical morning routine in preparation for going to school.

You must realize that there is no "right" list of categories to use. Use what makes sense for the individual client and situation. Worksheet 8-1 will give you the opportunity to rewrite a chronologically organized note into categories.

Please note that experienced therapists often combine Steps 2 and 3. However, it has been our experience over years of teaching documentation that students and new practitioners often get so caught up in describing the details of *what* the client did that they fail to convey the details of *how* the client performed a functional activity. Some of the examples in this chapter and throughout the book will have a distinct statement of the client's key deficits, while other examples will have that information embedded into the summary of what was observed. Either method is acceptable, as long as the reader has a clear picture of the client's functional performance.

STEP 4: BE PROFESSIONAL, CONCISE, AND SPECIFIC

The "O" section does not need to be written in complete sentences. Give complete information in the most concise form possible. Some details must be included. For example, ROM must be specified as active, passive, or assistive and must indicate the joint at which the movement occurred. You always must indicate ®, Ⓛ, or Ⓑ when discussing UEs or LEs. You must specify the level of assistance that was provided. The following are some examples of wording change that make your documentation more professional, concise, and specific.

Rather than saying:	*Resident flopped down onto the bed short of breath, closed her eyes, and moaned. Resident lay in bed with min Ⓐ to position herself.*
You might say:	*Resident observed to be fatigued with SOB following tx session and required min Ⓐ for positioning in bed.*

Rather than saying:	*Veteran had to use a trapeze to sit up.*
You might say:	*Supine → sit using trapeze.*

Rather than saying: *Client put the board in place to make a sliding board transfer.*
You might say: *Client positioned sliding board for transfer.*

When you are documenting test results, it is helpful to put them into a chart like the following one, rather than burying them in narrative:

Ⓛ **Hand Sensation**	
Hot/Cold	Intact
Sharp/Dull	Impaired over volar surface; intact over dorsal surface
Stereognosis	Absent

When you are first learning to write client observations, it is hard to decide what to include and what to leave out. At first, it is better to include too much data rather than taking a chance of omitting something important. As your observational skills become more refined, it will become second nature to include all of the important data, and the "O" section of your notes will begin to be more concise. Here is a client observation written by an inexperienced therapist. In an effort to include all of the necessary data, she wrote a note that was too wordy.

O: *Client participated in 30 minutes of Ⓡ UE strengthening in outpatient therapy gym to prevent future shoulder dislocation. Client is no longer required to wear the brace she wore previously after surgery, but she still holds Ⓡ UE in a protective position close to her body against her abdomen when she was seated. Client maintained same Ⓡ UE position when ambulating in gym. Client was asked to clasp hands together and raise arms above head x 30. Client was then instructed to cross her midline and touch her opposite shoulder with Ⓡ UE x 30. Client required 6 rest periods for completion. Client completed tasks Ⓘ. Client was then introduced to weight and pulley system. Client was asked to specify how much weight she thought she could do. She responded with 5#. Client did 30 repetitions of the pulley system with 5# in shoulder flexion to strengthen her rotator cuff to decrease the probability of dislocating her shoulder again. After strengthening exercise, client had 3 heat packs applied to shoulder to decrease pain.*

A more experienced therapist might have written:

O: *Client participated in 30 minutes of Ⓡ UE strengthening in therapy gym to prevent future shoulder dislocation. Client no longer required to wear postsurgical immobilizer but noted to hold Ⓡ UE in guarded position across her body when seated and during functional mobility. Client completed the following:*

- *Ⓑ clasped-hand shoulder flexion and extension x 30 repetitions*
- *Horizontal adduction Ⓡ hand to Ⓛ shoulder x 30 repetitions*
- *Ⓡ shoulder flexion pulleys with 5# wt. x 30 repetitions*

3 hot packs applied to Ⓡ shoulder to ↓ pain after tx.

You will notice, however, that there is another problem with this note besides the fact that the original note is wordy. It also sounds like a physical therapy note rather than an occupational therapy note. This note needs to have a functional component added in the opening statement of the "O" section. A statement from the client in the "S" about what she is unable to do with an injured rotator cuff and a statement in the "A" and/or "P" indicating functional problems/goals would suffice to make it a good occupational therapy note.

Notice that being more concise means knowing what information can be omitted without compromising the quality of the observation. It is possible to be too concise, omitting necessary information. For example, consider the following "O" from a community mental health center evaluation:

O: *Client evaluated in office using COPM. Client required 45 minutes to complete COPM. Client responded to directive questions regarding self-care, productivity, and leisure.*

This "O" does not provide much information. When additional information is added, we learn much more about the evaluation session with this client:

O: *Client participated in evaluation in office using the Canadian Occupational Performance Measure (COPM), which she completed in 45 minutes. She arrived 45 minutes late to the appointment, well groomed and neatly dressed. Questions regarding productivity and leisure were answered with clear enunciation and animated tone, but questions about self-care (particularly those about scar management) were declined or given short answers with sad tone and no eye contact. Client frequently touched scars on trunk during the evaluation.*

It is a matter of balancing the need to be complete with the need to be concise when writing the "O." Worksheet 8-2 will give you an opportunity to make an observation more concise without losing any of its informational content.

TIPS FOR MAKING YOUR DOCUMENTATION SOUND MORE PROFESSIONAL

There are several ways to make your documentation sound professional. The following are some tips to remember when writing your note:

- Focus on occupation.
- Focus on the client's response to the treatment provided rather than on what the therapist did.
- Write from the client's point of view, leaving yourself out.
- Be specific about assist levels.
- Avoid making a list of actions and assist levels.
- De-emphasize the treatment media.
- Make it clear that you were not just a passive observer in the session.
- Avoid judging the client.
- Use only standard abbreviations.

Let's look at some examples of each of these recommendations.

FOCUS ON OCCUPATION

Make certain that occupation is integral to the note. In a treatment session devoted to self-care activities, function is obvious. However, in a session devoted to addressing client factors such as strength or endurance, in a session where modalities are used, or in a co-treatment session, function must be addressed separately to justify skilled occupational therapy. For example, although the following note is an observation of a session that was devoted to performance components, it contains a statement about the functional intent of the exercises.

O: *Veteran participated in 30-minute OT session in room for AROM and strengthening of Ⓛ UE to regain ability to dress self. Client demonstrated Ⓛ UE AROM 90° and required verbal cues to avoid trunk substitution. Client performed self-ranging exercises from standing and seated position with SBA for balance and verbal instructions to correct errors. Client completed therapy putty exercises x 5 minutes using Ⓛ hand with minimal resistance putty to improve strength for ability to manipulate clothing fasteners.*

FOCUS ON THE CLIENT'S RESPONSE TO THE TREATMENT PROVIDED

Rather than saying: *Client was reminded about hip precautions.*
You might say: *Client required 4 verbal cues to keep hip in correct alignment when donning shoes.*

Rather than saying: *Client was asked orientation questions pertaining to the time of day.*
You might say: *When verbally cued to look at watch, client was unable to correctly identify time.*

Rather than saying: *Client reminded to relax.*
You might say: *UE tone moderately increased but relaxes with verbal cue for repositioning.*

Rather than saying: *Child was given a puzzle to play with.*
You might say: *Child able to place simple shapes into inset puzzle with min Ⓐ to reposition pieces.*

WRITE FROM THE CLIENT'S POINT OF VIEW

The focus of good professional writing is always on the client. Turn your sentences around so that the client is the subject of your sentence.

Rather than saying: *The OT put the client's shoes on for him.*
You might say: *Client unable to don shoes.*

Rather than saying: *OT instructed the client and family in energy conservation techniques.*
You might say: *Client and family instructed in energy conservation techniques and demonstrated understanding by incorporating techniques during ADL tasks.*

BE SPECIFIC ABOUT ASSIST LEVELS

When documenting assist levels, be sure to note **what part of the activity** the client needed physical assistance or verbal cues to perform.

For example:

- *Veteran doffed night garment with min Ⓐ **to untie strings in back.***
- *Child needed HOH assist **for accuracy in staying on line** when cutting with scissors.*
- *Client required verbal cues **to sit down** for safety when doffing socks.*
- *Consumer able to follow bus schedule with min verbal cues **to identify correct time.***
- *Resident completed supine → sit in bed with min verbal cues **to roll to** Ⓡ **side.***
- *When transitioning stand → w/c using a standard walker, pt. required min physical Ⓐ and min verbal cues **to bring walker completely back to w/c and reach back for armrest before sitting.***
- *Infant able to roll supine to prone with min tactile cues **to initiate movement.***
- *Pt. required 5 verbal cues **for sequencing of tasks** during morning ADL routine.*
- *Client required mod Ⓐ **to follow total hip precautions** while washing lower legs and feet with long-handled sponge.*

Worksheet 8-3 will give you practice in being specific about assist levels.

AVOID MAKING A LIST OF ACTIONS AND ASSIST LEVELS

In trying to be concise, sometimes inexperienced therapists make the mistake of writing an "O" that contains only a list of actions with assist levels. While this is a common error, it is incorrect. Simply writing a list of activities or assist levels does not show the skilled occupational therapy being provided. Consider this occupational therapist's observation:

O: *Client participated in 1-hr. OT session in shower room to ↑ activity tolerance and improve balance during showering. Client presents with shortness of breath upon exertion and ataxic movements of trunk and all extremities. Client was shown a smaller shower that simulated her home shower, to prepare for discharge in 1 week. Client A&Ox4.*
Client required min Ⓐ with verbal cues to sit in w/c to doff hosiery and to dry off Ⓑ LEs.
Client spontaneously rinsed soap off hands before gripping grab bar while showering.
Client used walker going to and coming from shower room.
Client tolerated standing Ⓘ during entire shower.
Client instructed in home showering.

Now let's take a look at the same observation, rewritten in a more useful format:

O: *Client participated in 1-hr. OT session in shower room to ↑ activity tolerance and improve balance during showering. Client presents with ataxic movements of trunk and all extremities following cerebellar CVA. Client completed shower in smaller shower stall that simulates her home shower to prepare her for safe and Ⓘ showering after discharge in 1 week.*
***Functional Mobility:** Pt. ambulated to/from shower room and completed standing portion of dressing/undressing with modified Ⓘ using standard walker for stability.*
***Cognition:** Client oriented x 4.*
***ADLs:** Client required min Ⓐ and verbal cues to sit down to doff hosiery and to dry Ⓑ LEs safely. Client rinsed soap off hands s̄ verbal cues prior to gripping grab bar during shower. Client tolerated standing with modified Ⓘ ~5 minutes during shower s̄ SOB. Client received skilled instruction in safe technique to use in her single shower stall and recommendations were provided re: grab bar placement. Client voiced understanding of all recommendations.*

DE-EMPHASIZE THE TREATMENT MEDIA

To improve a client's performance skills, you may use various media, such as equipment or activities that will help the client reach functional goals. However, when documenting your observations of these treatment sessions, you should de-emphasize the media used and focus instead on the performance skills needed for function. For example, an inexperienced therapist might write the following:

Client worked on placing pegs into a pegboard.

This statement may accurately describe what a casual observer would see, but as a trained professional, you need to look beyond the media used and see what the client was really accomplishing. The media used here are pegs and a pegboard, but what is the performance skill? Placing pegs into a pegboard is not a skill this client needs to be able to care for herself. However, the performance skills she practices during this activity may well be crucial to achieving independence. Suppose the therapist had written:

Client worked on tripod pinch using pegs and a pegboard.

Notice that in this example the therapist did not simply add the performance skill to the statement *"Client worked on placing pegs into pegboard to increase tripod pinch,"* but actually turned the sentence around so that the tripod pinch received the emphasis and the media was mentioned only for clarification. Suppose the therapist had written:

Client demonstrated multiple repetitions of tripod pinch to be able to grasp objects needed for ADL tasks.

In this case mention of the media becomes optional. She could also have written:

Client demonstrated multiple repetitions of tripod pinch using pegs and a pegboard to be able to grasp objects needed for ADL tasks.

Which of the three preceding examples do you think best describes the skilled instruction that is occurring in this treatment session? This may seem like a minor distinction, but it is important in demonstrating the need for skilled occupational therapist and the emphasis on functional outcomes in therapy.

One of the most common errors among inexperienced occupational therapists is focusing on the media used rather than on the performance skill and area of occupation that are being improved by use of the media. Consider this occupational therapist's observation:

O: *Client participated in 30-minute OT session at outpatient rehab clinic for standing balance activities. Client relies on wheeled walker for functional mobility and demonstrates decreased static and dynamic standing balance without walker for support. Client used ® UE to hit balloon and was able to reach to ® and Ⓛ sides approximately 7 out of 10 tries. Activity was continued for 3 minutes. Client requested rest break and sat for 30 seconds. Client then stood with mod Ⓐ to walker and hit balloon with Ⓛ UE for 3 minutes. Client was able to hit balloon approximately 6 out of 10 times and spontaneously switched to ® hand x 2 when balloon was to her far right. Client sat for another break and to switch activities. Client stood with CGA to toss beanbags with ® hand for 4 minutes. Client scored 240 points with ® hand by throwing beanbags at target. Once all beanbags were thrown, client sat for a 30-second break, Client stood with CGA for balance to toss beanbags with Ⓛ hand for 30 seconds. Client scored 150 points with Ⓛ hand by throwing beanbags at scoring target. Once all beanbags were thrown, client sat and session was ended.*

When this note is rewritten to focus on the performance skills, notice the difference in professionalism and the way the note reads:

O: *Client participated in 30-minute OT session at outpatient rehab clinic to address standing balance needed for ADL and IADL tasks. Client relies on wheeled walker for functional mobility and demonstrates decreased static and dynamic standing balance without walker for support. Client stood with walker with mod Ⓐ for dynamic standing balance necessary for Ⓘ showering, using a balloon toss activity. Client held walker with Ⓛ hand and used ® UE to reach both ® and Ⓛ sides approximately 7/10 attempts. Client sustained activity for 3 minutes continuously before requiring a 30-second seated rest break. Client stood with walker again with mod Ⓐ for 3 minutes of continuous activity involving weight shifting and balance. Client demonstrated ability to reach to ® and Ⓛ sides to reach for moving object approximately 6/10 times. Client demonstrated ability to spontaneously weight shift 2 times to reach object. Client required another 30-second seated rest before next activity. Client worked on dynamic standing balance using beanbag toss activity with target. Client stood with walker for 4 minutes of dynamic balance activity with CGA, then sat for a 30-second rest. Client stood again with CGA for 3½ minutes of continuous dynamic balance activity.*

Refer to Worksheet 8-4 for practice in de-emphasizing the treatment media.

MAKE IT CLEAR THAT YOU WERE NOT JUST A PASSIVE OBSERVER IN THE SESSION

This will be a critical factor in reimbursement. Although you should write from the client's point of view as described previously, we do not get paid to watch a client do something. To show that the skill of an occupational therapist is needed, you must be actively involved in intervention, such as evaluating or modifying the activity; otherwise it will be considered unskilled.

Rather than saying: *Client compensated for shoulder flexion by leaning forward with entire body during prehension activities.*

You might say: *Client required skilled instruction to avoid compensation at the shoulder during prehension activities.*

Rather than saying: *Client performed Home Exercise Program.*

You might say: *Client's performance of Home Exercise Program was assessed for accurate movement patterns and modified to accommodate for progress.*

AVOID JUDGING THE CLIENT

Rather than saying: *Client was compliant/Client was cooperative.*

You might say: *Client demonstrated ability to follow 3-step directions and sequence WFL.*

When you are working with a client who is difficult or whose opinions and behavior you do not agree with, it is easy to judge the client and to reflect your judgments in your observation. The following is a note written by a student who was in a difficult situation. The client "went off" on the student, refusing a sponge bath, lying about having already bathed, throwing her washcloth across the room so the student would have to pick it up, refusing to put on her slacks, and announcing that therapy was "stupid." In spite of all this, the student wrote an observation that was nonjudgmental of the client:

> *Client required max encouragement to participate in 30-minute therapy session this am. Client completed sit → stand & ambulated to sink Ⓘ. Client modified Ⓘ at sink c̄ simulated bathing activity using long-handled sponge. Client retrieved washcloth from floor using a reacher with modified Ⓘ. Client able to don/doff socks and shoes c̄ adaptive equipment p̄ set-up. Client retrieved gown and socks modified Ⓘ c̄ reacher. Client declined to don slacks.*

USE ONLY STANDARD ABBREVIATIONS

You may only use the abbreviations **approved by your facility**. Please note that the list of abbreviations provided in Chapter 4 is for purposes of learning to document using the exercises in this workbook. Do not use any other abbreviations, even if they seem common to you. This is particularly important as many students have grown up in an age where abbreviations are commonly used in texting and other social media communications. If you try to read a note containing abbreviations with which you are unfamiliar, you will understand instantly how important this is. Remember that your documentation must be read by those unfamiliar with the "shorthand" that health professionals use so freely. Suppose your chart is being read by someone who is from a different background, such as an insurance clerk, attorney, or committee at the Lion's Club who is considering funding a piece of equipment for your client. To make your note understandable to all readers, be judicious in applying abbreviations and keep them very standard. A good rule to follow: **When in doubt, write it out!**

SUMMARY

Good documentation is based on accurate observation, which is based on knowing what to look for. For an experienced therapist, this becomes second nature. For a student therapist, it is helpful to review the guidelines in this manual and to check your observations against what your supervising therapist observed during the treatment session to be sure you are noticing the items that matter most.

REFERENCES

American Occupational Therapy Association. (2014). *Occupational therapy practice framework: Domain & process* (3rd ed.). Bethesda, MD: AOTA Press.

Muir, S. (2015). *Documenting function*. Session presented at Missouri Occupational Therapy Association Annual Conference, Kansas City, MO.

Sames, K. (2015). *Documenting occupational therapy practice* (3rd ed.). Upper Saddle River, NJ: Prentice Hall.

WORKSHEET 8-1

Using Categories

Consider the following chronological observation:

O: *Child participated in 60-minute OT session at daycare to address feeding skills and reach/grasp/release during play. Child demonstrated strong Ⓡ hand preference, flexed position of Ⓛ UE, and did not spontaneously initiate use of Ⓛ UE as a functional assist during self-care or play. With min Ⓐ for facilitation of extension at elbow, child demonstrated ability to use Ⓛ UE to reach, grasp, and release 5 objects with 1-2 verbal cues per object and restriction of Ⓡ UE movement. Child was able to feed self with modified Ⓘ c̄ ~50% spillage, but demonstrated significant limitations in chewing action p̄ ~3 rotary chews & swallowing ~90% of food s̄ chewing. Child required verbal cues throughout session to maintain attention to task. Child wore soft spica thumb splint for entire session.*

How would you divide this information into categories to make it easier to read? Choose three to four categories and redistribute the information above into the categories you have chosen.

WORKSHEET 8-2

Being More Concise

Revise the following note to be complete but more concise.

O: *Pt. participated in 60-minute OT session bedside to complete morning ADL routine. Pt. presented with decreased standing balance and safety awareness. Pt. ambulated ~36 inches to shower c̄ SBA for safety. Pt. instructed to complete shower while sitting. Pt. performed shower c̄ SBA to manage IV line. Pt. able to wash upper and lower body with SBA and dry entire body with SBA after completing shower. Pt. required ~20 minutes to complete shower. Pt. then ambulated ~36 inches to chair and sat. Pt. needed verbal cues to remain seated while donning underwear and pants. Pt. able to dress upper body modified ① and lower body p̄ verbal cues for sitting. Pt. demonstrated good sitting balance, but needed SBA for standing balance. Following shower, client stated he would like to take a nap and was assisted back to bed.*

WORKSHEET 8-3

Being Specific About Assist Levels

When noting assist levels in your observation, it is not enough to note just the level of assistance required. You also need to note the part of the task that required assistance.

For example:

- *Resident donned pants with min Ⓐ* **to pull up over hips.**
- *Client propelled w/c from room to OT clinic but required verbal cues* **to avoid running into other clients.**

Rewrite the statements below to provide a part of the task that required assistance. Since you have not seen the client, you cannot know what part really required assistance. In the real world of professional behavior, making things up is fraud, so please keep in mind that the client you are about to imagine is just an exercise in creativity. For this exercise, you will create a client in your mind and imagine that client doing the task described. As you watch your client in your mind, notice what parts of the task required assistance, and modify the sentences below accordingly.

1. *Client completed supine → sit with min Ⓐ; bed → w/c with mod Ⓐ.*

2. *Client required SBA in transferring w/c ↔ toilet.*

3. *Client retrieved garments from low drawers with min Ⓐ.*

4. *Client required max Ⓐ to brush hair.*

5. *Client completed dressing, toileting, and hygiene with min Ⓐ.*

WORKSHEET 8-4

De-Emphasizing the Treatment Media

Rewrite the following statements to emphasize the skilled occupational therapy that is actually occurring in the treatment session.

1. *Client played catch using Ⓑ UEs to facilitate grasp and release patterns.*

2. *Resident put dirt into pot to halfway point, added seedling, and filled remainder of pot with dirt transferred by cup. Resident completed 3 more pots while standing 8 minutes before requiring a 5-minute rest. Resident resumed standing position to water completed pots for approximately 5 minutes.*

3. *Client painted some sun catchers in crafts group to be able to see that she could do something successfully.*

4. *Pt. cut out magazine pictures that indicated her emotions and glued them onto construction paper.*

5. *Child picked up beans with tweezers and placed in pill bottle to work on tripod grasp in preparation for handwriting.*

9

Writing the "A"—Assessment

The third section of the note is the *assessment*, which contains the therapist's appraisal of the client's progress, occupational limitations, and expected benefit from occupational therapy intervention. In the assessment section of the note, you will use your clinical reasoning to interpret the meaning of the data you have presented in the "S" and "O" sections. You will describe what it means in your professional judgment and its potential impact on the client's ability to engage in meaningful occupation.

In the assessment section of your note, you will primarily note the 3 Ps: *problems*, *progress*, and rehab *potential*. You might also point out inconsistencies, discuss emotional components, or present some reason that something was not done as planned. Finally, the assessment section is where you justify continuation of occupational therapy services.

> The assessment is the "heart" of your note. If you could write only six lines, the assessment section of your note would contain the six lines you would choose. This is the section that demonstrates your clinical reasoning as an occupational therapy practitioner.

ASSESSING THE DATA

To assess the data, go through the information presented in the "S" and the "O" sentence by sentence, and ask what the information means for the client's ability to engage in meaningful occupation. Note what problems, progress, and potential for rehabilitation you see.

PROBLEMS

Some notes will show progress and/or rehab potential and some will not, but almost all notes will show problem areas. The problem areas are what keep a client in active treatment. Problems may include the following:

- Safety risks:
  - *Attempt to stand without locking w/c brakes raises safety concerns for falls during ADL transfers.*
  - *Poor problem solving when using the stove raises safety concerns for staying home alone.*
  - *Limited coping strategies for dealing with stress raise concerns for continuing to demonstrate self-destructive behaviors.*

Gateley CA, Borcherding S. *Documentation Manual for Occupational Therapy: Writing SOAP Notes, Fourth Edition (pp 99-113).* © 2017 SLACK Incorporated

- Inconsistencies between client report and objective findings:
  - *Although client reports anticipating no difficulty in returning to prehospitalization level of homemaking activity, her left-side neglect could cause significant in-home safety risks.*
  - *Although client expresses willingness to do ADL tasks, motor planning problems create a barrier to ADL task performance.*
  - *Although client verbalizes a desire to progress to the next level of responsibility, ↓ behavioral control when reward incentives are unavailable limits this progress.*
- Contributing factors that can be influenced by occupational therapist intervention:
  - *Left-side weakness interferes with standing balance in tub.*
  - *Left-side neglect necessitates verbal cues to attend to left side during ADL tasks.*
  - *Deficits in cognitive processing create a need for constant verbal cues to perform kitchen tasks safely.*

The most common problem area that you will be assessing is the impact of a contributing factor on the ability to engage in occupation. When therapists are first learning to write SOAP notes, they may find it difficult to distinguish observations from assessments. In Chapter 5, you learned multiple formats for writing functional problem statements. In the "A" section of a SOAP note, you should use the following format that calls for **making the limiting factor the subject of the sentence**, and then telling how that factor affects a client's ability to engage in an area of occupation:

Contributing Factor	Impact	Ability to Engage in Occupation

You may want to refer back to Chapters 1 and 5 to review the aspects of occupational therapy's domain as described in the *OTPF-III* (American Occupational Therapy Association [AOTA], 2014b) to identify the contributing factors. For example:

- Client factors: ROM, strength, edema, sensation, etc.
  - *Deficits in UE strength and activity tolerance limit client's ability to complete basic self-care tasks.*
  - *Lack of forearm supination and active elbow flexion against gravity interfere with child's ability to perform age-appropriate developmental play activities.*
  - *Pain in Ⓛ shoulder limits client's ability to carry out child-care and household management tasks.*
- Performance skills: Balance, coordination, cognition, behavior, social interaction, etc.
  - *Deficits in attention span make IADLs difficult and potentially unsafe.*
  - *Inability to manage anger results in difficulty finding work and establishing successful intimate relationships.*
  - *Decreased fine motor coordination affects child's ability to write name.*
- Performance patterns: Habits, routines, etc.
  - *Perseveration with lining up toys limits child's social interaction with peers at school.*
  - *Client's gambling habits result in lack of financial resources to pay monthly rent.*
  - *Client's routine of watching television for 12+ hours daily limits performance of household management tasks.*
- Context and environment: Natural environment, built environment, socioeconomic status, social environment, etc.
  - *Extraneous noises in classroom limit child's ability to attend to written work.*
  - *Narrow doorways in home inhibit client's ability to access the bathroom from w/c level for toileting and bathing.*
  - *Lack of financial resources affects client's ability to purchase clothing necessary to obtain employment.*

In addition to the potential contributing factors listed above from the domain of occupational therapy, you should also consider activity and occupational demands that affect a client's participation in occupation. The *OTPF-III* defines these demands as "the components of activities and occupations that...depending on the context and needs of the client...can be deemed barriers to or supports for participation" (AOTA, 2014b, p. S32).

- Activity and occupational demands: Space demands, social demands, sequencing and timing requirements, required body functions and structures, etc.
  - *Need for assistance during multi-step sequences limits independence with self-catheterization.*
  - *One-handedness following traumatic amputation of Ⓡ hand limits ability to tie shoes.*

- ■ ***Inability to tolerate close proximity of classmates during circle time*** *interferes with child's ability to partici-pate in group classroom activities.*

Notice that in each example given, **the contributing factor is the subject of the sentence**, and then it is followed by the negative impact it has on a specific area of occupation. This is not the only way to write an assessment of problem areas, but the formula is a good one when you are first learning to help you refrain from simply repeating an objective statement. Refer to Worksheet 9-1 for practice using this formula of writing assessment statements.

Progress

Think about whether the occupational therapy treatment being provided is effective. What improvements have you observed? This may be progress that you observe within a single session or progress as compared to a previous session. For example:

- ◆ *Weighted utensils decrease intention tremors by ~50% when eating.*
- ◆ *Brady's ability to prepare for outing, respect rules by following directions, interact socially with staff, and control his behavior indicate progress toward community re-entry.*
- ◆ *Ten-degree ↑ in AROM in Ⓛ elbow this week allows client to don shirt modified Ⓘ.*
- ◆ *Infant's ability to maintain seated position indicates improved postural control needed for engagement in play activities.*
- ◆ *Patient's ability to attend to ADL tasks for 3 minutes today is significantly improved from baseline attention span of 60 seconds.*
- ◆ *Client's spontaneous participation in group discussion shows good progress in developing social interaction skills.*
- ◆ *Improved prehension skills now enable child to zip coat.*

Sometimes progress is indicated by stating that previous goals have been met or modified:

- ◆ *STG #2 (buttoning ½-inch buttons x 3 on shirt) met this week.*
- ◆ *STG #3 upgraded to "complete grooming tasks, <u>standing</u> for at least 3 minutes at sink."*
- ◆ *STG #4 changed to "attend at least 2 group sessions daily."*

Sometimes you may need to explain why there has been a lack of progress:

- ◆ *Acute infection has resulted in patient being more dependent in ADL tasks this week.*
- ◆ *Client's need to care for terminally ill spouse has resulted in sporadic attendance of therapy sessions this month.*
- ◆ *Child's progress toward handwriting goals has been limited due to recent Ⓡ radius fracture and casting of domi-nant Ⓡ UE.*
- ◆ *Anesthesia from an earlier medical procedure impaired client's ability to remain alert during OT session.*

Potential

In addition to problems and progress, the "A" section is also where you should comment on the client's potential for success in rehabilitation:

- ◆ *Ability to understand instructions and desire to return to living independently indicate good potential to return to prior living situation.*
- ◆ *Patient's ability to recall and demonstrate 3/3 hip precautions shows good potential to follow hip precautions after discharge.*
- ◆ *Patient's intact cognitive skills indicate good potential for learning compensatory strategies for ADLs and IADLs.*
- ◆ *Participation in groups, including not interrupting, asking questions appropriately, and sharing experiences, indicates good potential to form successful social relationships.*
- ◆ *Student's progress in ability to use scissors indicates good potential to meet goals stated in IEP.*

Note: The assessment section is NOT the place to introduce new data. **Do not put anything in your "A" that has not been discussed in the "S" or "O."** If you find yourself wanting to make a statement in the "A" that is not supported by the data in your "S" or "O," ask yourself what you might have observed to support the assessment statement. Then decide whether you need to add it to your "S" or "O."

Justifying Continuation of Occupational Therapy Services

After you have documented the client's problems, progress, and potential, you should end the "A" section of your note with a justification of continued occupational therapy services. One very useful way of justifying continued occupational therapy treatment for your client is to end the "A" with the statement *"Client would benefit from..."* and complete the sentence with a justification of continued treatment that requires the skill of an occupational therapy practitioner. Not every therapist ends the "A" with this method, but for purposes of learning, we will use this method. This helps to make certain that justification for continued treatment is present in the note, and is a good method for setting up the plan. Following are some examples:

- *Resident would benefit from environmental cues to orient him to the environment.*
- *Consumer would benefit from continued instruction in problem-solving and anger management techniques needed for successful personal and social relationships.*
- *Client would benefit from further instruction in IADL tasks along with visual perceptual and problem-solving activities to increase safety.*
- *Veteran would benefit from activities that encourage trunk rotation to facilitate transfers and dressing skills.*
- *Consumer would benefit from continued mental health education including recognition of his delusions, need for medication, how it can help him, and why it is essential to his recovery.*
- *Client would benefit from instruction in use of reacher, sock aid, and long-handled shoehorn to aid in LE dressing.*
- *Resident would benefit from skilled instruction in sequencing of tasks to increase safety while performing ADL tasks.*
- *Client would benefit from instruction in energy conservation techniques to perform meal preparation and clean-up.*
- *Child would benefit from continued use of modalities which ↓ tactile defensiveness as well as establishment of home program for parents to carry out with child.*
- *Infant would benefit from therapeutic exercises on therapy ball to encourage trunk extension needed for postural control during play activities.*

Make sure that you are **specific** with your description of what the client would benefit from and why it is important. A common mistake by students and new therapists when learning to write the "A" is making the vague statement that the client would benefit from more of the same techniques that have already been provided without specifying the targeted outcome. **Don't just say the client needs more of the same intervention.** This is particularly important with the increased level of scrutiny by third party payers as they review claims to determine if occupational therapy services will be reimbursed. Ask yourself **what else** the client needs to work on.

Too vague: *Client would benefit from continued ADL training.*
Better: *Client would benefit from instruction in use of tub bench and handheld shower to increase safety during bathing.*

Too vague: *Student would benefit from continued visual perceptual activities.*
Better: *Student would benefit from visual memory activities to improve ability to copy math problems from board to paper.*

When you justify the need for continued occupational therapy services, it is necessary to document the reason the service must be provided by an occupational therapist or occupational therapy assistant rather than by another professional or by nonprofessional personnel. The *Scope of Practice* (AOTA, 2014c) and *Guidelines for Supervision, Roles, and Responsibilities during the Delivery of Occupational Therapy Services* (AOTA, 2014a) outline the services that require an occupational therapy practitioner.

> Occupational therapists are responsible for all aspects of occupational therapy service delivery and are accountable for the safety and effectiveness of the occupational therapy services and service delivery process... Occupational therapy assistants deliver occupational therapy services under the supervision and in partnership with occupational therapists. (AOTA, 2014a, p. S16)

Occupational therapists provide the following services:

- Evaluating clients, identifying problems, establishing goals, and developing intervention plans
- Reviewing the effectiveness of the intervention and modifying the intervention plan as needed

Occupational therapists *and* occupational therapy assistant provide the following services:

- Modification of functional activities and/or instruction in compensatory techniques
- Instruction in the use of adaptive equipment for functional activities
- Health promotion and wellness activities to enhance occupational performance
- Training in ADLs, IADLs, and community/work reintegration
- Provision of individualized education to clients, family members, and caregivers
- Modification of environments to enhance occupational performance
- Fabrication of splints and other orthotic devices
- Training in use of prosthetic devices
- Training in assistive technology and adaptive devices
- Management of feeding and swallowing deficits
- Application of physical agent modalities to enhance occupational performance
- Management of wound care and use of manual therapy techniques
- Driver rehabilitation and community mobility
- Therapeutic exercises and activities to develop, remediate, or compensate for deficits in performance skills

Skilled occupational therapy is **not** evident when the occupational therapist or occupational therapy assistant provides the following services:

- Continuing treatment after goals are reached or no further significant progress is expected
- Providing routine strengthening or exercise programs if there is no potential for functional improvement
- Carrying out daily programs after the adapted procedures are in place and no further progress is expected
- Presenting information in the form of handouts or videos without having the client or caregiver perform the activity (e.g., energy conservation techniques; donning of postsurgical corset)
- Providing services to a client who has poor rehabilitation potential
- Duplicating services with another discipline
- Carrying out a maintenance program, unless the occupational therapy practitioner clearly documents that "skilled services are necessary to maintain an individual's condition or prevent or slow their decline" (AOTA, 2013)

Wording is critical to documenting the necessity for continued skilled occupational therapy. The occupational therapy practitioner **provides skilled instruction** to clients rather than **assisting** them. For example, an occupational therapist may provide instruction in methods of energy conservation and work simplification instead of helping the client perform a strenuous task. Occupational therapists **design** home programs and occupational therapists or occupational therapy assistants may **provide instruction** in home programs, which will then be carried out by clients, aides, or family members.

Why should a client's funding source reimburse you to watch a client carry out the home exercise program that he performs daily on his own? If you are **evaluating** his ability to do all the components of it correctly, or **modifying** it to compensate for recent progress, then your professional skill is clearly required. Analyze your clinical reasoning and then document the principles and strategies used during a treatment session in justifying the continuation of skilled occupational therapy services. Refer to Worksheet 9-2 for practice in determining which services would justify continued occupational therapy treatment.

Remember that the justification for continued treatment must support the frequency and duration of the plan that you will establish in the "P" section of your note. If the last sentence of your "A" reads, *"Client would benefit from information on energy conservation techniques,"* do not expect the payer to approve more than one more treatment session.

If this is your last session, complete the sentence with what the client would benefit from after discharge. For example:

- *Following discharge from rehab unit, client would benefit from home health OT to assess need for home adaptations to accommodate use of w/c for ADLs and IADLs.*
- *Client would benefit from continued PROM provided by restorative aide to prevent ® UE contracture and skin breakdown.*
- *Child would benefit from OT re-evaluation in 6 months to determine if fine motor skills are developing at an age-appropriate level.*

WRITING THE ASSESSMENT

As you read carefully through the material in your "S" and "O," it is sometimes helpful to make a quick list of things you want to discuss in the "A" section of your note. For example, consider this "S" and "O":

S: *Client stated that he gets bored during the day when he has nothing to do, and said, "I wish I had a car so I could get out easier."*

O: *Client participated in 90-minute OT session in his home, on city bus, and at grocery store for community reintegration following discharge from inpatient facility. Client deficits include limited problem-solving and money management skills. Client demonstrated home management skills and ability to care for pets by simulation. Client was able to identify which bus to catch to go to grocery store, but needed reassurance that his choice was correct. At the grocery store, client independently chose lunch meat and fruit for lunches this week, but needed SBA for payment.*

The therapist identified the following problems, progress, potential, and need for continued services:

- Problems:
    - Client is anxious about whether his bus choice is really correct.
    - Client is still unable to manage money independently.
- Progress:
    - Client is able to simulate care of home and pets.
    - Client is able to choose the correct bus to get to the grocery store.
    - Client is willing to choose healthier foods at the store this visit.
- Potential:
    - In this therapist's professional judgment, the progress shown to date is also a good indicator of rehab potential for this client.
- Need for Continued Services:
    - Client still needs to improve community mobility and money management skills to increase functional independence.

A: *Anxiety level in selecting the correct bus and need for assistance in managing money continue to limit client's functional independence. Client's ability to demonstrate home and pet care activities as taught earlier shows good progress toward being able to live independently in the community. Ability to identify correct bus and willingness to choose healthier food items also indicate progress and potential to transition to less caregiver support. Client would benefit from continued instruction in going new places in the community and instruction in money management to increase his ability to shop without caregiver support.*

Here are a few more examples of what the completed assessment of a note might look like:

A: *Inability to don Ⓛ LE prosthesis Ⓘ currently limits Ⓘ in transfers and mobility needed for functional toileting. Ability to don prosthesis today with min Ⓐ indicates progress from mod Ⓐ needed yesterday. Recent progress and motivation are good indications of potential to be Ⓘ with management of prosthesis. Client would benefit from additional skilled instruction in use of pulley-like fasteners installed this date on prosthesis to allow one-handed closure.*

A: *Fear, isolation, and decreased activity tolerance limit Dominique's independent living skills and are the focus of current treatment. Emerging willingness to initiate conversation with others and to initiate daily bathing and grooming indicate good progress toward goals. She has good potential to return to the level of independence she had prior to her recent psychotic episode. Dominique would benefit from continued skilled instruction in self-care skills as well as increased socialization and physical activity to be successful with community re-entry.*

A: *Child's Ⓛ neglect continues to limit her independence in self-care and play tasks. Spontaneous use of Ⓛ hand as a functional assist 60% of the time demonstrates progress from less than 50% spontaneous use during prior visits. She would benefit from facilitation of more bilateral activities to ↑ use of Ⓛ hand during play, as well as establishment of a home program for foster parents to carry out in between bi-weekly visits.*

A: *Client's spontaneous actions in groups, willingness to share verbally, and improved dress and hygiene indicate an improved mood this week. Progress also noted in unprompted attendance, which is up this week from 2/8 to*

6/8 groups attended. Goals #1 (assertion) and #2 (communication) are met as of this date. Recent progress indicates excellent potential for successful community re-entry. Inability to identify preferred leisure tasks continues to limit client's ability to plan daily activities, both individually and involving interaction with others. Goal #3 (leisure skills) will be continued through discharge. Client would benefit from continued instruction and opportunities in formulating a plan for use of leisure time.

Notice in the last example that the problems, progress, and rehab potential do not have to be in a particular order. Sometimes it makes more sense to identify the progress first and then comment on the remaining problems that justify continued services. Let's walk through one more example in a step-by-step manner.

MRS. W'S STROKE

Mrs. W is a 62-year-old woman who had a stroke 3 weeks ago. She lives with her husband of 40 years in a one-story home. Her husband works full time as an account manager at a local bank. She has good return in her involved LE and is getting some return in her UE as well. She intends to return home to live with her husband and will be alone during the day while he is at work. (You met Mrs. W in Chapter 7 when you chose a subjective statement for her treatment session.)

S: *Client says she has difficulty moving Ⓡ UE, although she does not know why it will not move. She reports, "It really doesn't hurt. It's just tight."*

O: *Client participated in 30-minute OT session in rehab gym for UE activities to ↑ independence in ADL tasks. Pt. presents with ↓ AROM in Ⓡ shoulder, ↓ activity tolerance, ↓ Ⓡ UE strength, and ↓ dynamic standing balance.*

ADLs: In room, client was instructed in safety techniques and adaptive equipment use in toileting. Client needs Ⓑ grab bars in bathroom for safe sit ↔ stand transition during toileting. Client attempted to stand by pulling on walker and one grab bar. Client was educated on safety issues and the use of Ⓑ grab bars; she verbalized understanding of recommendations.

Performance Skills: Client required CGA for balance during sit ↔ stand. To address activity tolerance, dynamic standing balance, and ↑ AROM in Ⓡ shoulder, client moved canned goods from counter to cupboard for 5 minutes before needing a 2-minute seated rest break. After resting, she participated in activities to ↑ dynamic standing balance by pouring liquid from a pitcher while standing with CGA for balance. After a 1-minute seated rest, client continued activities to ↑ dynamic standing balance and safety by retrieving objects from floor using reacher while ambulating c̄ wheeled walker and CGA.

Client Factors: Ⓡ shoulder abduction AROM < 90°. Ⓡ shoulder abduction PROM WFL.

How would you assess this information? What **problems** can you identify? Safety risks? Are there performance skills that are not WFL that occupational therapy might affect? Do you see evidence of **progress**? Is there any indication of the client's rehab **potential**? What would this client **benefit from**?

The therapist identified the following problems, progress, potential, and need for continued services:

- Problems:
  - Client is unsafe during toilet transfer.
  - Client has ↓ AROM in Ⓡ shoulder, ↓ activity tolerance, and ↓ dynamic standing balance.
- Progress:
  - Client verbalized understanding of safety instructions.
- Potential:
  - Ⓡ UE PROM is WNL
  - In this therapist's professional judgment, the client has good potential to return home independently.
- Need for Continued Services:
  - Client needs to improve AROM, strength, and activity tolerance and also needs instruction in safety and energy conservation techniques.

In preparing an assessment of the data in this note, this therapist identified two main problem areas: the safety of transferring to/from the toilet, and the client factors that were not WFL. This therapist was particularly concerned about the safety issues and addressed those first. She also noted the rehabilitation potential that would be helpful to a reviewer in deciding whether the client's progress is sufficient to justify the expense of treatment.

A: *Impulsivity and ↓ dynamic standing balance pose safety concern during sit → stand transfer for toileting. Verbalization of understanding safety instructions demonstrates progress and indicates that the client has the potential to progress to independence.*

Next she addressed the clinical reasoning behind devoting time to addressing client factors, in the light of her rehab potential.

A: *Impulsivity and ↓ dynamic standing balance pose safety concern during sit → stand transfer for toileting. Verbalization of understanding safety instructions demonstrates progress and indicates that the client has the potential to progress to independence.* **Client's ↓ AROM in Ⓡ shoulder, ↓ activity tolerance, and ↓ dynamic standing balance all interfere with ability to complete ADL tasks safely and independently.**

She completes the assessment by justifying continued treatment.

A: *Impulsivity and ↓ dynamic standing balance pose safety concern during sit → stand transfer for toileting. Verbalization of understanding safety instructions demonstrates progress and indicates that the client has the potential to progress to independence. Client's ↓ AROM in Ⓡ shoulder, ↓ activity tolerance, and ↓ dynamic standing balance all interfere with ability to complete ADL tasks safely and independently.* **Client would benefit from Ⓡ UE AROM and strengthening exercises along with continued skilled instruction in safety issues and energy conservation techniques.**

In this case, the therapist decided that the client factors could be addressed in two different ways, both by working on ↑ AROM, strength, and activity tolerance, and by teaching some energy conservation techniques. We know that payment for ongoing treatment of range and strength is often denied. In Chapter 10, you will see how this therapist plans to provide the services this client would benefit from in a cost-effective manner.

REFERENCES

American Occupational Therapy Association. (2013). Jimmo v. Sebelius: The so-called Medicare "Improvement Standard" deemed illegal, skilled maintenance care now covered. Retrieved from http://www.aota.org/advocacy-policy/federal-reg-affairs/news/2013/ improvement-standard.aspx.

American Occupational Therapy Association. (2014a). Guidelines for supervision, roles, and responsibilities during the delivery of occupational therapy services. *American Journal of Occupational Therapy, 68*(Suppl.), S16-S22. doi: 10.5014/ajot.2014.686S03

American Occupational Therapy Association. (2014b). *Occupational therapy practice framework: Domain & process* (3rd ed.). Bethesda, MD: AOTA Press.

American Occupational Therapy Association. (2014c). Scope of practice. *American Journal of Occupational Therapy, 68*(Suppl.), S34-S40. doi: 10.5014/ajot.2014.686S04

WORKSHEET 9-1

Writing About Problems in the Assessment

You will be rewriting some statements to make them more effective assessment statements using the following formula:

Contributing Factor	Impact	Ability to Engage in Occupation

For example, this statement is an observation:

Client's activity tolerance for lower body dressing was < 2 minutes secondary to SOB from COPD.

It tells you what the therapist observed while providing intervention. To make it into an assessment statement, you would need to change the emphasis by turning the statement around to **make the contributing factors the subject of the sentence** and by adding the impact that those factors have on her independence in dressing. Using the formula above, you might write:

Client's SOB and activity tolerance < 2 minutes limits client's ability complete lower body dressing.

Rewrite the following observation statements into **assessment** statements using the formula given above.

1. *Client demonstrated difficulty with laundry and cooking tasks due to memory and sequencing deficits.*

2. *Decreased level of arousal noted during morning dressing activities, requiring redirection to task.*

3. *Client unable to follow hip precautions during morning dressing due to memory deficits.*

4. *Client problem solved poorly while performing lower body dressing, as evidenced by multiple attempts required to button pants and don socks successfully.*

WORKSHEET 9-2

Justifying Continued Treatment

Which of the following require the skills of an occupational therapist?

_____ Evaluation of a client

_____ The practice of coordination and self-care skills on a daily basis

_____ Establishing measurable, behavioral, objective, and individualized goals

_____ Developing intervention plans designed to meet established goals

_____ Analyzing and modifying functional activities through the provision of adaptive equipment or techniques

_____ Determining that the modified tasks are safe and effective

_____ Routine exercise and strengthening programs

_____ Teaching the client to use the breathing techniques he has learned while performing ADLs

_____ Providing individualized instruction to the client, family, or caregiver

_____ Modifying the intervention plan based on a re-evaluation

_____ Donning/doffing of a client's resting hand splint on a regular schedule throughout the day

_____ Providing specialized instruction to eliminate limitations in a functional activity

_____ Developing a home program and instructing caregivers

_____ Making changes in the environment

_____ Teaching compensatory skills

_____ Gait training

_____ Adding instruction in lower body dressing techniques to a current ADL program

_____ Presenting informational handouts without having the client perform the activity

_____ Teaching adaptive techniques such as one-handed shoe tying

WORKSHEET 9-3

Writing the Assessment—Ellie's Development

Ellie was born prematurely at 24 weeks gestation. She is currently almost 7 months old, with an adjusted age of 3 months. She was referred to occupational therapy while in the NICU for stimulation of normal developmental sequence and continues to receive occupational therapy services because she is considered a high-risk infant.

S: *Parent reports that infant is gaining ~1 oz. per day and will probably be able to discontinue O_2 "in a couple days."*

O: *Infant participated in 30-minute OT session in home to assess visual skills and to ↑ mobility skills related to play (head righting, rolling supine → side lying, and push-up in prone). Infant presents with low proximal and distal tone and poor head control. Infant oriented to black & white illuminated design by turning head. In supine, infant demonstrated visual tracking in horizontal plane 20° past midline. Infant unable to roll, right head, or push up in prone Ⓘ to engage with caregiver or toys, but with facilitation of weight shift and proximal stability, infant could perform activities after about 20 seconds and hold position. Infant became fatigued and "fussy" after 20 minutes of treatment, with four 1-minute rest breaks.*

How would you assess this information? What **problems** can you identify? Are there any contributing factors that occupational therapy might affect? What influence do the limiting factors above have on Ellie's ability to engage in occupation that is appropriate for her age? Do you see evidence of **progress**? Is there any indication of Ellie's rehab **potential**? What would she **benefit from**?

The therapist who is working with Ellie was concerned about the following:

- Inability to perform age-appropriate mobility skills Ⓘ during play
- Became fatigued after 20 minutes
- Lack of head righting responses
- Needs O_2

She was encouraged by the following:

- Need for O_2 is decreasing and she is gaining weight
- Ability to hold position if facilitated
- Ability to orient to a black and white image and to visually track horizontally

Write an assessment to add to the "S" and "O" given above.

A:

WORKSHEET 9-4

Writing the Assessment—Ms. D's Social Skills

Ms. D is a 35-year-old woman who has a diagnosis of bipolar disorder, although in a prior admission, she was diagnosed with schizophrenia. One of her goals is to talk to the mental health center staff about her problems rather than acting out her feelings. Today she was seen in social skills group with five other clients who also need help with relationship issues.

S: *Client reports that she understands the purpose of social skills group. She expressed a desire to attend all of the groups, saying that they are "fun."*

O: *Client participated in 60-minute social skills group focusing on friendship. Client appeared unkempt, with hair not combed and shirt rumpled. Client engaged in conversation with the other clients and the facilitator. Client interrupted others on 5 occasions. Client spontaneously verbalized her experiences with past friendships and her ideas of useful ways to make new friendships, but had to be redirected to the topic twice during discussion.*

1. What problems do you see in the above "S" and "O"?

2. What areas of occupation do these problems affect?

3. What evidence of progress and/or potential do you see?

4. What would this client benefit from?

5. Write a complete assessment statement for this note.

Writing the "P"—Plan

The last section of a SOAP note is the *plan*. In this section, you document the anticipated frequency and duration of your services and the specific interventions that will be used to achieve the client's goals. The plan should relate to the information presented in the "O" and the "A" and should address your assessment of what the client would benefit from. The "P" will inform your reader of your priorities regarding intervention strategies.

> Note: In an initial evaluation report, the "P" section will also contain the long-term and short-term goals. This will be covered in Chapter 12 when you learn more about intervention planning.

In some settings, you will see the "P" simply written as *"Continue plan of care."* For purposes of learning in this manual, that is NOT a sufficient plan. Your "P" should include the following:

- Frequency (how often; may also include length of session in some settings)
  - *Infant will be seen **2x/wk**...*
  - *Continue OT **daily**...*
  - *Client will be seen **30 minutes bid**...*
- Duration (how long occupational therapy will continue)
  - *Infant will be seen 2x/wk for **2 months**...*
  - *Continue OT daily for **3 days**...*
  - *Client will be seen 30 minutes bid for **1 week**...*
- Purpose of continued therapy and/or specific interventions (also include referral to other professionals or agencies if appropriate)
  - *Infant will be seen 2x/wk for 2 months **to address feeding skills. Treatment to include oral desensitization and caregiver training in use of adaptive bottles.***
  - *Continue OT daily for 3 days **for skilled instruction in ADLs and IADLs. Sessions will focus on education in postsurgical hip precautions and adaptive equipment to maximize safety and independence in preparation for return to independent living situation. OT will also contact social worker to explore options for home assistance with laundry and housekeeping. Referral also made to local Independent Living Center for assistance in obtaining necessary adaptive equipment due to client's limited insurance and financial resources.***
  - *Client will be seen 30 minutes bid for 1 week **to address visual perceptual and cognitive skills necessary for safe performance of ADLs and IADLs. Environmental modifications will be made to improve visual scanning to Ⓛ side during basic ADLs. Telephone book activity planned for afternoon session tomorrow.***

Gateley CA, Borcherding S. *Documentation Manual for Occupational Therapy: Writing SOAP Notes, Fourth Edition* (pp 115-121).
© 2017 SLACK Incorporated

In each of the previous examples, another therapist could read your "P" and know exactly how to proceed with this client's treatment. Consider the following situations in which this would be crucial to providing quality care for your client:

- In acute care and rehabilitation settings, treatment may be provided 7 days per week and the client will encounter multiple occupational therapists during his or her hospital stay. Writing a thorough "P" ensures that the next therapist to see the client will use the client's therapy time efficiently to work toward meeting goals.

- In any setting where an occupational therapy assistant will be providing services, a thorough "P" is critical for communication between the occupational therapist and the occupational therapy assistant.

- Unexpected therapist absences happen in any setting. The "P" section of your note should allow another therapist to continue the client's treatment without interruption.

Note: There are a two common errors in the "P" that students often make when they are first learning to document:

1. The first error is to keep using the words **plan to assess** in the "P" of the SOAP note. From an insurance reviewer's standpoint, most of your assessment should have taken place during the initial evaluation, and the expectation is that future sessions will focus on **intervention**. Unless you have specific assessments that you plan to complete in future sessions, such as standardized visual perceptual or cognitive tests, your "P" should focus on your planned interventions. It is implied that ongoing assessment is part of every session.

2. The second error is to list interventions in the "P" that are **not relevant for the client's current setting**. For example, if you are an occupational therapist in an acute care setting, your plan should not include interventions that will occur in the home, health, or outpatient setting. You should only document what you can address in the current setting in which you are treating the client.

Here are some more examples of a "P":

- *Resident to be seen for 2 more weeks for ½-hr. bid sessions for skilled instruction in meal preparation and clean-up. Focus will be on independent use of microwave using wheeled walker for mobility.*

- *Child will continue to be seen 1x/wk for 30-minute sessions until IEP review to ↑ fine motor skills for better classroom performance. OT sessions to address handwriting and cutting skills.*

- *Client will continue to be seen in groups 5x/wk for 1 week to work on social participation. Group sessions to address assertion skills and anger management techniques.*

- *Consumer will continue sheltered workshop program 5 days/wk for 1 month to ↑ work skills. Target behaviors are improved attention to task and ability to follow 2-step directions.*

- *Continue 1-hr. daily sessions for 1 week for skilled ADL training. One-handed dressing techniques for donning shirt will be taught and buttonhook will be introduced.*

You must use your clinical judgment when determining frequency and duration of services. In many cases, there are expected norms of frequency and duration based on setting, funding source, or physician's order. For example:

- In a school setting, the frequency of services will be determined in the child's annual IEP meeting date and will remain the same until the IEP is modified.

- In an acute care setting, patients who have had orthopedic surgery likely will have occupational therapy services once or twice daily for the duration of the hospital stay, but this may vary depending on each surgeon's protocol for therapy services. Total length of stay is often just a few days. As soon as the patient is medically stable, he or she will be discharged to a different setting such as inpatient rehabilitation, home with home health therapy services, skilled nursing, etc.

- Patients who are admitted to a hospital for general medical issues such as pneumonia or other illness often have only one or two occupational therapy sessions to assess ability to return home. Again, the patient's total length of stay will likely be just a few days before discharging to a different setting.

- Patients in an inpatient rehabilitation facility must receive 3 hours of therapy per day. Patients typically have occupational therapy for 60 or 90 minutes daily (generally split between 2 sessions), depending on the amount of physical therapy and speech therapy services that they are receiving. Length of stay may vary from a few to several weeks depending on setting and severity of impairments.

- Residents of long-term care facilities may receive occupational therapy services a few times per week or daily depending on the individual situation and client needs. Total duration of therapy services may last from a few to several weeks depending on severity of impairments and client progress.

♦ Home health clients may have just a few occupational therapist visits to assess home safety or may continue occupational therapy services a few times a week for several weeks to address functional deficits.

♦ Clients in an inpatient psychiatric setting may have both individual and group sessions on a daily basis during their stay, which may last a few days to a few weeks.

♦ In an outpatient setting, a physician may write orders that specify the frequency and duration of occupational therapy services, typically from a few to several weeks. Funding sources in outpatient settings often require updates approximately every 30 days.

♦ Early intervention services typically range from monthly consultation to direct services one or more times weekly, and duration of therapy services may last a few to several months.

Funding sources may dictate the number of occupational therapist visits that will be paid, such as 60 minutes weekly for 8 weeks. Insurance companies may also limit the total number of therapy visits they will pay in a calendar year. For example, it is common to see a limit of 60 outpatient visits per year for combined occupational therapy, physical therapy, and speech therapy visits. In such cases, it is important to communicate with other team members and the client to determine the optimal frequency and duration of therapy visits.

Please note that these examples are not standards. They are simply provided to demonstrate that the frequency and duration of services will vary greatly among settings and situations. You must be familiar with the expectations of your particular setting.

COMPLETING THE PLAN FOR MRS. W

Now let us write a plan for the note on Mrs. W that we assessed in the last chapter. As you recall from Chapter 9, Mrs. W is a 62-year-old woman who had a stroke 3 weeks ago. She has good return in her involved LE and is getting some return in her UE as well. She intends to return home to live with her husband and will be alone during the day while he is at work.

S: *Client says she has difficulty moving ⓡ UE, although she does not know why it will not move. She reports, "It really doesn't hurt. It's just tight."*

O: *Client participated in 30-minute OT session in rehab gym for UE activities to ↑ independence in ADL tasks. Pt. presents with ↓ AROM in ⓡ shoulder, ↓ activity tolerance, ↓ ⓡ UE strength, and ↓ dynamic standing balance.*

***ADLs:** In room, client was instructed in safety techniques and adaptive equipment use in toileting. Client needs ⓑ grab bars in bathroom for safe sit ↔ stand transition during toileting. Client attempted to stand by pulling on walker and one grab bar. Client was educated on safety issues and the use of ⓑ grab bars; she verbalized understanding of recommendations.*

***Performance Skills:** Client required CGA for balance during sit ↔ stand. To address activity tolerance, dynamic standing balance, and ↑ AROM in ⓡ shoulder, client moved canned goods from counter to cupboard for 5 minutes before needing a 2-minute seated rest break. After resting, she participated in activities to ↑ dynamic standing balance by pouring liquid from a pitcher while standing with CGA for balance. After a 1-minute seated rest, client continued activities to ↑ dynamic standing balance and safety by retrieving objects from floor using reacher while ambulating c̄ wheeled walker and CGA.*

***Client Factors:** ⓡ shoulder abduction AROM < 90°. ⓡ shoulder abduction PROM WFL.*

A: *Impulsivity and ↓ dynamic standing balance pose safety concern during sit → stand transfer for toileting. Verbalization of understanding safety instructions demonstrates progress and indicates that the client has the potential to progress to independence. Client's ↓ AROM in ⓡ shoulder, ↓ activity tolerance, and ↓ dynamic standing balance all interfere with ability to complete ADL tasks safely and independently. Client would benefit from ⓡ UE AROM and strengthening exercises along with continued skilled instruction in safety issues and energy conservation techniques.*

In the "A" section, the therapist has already justified the main things she intends to do and indicated the client's rehabilitation potential. Now she needs to be specific about how often the client will be treated and for what length of time. She first specifies the frequency and duration of treatment:

P: *Continue to treat client 5x/wk for 1 week...*

She could have specified the length of the treatment sessions (e.g., "*for 1 hr. sessions*"), but this therapist chose not to do that in this particular note. Next she specifies how she plans to use the treatment time:

P: *Continue to treat client 5x/wk for 1 week **for skilled instruction in safe transfers and toileting...***

Since she anticipates discharge in 1 week, she has to prioritize her time. She chooses to work on balance and energy conservation as a part of functional mobility during ADL activities. Since she has already written in the "A" that the client would benefit from additional AROM and strengthening exercises, she now needs to specify how she plans to address this need as well:

P: *Continue to treat client 5x/wk for 1 week for skilled instruction in safe transfers and toileting. **Plan to address dynamic standing balance and to provide skilled instruction in energy conservation techniques. Home program for AROM and strengthening exercises for Ⓡ shoulder will be taught.***

This note is now complete. This therapist has demonstrated clinical reasoning in planning for discharge in advance of the discharge date. In later notes, she will indicate the client's progress in learning the home program since simply handing the client a set of printed exercises is not considered a skilled or billable service. The client's progress in learning the home program will also confirm that the therapist's assessment of the client's rehabilitation potential was on target.

WORKSHEET 10-1

Completing the Plan for Ellie

In the last chapter, you wrote an assessment for a treatment note on Ellie's development. Now you will complete that note by adding a plan. As you recall from Chapter 9, Ellie is a 7-month-old infant (adjusted age of 3 months following premature birth at 24 weeks gestation). She was seen in the NICU and continues to receive occupational therapy services because she is considered a high-risk infant.

In the last sentence of your "A," you have established what you want to do. In your "P," state how often you plan to see Ellie, how long each session will last, how long you plan to continue your intervention before re-evaluating or discontinuing treatment, and how you plan to use your time.

S: *Parent reports that infant is gaining ~1 oz. per day and will probably be able to discontinue O$_2$ "in a couple days."*

O: *Infant participated in 30-minute OT session in home to assess visual skills and to ↑ mobility skills related to play (head righting, rolling supine → side lying, and push-up in prone). Infant presents with low proximal and distal tone and poor head control. Infant oriented to black & white illuminated design by turning head. In supine, infant demonstrated visual tracking in horizontal plane 20° past midline. Infant unable to roll, right head, or push up in prone Ⓘ to engage with caregiver or toys, but with facilitation of weight shift and proximal stability, infant could perform activities after about 20 seconds and hold position. Infant became fatigued and "fussy" after 20 minutes of treatment, with four 1-minute rest breaks.*

A: *Decreased postural control and need for facilitation of weight shift limits infant's ability to perform early mobility skills needed for play. Limited mobility combined with her tolerance for less than 20 minutes of activity and the need for frequent rest breaks limit her ability to explore her environment and reach developmental milestones at a typical age. Ability to perform transitional movements with facilitation, orientation to black and white design, and ability to track in horizontal plane show good progress and potential for future developmental gains. Infant would benefit from continued OT services to stimulate developmental skills and from parent education in a home program.*

P:

WORKSHEET 10-2

Completing the Plan for Ms. D

As you recall from Chapter 9, Ms. D is a 35-year-old woman who has a diagnosis of bipolar disorder, although in a prior admission, she was diagnosed with schizophrenia. One of her goals is to talk to the mental health center staff about her problems rather than acting out her feelings. Today she was seen in social skills group with five other clients who also need help with relationship issues.

You have noted in the last sentence of your assessment some of the areas of intervention that you think might benefit Ms. D. Now you will fill in the specifics of your plan.

S: *Client reports that she understands the purpose of social skills group. She expressed a desire to attend all of the groups, saying that they are "fun."*

O: *Client participated in 60-minute social skills group focusing on friendship. Client appeared unkempt, with hair not combed and shirt rumpled. Client engaged in conversation with the other clients and the facilitator. Client interrupted others on 5 occasions. Client spontaneously verbalized her experiences with past friendships and her ideas of useful ways to make new friendships, but had to be redirected to the topic twice during discussion.*

A: *Client's unkempt appearance, interrupting behaviors, and need for redirection to topic of conversation interfere with her ability to engage in social participation with peers. Her expressed interest in groups and her willingness to engage in conversation and share her ideas show good potential to develop relationships and to express herself verbally in place of acting out. Client would benefit from participating in groups where conversational skills are stressed, from further facilitation of attention to social cues, and from instruction in ADLs stressing hygiene and appearance.*

P:

11

Making Good Notes Even Better

Now that you have learned to write effective SOAP notes, it is time to review your work and take your skills to the next level. We will begin by reviewing problem statements and goals, and then we will review each of the SOAP categories. As we review, you will have an opportunity to refine your skills beyond the basics learned so far by completing the worksheets at the end of this chapter.

PROBLEM STATEMENTS

As you recall, a problem list is developed from your initial assessment. Problems are defined as areas of occupation that are not within functional limits (WFL) and that you plan to address through occupational therapy intervention. Problem statements need both a *contributing factor* (client factor, performance skill, contextual limitation, etc.) and a related *area of occupation*. Remember that the best problem statements also give a way of measuring the extent of the problem (such as "*needs mod assist*"). Also remember that those clients who use our services are more than an assist level, and we make a statement in terms of what the client is **unable to do** or **needs assistance in doing** rather than saying that the client is a particular assist level.

WRITING MEASURABLE OCCUPATION-BASED GOALS AND OBJECTIVES

You have a method for writing goals that will ensure that all the necessary components are present:
- C—Client   Client will perform.
- O—Occupation   What occupation?
- A—Assist Level   With what level of assistance/independence?
- S—Specific Condition   Under what conditions?
- T—Timeline   By when?

Remember that sometimes the order of the elements must be rearranged so that your goal statement does not sound awkward, but you should **always keep the "C" and the "O" together** to ensure that the emphasis of the goal is on the occupation. Another tip you learned about writing observations is to de-emphasize the treatment media. That is also important in goal writing. Consider the following goal:

Client will place 8 half-inch screws and washers on a block of wood with holes by the next treatment session.

This goal emphasizes the treatment media and is not occupation-based. Written in a different way, the targeted occupation of work becomes evident and the treatment media becomes the **specific condition** rather than the focus of the goal:

By the end of the 2nd treatment session, client will complete work simulation task by placing 8 half-inch screws into a block of wood in < 5 minutes.

Gateley CA, Borcherding S. *Documentation Manual for Occupational Therapy: Writing SOAP Notes, Fourth Edition (pp 123-151)*. © 2017 SLACK Incorporated

THE SOAP STRUCTURE

"S"—SUBJECTIVE

In this section, you report anything significant that the client says about his or her treatment. If the client is unable to speak, report on his or her nonverbal communication, if any. In the case of a young child, a confused client, or a client who is unable to communicate, you may use what the primary caregiver says.

"O"—OBJECTIVE

Writing Good Opening Lines

This section begins with opening lines that explain where the session took place, for how long, and the purpose of the session. It is essential that you indicate that the client and/or caregiver was an **active participant** and that you show your professional skill as an occupational therapist in the first few sentences of the "O." Because you can never assume that another therapist or insurance reviewer has read all of your previous notes, it is also important to **clearly indicate the client's primary impairments** that were the focus of the session. For example, suppose you are treating a client whose contractures are compromising his positioning. Instead of saying, "*Client seen for positioning*," you might introduce your "O" by saying one of the following:

- *Caregivers participated in 15-minute bedside OT session for education on positioning client to prevent skin break-down. Client presents with severe Ⓑ hip flexor, elbow flexor, and finger flexor contractures related to spastic quadriplegic cerebral palsy.*
- *Pt. participated in 30-minute session in home to select positioning strategies to improve seated posture for meal-times. Client has custom molded seating system in manual w/c to address low trunk tone and spasticity of all extremities related to spastic quadriplegic cerebral palsy.*

In another scenario, suppose your client is ambulating as a part of IADLs. Since this might potentially be seen as a duplication of services with physical therapy, you would need to be careful about the words you use. Instead of saying, "*Client seen for ambulation*," you might say:

- *Client participated in 30-minute IADL session in rehab kitchen to increase dynamic standing balance and attention to Ⓛ UE for safety when ambulating around kitchen to prepare meals. Client presents with decreased strength, sensation, and proprioception of Ⓛ LE and Ⓛ UE following recent Ⓡ CVA.*

Being Specific About Assist Levels

Remember that you also need to be specific about **the part of the task** that required assistance, rather than reporting only the level of assistance needed.

Not specific enough: *Client supine → sit max Ⓐ, sit → stand mod Ⓐ.*

Specific: *Client supine → sit with max Ⓐ to lift body weight, sit → stand with mod Ⓐ for balance and to maintain TTWB precautions.*

There is a difference between telling **why** the assist was needed, for example:

Client needed mod Ⓐ to transfer w/c → bed due to flaccid left side.

and **the part of the task** that required assistance, for example:

Client needed mod Ⓐ to stand and pivot when transferring w/c → bed.

When writing about assist levels in your "O," please specify **what part of the task** required assistance.

Writing a Complete and Concise "O"

In the objective section of the note, you report what you observed while providing treatment for the client, either chronologically or in categories. As you gain skill in documentation, you become more aware of what to include and what to omit to be concise. Below is an observation that is very concise. Read it and spend a few minutes deciding what it needs to make it better before reading on.

O: *Client participated in 60-minute session in room for ADLs and transfer training.*
ADLs: *Client donned robe with set-up. Client donned/doffed socks with set-up.*
Mobility: *Bed → chair with CGA; supine → sit Ⓘ.*

This note does not have enough information. It is too concise. There is no indication of what the client's deficits are, and there needs to be some indication that skilled occupational therapy was provided. You could start with an opening statement that shows why your skill as an occupational therapist is needed in this situation. As it stands, it is apparent that someone observed the client dress and transfer and recorded assist levels, but a rehabilitation aide or nursing staff could have done this.

In addition, the time required to do the activities documented in this note could be very short. If this is a 1-hour treatment session, what else was done? If the client was slow to do the things recorded, what caused so few activities to take so long? Is there a cognitive problem? Is there a coordination, safety, or motor planning problem? Were adapted techniques or adaptive equipment used to allow the client to be independent?

Finally, with this client's documented level of independence, there is nothing in this note to justify further skilled occupational therapy. Unless this is the client's last session, information needs to be provided that will justify continued treatment.

"A"—Assessment

This is your professional opinion about the **meaning** of what you have just observed. In assessing your data, you will pay special attention to evidence of *problems*, *progress*, and rehab *potential*. The assessment ends with a statement of what the client would benefit from.

Writing Effective Assessment Statements

When occupational therapists are first beginning to write SOAP notes, it is sometimes difficult to decide what is an observation and what is an assessment. Anything you see a client do is an observation. Its meaning in terms of your client's ability to function in some area of occupation is your assessment. Sometimes the difference between an observation and an assessment is one of emphasis. Remember the formula that puts the **contributing factor as the subject of your sentence**:

Contributing Factor	Impact	Ability to Engage in Occupation

- Identify the contributing factor (e.g., ↓ *AROM*; *inability to sequence*; or *narrow doorways*) and make it the subject of your sentence to give it the emphasis it needs in this section of your note.
- Decide whether the area of difficulty you observed today is an indicator of a broader area of occupation. For example, is the decreased AROM you observed during grooming also a problem in other ADL tasks? Will the client's inability to balance a checkbook also cause problems with other money management tasks? Do the problems you observed today put his or her safety at risk?
- Make certain your assessment statement tells how the problem areas affect the client's ability to engage in meaningful occupation. After each problem you note (e.g., limited AROM, sequencing deficits, unstable balance), ask yourself "**So what?**" So he or she is unable to do that—what difference does that make? The answer to your "So what?" question is your assessment of the situation.

Let's consider some examples of how an observation statement would be worded differently than an assessment statement. For example, suppose you are working with a client who tells you she plans to return home to live alone in her farmhouse. You have worked on teaching her some energy conservation techniques, but she forgets to incorporate those into her morning dressing routine. What is the basic or core problem for this client? Why does it matter? The following statement is an **observation** of the client's behavior:

> *Pt. was unable to use energy conservation techniques during morning dressing due to memory deficit.*

However, phrased differently, it becomes an **assessment** of what was observed:

> *Memory deficit interferes with client's ability to retain instructions in compensatory techniques such as energy conservation, which limits her ability to safely perform self-care tasks needed to return to prior ① living situation.*

Note that in this assessment statement, the occupational therapist has identified the basic or core problem as the client's inability to retain instructions she has been given. This might be followed by a recommendation to use memory cues of some kind. Otherwise, why should a payer continue to pay for instruction that will not be remembered? You might also want to consider her safety in living alone if her short-term memory is impaired.

According to the formula, the assessment does not repeat what was observed. Instead, it begins with the contributing factor that is a problem, **broadens the scope of the performance area to include related tasks**, and answers the question "So what? Why does this matter in this client's life?" Let's look at another example. The following is an **observation** of what the occupational therapist saw today:

Client's problem solving was functional and accurate with verbal prompts.

An **assessment** of this situation would sound like this:

Client's need for multiple verbal prompts to solve social problems limits his ability to respond appropriately in unstructured social situations and to enter into successful relationships with others. Ability to problem solve with verbal prompting indicates good potential to reach stated goals.

Note that in the observation statement, there was no area of occupation mentioned. In the assessment statement, the occupational therapist addressed the areas of occupation that are affected by the client's ↓ problem-solving skills.

Let's look at one last example. The statement is an **observation** because it tells **what the client did**:

Client tolerated vestibular and proprioceptive input well today as evidenced by his choosing the activity.

Yes, the client choosing the activity is an indication of his tolerance, and that is good clinical reasoning, but there are more important things to **assess**. One is his progress in tolerating input, and the other is the affect that this progress has on his ability to engage in occupation

Client's choices of activities with proprioceptive and vestibular components indicate progress in sensory tolerance necessary for attention to task in the classroom.

Sweeping Assessment Statements

In the face of a busy schedule, time constraints, and productivity expectations, it is tempting to make concise and sweeping assessment statements, such as the following:

A: *Poor postural stability interferes with ADL performance. Improvement since last note shows good rehab potential. Client would benefit from continued activities to increase postural stability and ability to do personal ADL tasks.*

A: *Decreased strength and coordination prevent client from completing ADLs Ⓘ. Client's ability to follow instructions shows good rehab potential. Client would benefit from continued activities to increase strength, coordination, and fine motor skills.*

A: *Deficits in upper body strength, fine motor, and feeding limit Jordan's ability to be Ⓘ in home and classroom activities.*

While these are accurate, they are limited and would benefit from some elaboration. An elaboration on Jordan's note might read:

A: *Deficits in upper body strength limit Jordan's ability to be Ⓘ in eating and dressing. Decreased fine motor skills impede typical classroom activities such as holding a pencil or crayon and manipulating small items. Recent emergence of supinated digital grasp on crayon indicates improvement from previous pronated mass grasp. Jordan's motivation to engage in classroom activities with peers indicates good potential for future progress in deficit areas. Jordan would benefit from continued upper body strengthening, reach-grasp-release activities, and feeding activities to reach developmental milestones more expediently.*

Here are two more examples of thorough assessments:

A: *Decreased cheek and lip range diminishes pressure in mouth needed for swallow, which results in inadequate swallow reflex. Poor suck and swallow pattern due to decreased oral musculature may lead to inadequate nutritional intake. Decreased head control with upright posture indicates poor head-righting skills, which will hinder Hannah during feeding. Demonstration of visual tracking in different planes indicates good rehab potential. Hannah would benefit from continued skilled OT for oral motor stretches, increased head control, increased oral motor skills, and a home program for prone position activities.*

A: *Ability to complete simple to complex bilateral eye coordination and visual scanning tasks in static position without verbal cues demonstrates improvements since last session. Eye coordination and visual scanning deficits during dynamic movement pose safety concerns during functional mobility for IADLs. Ability to perform Ⓛ shoulder AROM with ↓ pain indicates improvement since last session. Client would benefit from further skilled OT in complex bilateral eye coordination and visual scanning activities during dynamic movement, and increased AROM in Ⓛ shoulder without pain to increase functional performance during ADL and IADL tasks.*

"P"—PLAN

Your plan contains a statement of the frequency, duration, and purpose of future occupational therapy visits for your client, as well as any necessary referrals to other care providers or agencies. Good plans also include a description of the intervention strategies that will address the client's goals.

Too concise: *Continue plan of care.*

Thorough: *Pt. will be seen for one more OT visit prior to discharge home to focus on safe ADL and IADL transfers. Client and spouse will be instructed in use of tub transfer bench and pt. will practice car transfers in simulated car in rehab gym. Recommend that family contact local equipment consortium to explore availability of tub transfer bench before pursuing out-of-pocket purchase.*

A COMPLETE SOAP NOTE

Let's look at a complete SOAP note that meets the criteria described in the last several sections.

S: *Client reported that she bent to the floor to pick up her makeup case this morning. She stated, "I just have a hard time remembering not to bend down." Daughter reports she will provide increased supervision to help client remember to follow hip precautions.*

O: *Client participated in 45-minute session in dining room with daughter present for skilled instruction in maintaining hip precautions during household management tasks. Client presents with short-term memory deficits from early stage age-related dementia. Client ambulated to dining room SBA for balance using wheeled walker. Client retrieved snack from refrigerator and utensils from drawer c̄ SBA for safety. Client required 4 verbal cues to remember hip precautions for stand → sit and when turning with wheeled walker. Following skilled instruction, client able to retrieve items from floor using a reacher. Education provided to client and daughter on hip precautions and safety during both basic and instrumental ADL tasks. Client and daughter both voiced understanding.*

A: *Client's inability to remember hip precautions during household management tasks without verbal cues puts her at risk for re-injury. Supportive daughter and ability to use adaptive equipment properly after instruction indicate good potential for reaching stated goals. Client would benefit from further skilled instruction in maintaining hip precautions during ADL tasks, sit ↔ stand, and transitional living skills.*

P: *Continue tx 3x/wk for 1 wk to work on incorporating hip precautions into ADL and IADL tasks. Instruction of reacher will be continued, and written reminders (text & pictures) will be posted in prominent locations, including bathroom, bedroom, and kitchen.*

REVISING NOTES

The following note will help you apply the principles described earlier in this chapter. Jenna is a preschool child who is receiving occupational therapy twice weekly to increase her tolerance for sensory input. As you read each section of the note, consider what it needs to make it better.

"S"—SUBJECTIVE

S: *Grandma came in and stated, "Jenna was excited this morning to come see you girls." She also commented that Jenna tolerated a few seconds of tooth brushing this morning. Throughout session, Jenna stated several times, "wipe my hands" or "wipe my arms" when foam got on them for too long. She also cried out and yelled "stop" when she had enough of the oral ranging exercise.*

Revisions:

- The first sentence is irrelevant unless the child usually resists attending.
- The fact that the grandmother came in is irrelevant because we have her report.
- The "S" could be much more concise yet still effective.

S: *Grandmother reports that Jenna now tolerates a few seconds of tooth brushing. Jenna asked for hands/arms to be wiped off and asked for oral ranging exercises to be stopped when her tolerance had been reached.*

<h1 style="text-align:center">"O"—Objective</h1>

O: *Child was seen in the clinic to decrease oral defensiveness.*

*   **Proprioception/Deep Pressure:** The therapist began the session with a variety of proprioception and deep pressure activities to allow Jenna to have a better sense of her position in space. Jenna chose to bounce on the big therapy ball first, needing CGA. Jenna then began jumping and sliding, which added a vestibular element. These activities prepped her to engage attentively to the remainder of the session.*

*   **Sensory:** The therapist presented Jenna with foam, water, and foam stick-ups to play with. Jenna was hesitant to play with or touch any of the objects, but after prompting, Jenna actually touched the foam but immediately wanted her hands wiped off. Touching this texture is the beginning of a desensitization process that will assist her to be more tolerant of different textures for the purpose of feeding and hygiene.*

*   **Oral Motor:** The therapist introduced the idea of Jenna feeding the babies food in hopes of imitation. However, when Jenna put the spoon to her own moth, she began spitting. The therapist followed up this activity with completing oral resistive exercises of elongating and protruding the lips as well as stretching the cheek muscles. The intention is to increase length and range for speech and feeding. Jenna had an adverse reaction to this.*

Revisions:

- Opening statements needs to indicate active client participation and need to specify duration and purpose of session.
- Delete what the therapist did and reword to focus on the client.
- De-emphasize the treatment media in the first category and talk about the purpose. Keep this brief, since it is only prep for the sensory and oral-motor work, or make it part of the introduction.
- In the opening statements, talk about sensory as well as oral motor to clearly indicate client's deficits.
- Make the note more concise.
- Avoid mixing "A" material into the observation.
- When talking about desensitizing, tell how much the client could tolerate, to measure progress.

O: *Child participated in 45-minute session in clinic to address sensory processing skills in preparation for accepting a wider range of textures during feeding and hygiene activities. Child presents with both oral and tactile defensiveness and demonstrates strong avoidance behaviors. Child tolerated 10 minutes of proprioception/deep pressure and vestibular input in preparation for engaging her attention in the therapy activities.*

*   **Tactile:** Child presented with foam, water, and foam stick-ups to desensitize her to textures used in feeding/ hygiene, but was hesitant to touch any of the objects. After prompting, child touched the foam but immediately wanted it wiped off.*

*   **Oral Motor:** Child fed a baby doll as an intro to self-feeding. When putting the spoon to her own mouth, child began spitting. Child tolerated 45 seconds of oral resistive activities used to elongate and protrude the lips and stretch the cheek muscles for speech and feeding.*

<h1 style="text-align:center">"A"—Assessment</h1>

A: *Child has increased tolerance for proprioception activities, which has led to an increased ability for her to concentrate on one activity at a time. However, her unwillingness to engage in sensory activities with wet and semi-wet media is still a concern in relation to eating. Hopefully with continued desensitization and oral resistive exercise, Jenna will have decreased oral/tactile defensiveness.*

Revisions:

- We do not see any indication of ability to concentrate on one activity at a time. This is not a problem with the "A," but a change that would need to be made in the "O" so that we can assess it in the "A."
- The second sentence is good with a little revision. It is a sweeping assessment statement and covers a lot of material. Is there more that could be said about the session than this? Are there any other problems? What about the problems tolerating the oral resistive exercises? Is there any progress?
- The third sentence needs to be changed to what she would benefit from rather than what the therapist hopes.

A: *Child's reluctance to engage in sensory activities with wet or semi-wet media continues to interfere with eating and hygiene. Increased tolerance (from 8 to 10 minutes) of proprioceptive activities has resulted in an increased ability to concentrate on one activity at a time. Ability to tolerate 45 seconds of oral resistive activities, willingness to bring spoon to her mouth, and tolerance for a few seconds of tooth brushing also indicate progress. Client would benefit from continued desensitization and oral resistive exercises to decrease tactile defensiveness.*

"P"—Plan

P: *Continue plan of care.*
Revisions:
- There is no mention of frequency, duration, or purpose.
- There is no evidence of clinical reasoning that upcoming sessions will address issues that continue to limit this child's functional performance.

P: *Child will continue to be seen for 30-minute sessions 2x/wk for 3 months to increase tolerance of certain tactile media and to decrease oral defensiveness. Focus will be on increasing tolerated food textures and improving oral range needed for self-feeding. Grandmother will be instructed in home activities to enhance Jenna's development of sensory processing skills.*

The page that follows is a summary of everything you have learned about writing SOAP notes in occupational therapy. A copy of this page is provided at the back of this manual in a cardstock pullout. Pull it out and carry it with you to use as a quick-reference guide.

A Quick Checklist for Evaluating Your Note

Use the following summary chart as a quick-reference guide to be sure that your note contains all of the essential elements.

	S:
☐	Use something significant that the client says about his or her treatment or condition.
	O:
☐	Begin with 1 or 2 statements about the length, setting, and purpose of the treatment session, using wording that indicates active participation by the client and clearly describes the client's primary deficits targeted in the session.
☐	Follow the opening statement with a summary of what you have observed, either chronologically or using categories.
☐	Be professional, concise, and specific.
☐	Focus on occupation.
☐	Focus on the client's response to the treatment provided rather than on what the therapist did.
☐	Write from the client's point of view, leaving yourself out.
☐	Be specific about assist levels.
☐	Avoid making a list of actions and assist levels.
☐	De-emphasize the treatment media.
☐	Make certain that it is clear that you were not just a passive observer in the session.
☐	Avoid judging the client.
☐	Use only standard abbreviations.
	A:
☐	Go sentence by sentence through the information presented in the "S" and the "O," asking yourself what it means for the client's ability to engage in meaningful occupation. Note what problems, progress, and potential for rehabilitation you see.
☐	Remember the formula that puts the contributing factor as the subject of your sentence:

Contributing Factor	Impact	Ability to Engage in Occupation

☐	End the "A" with "*Client would benefit from…*," justifying continued skilled occupational therapy and setting up the plan. Be sure that you don't just simply say the client needs more of the same. Think about what else the client needs based on the deficits you observed in this session.
☐	Be sure that the timelines and activities you are putting in your plan match the skilled occupational therapy you say your client needs.
	P:
☐	Specify the frequency and duration of future occupational therapy sessions (e.g., 2x/wk for 4 wks).
☐	Describe the purpose of future occupational therapy sessions in the client's current setting.
☐	Include a brief description of the intervention strategies that will address the client's goals.
☐	If appropriate, indicate referral to other health care providers or agencies.

If you have read the text carefully, you will know what each item means. For a more complete explanation, refer to the chapter that provides information in detail.

S:
- Use something significant that the client says about his or her treatment or condition, describe any nonverbal communication that took place, and/or provide any relevant caregiver report. If there is nothing significant, ask yourself whether you are using your interview skills effectively to elicit the information about the client's perspective.

O:
- Begin with statements about the length, setting, and purpose of the treatment session, using wording that indicates active participation by the client and describes the client's primary deficits:
  Client participated in 45-minute OT session in rehab kitchen for meal preparation activity. Client exhibits Ⓛ visual neglect and Ⓛ UE hemiparesis, and uses a manual wheelchair for functional mobility during IADLs.
- Focus on the client's response rather than on what you did:
  Client able to don socks using sock-aid after demonstration.
- Write from the client's point of view, leaving yourself out:
  Client repositioned with max Ⓐ rather than *Therapist repositioned client.*
- Be specific about assist levels:
  Client required min Ⓐ for hand placement during pivot transfer to toilet.
- De-emphasize the treatment media:
  Client worked on tripod pinch using pegs to grasp objects needed for ADLs.
- Make certain that it is clear that you were not just a passive observer in the session. Don't just make a list of all the assist levels and think that is enough.
- Avoid judging the client. For example, say he *"...didn't complete the activity."* Don't add *"...because he was stubborn."*

A:
- Go sentence by sentence through the information presented in the "S" and the "O," asking yourself what it means for the client's ability to engage in meaningful occupation. Note what **problems**, **progress**, and **potential** for rehabilitation you see.
- Remember the formula that puts the contributing factor as the subject of your sentence:

Contributing Factor	Impact	Ability to Engage in Occupation

Example: *Deficits in UE AROM & strength limit client's ability to complete basic self-care tasks.*
- End the "A" with *"Client would benefit from...,"* justifying continued skilled occupational therapy and setting up the plan:
  Client would benefit from skilled instruction in energy conservation techniques, continued strengthening of UE, and compensatory techniques for performing IADLs one-handed.

P:
- Specify frequency, duration, and purpose of future sessions and give a brief description of planned interventions.
  Infant will be seen 2x/wk for 2 months to address feeding skills. Treatment to include oral desensitization and caregiver training in use of adaptive bottles.

WORKSHEET 11-1

Writing Problem Statements

Consider the following problem statements. Decide what is needed to make each one a better problem statement, then rewrite the sentence into a better format.

1. *Pt. unable to dress LE Ⓘ due to trunk instability.*

2. *Child doesn't tolerate very much classroom activity due to ↓ activity tolerance.*

3. *Consumer acts out.*

WORKSHEET 11-2

Writing COAST Goals

Remember that you should de-emphasize the treatment media in both your observations and your goal statements. Rewrite the following goal statements to emphasize change in occupational performance that you want to see and to de-emphasize the treatment interventions.

1. *Client will make a clock independently using the appropriate materials by anticipated discharge in 1 week.*

2. *Consumer will stay in his chair without reminders and spend at least 30 minutes lacing the leather billfold during the 45-minute craft group session within 2 weeks.*

WORKSHEET 11-3

SOAPing Your Note

Indicate in which section of the SOAP note you would place each of these statements.

_____ *Client supine → sit in bed Ⓘ.*

_____ *Client moved kitchen items from counter to cabinet Ⓘ using Ⓛ hand.*

_____ *Decreased coordination, strength, sensation, and proprioception in Ⓛ hand create safety risks in home management tasks.*

_____ *Client reports that his fingers are stiff this morning and that he is having trouble handling small items like buttons.*

_____ *↑ of 15 minutes in activity tolerance for UE activities permits client to prepare a light meal Ⓘ.*

_____ *Child participated in 60-minute eval. of hand function in OT clinic.*

_____ *Decreased proprioception and motor planning limit Ⓘ in upper body dressing.*

_____ *Continue retrograde massage to Ⓡ hand for edema control.*

_____ *Correct identification of inappropriate positioning 100% of time indicates memory WFL.*

_____ *Client reports that she cannot remember hip precautions.*

_____ *Veteran would benefit from further instruction to incorporate total hip precautions into lower body dressing, bathing, and toileting.*

_____ *Client's improvement with repetition indicates good potential for successful access of augmentative communication device using eye gaze.*

_____ *Client did not make eye contact during group session.*

_____ *Client wrote check for correct amount to pay electric bill with 2 verbal cues.*

_____ *Client's request to take breaks demonstrates awareness of her limitations in endurance.*

_____ *Client completed weight shifts of trunk x 10 in each of anterior, posterior, left, and right lateral directions in preparation for standing to perform IADLs.*

_____ *3+ muscle grade of Ⓡ wrist extension this week shows good progress toward goals.*

_____ *Continue OT 3x/wk for 2 weeks to address cognitive impairments that affect safe performance of IADLs.*

_____ *Unkempt appearance in mock interview situation indicates poor judgment and self-concept.*

WORKSHEET 11-4

Writing the "S"—Subjective

The subjective section of your note contains the client's perception of the situation.

Inexperienced therapists sometimes list anything important the client has said about his or her condition. In the example below, all of the information is relevant, but does not form a coherent whole. This is not wrong and is better than reporting irrelevant data, but it is less skillful than reporting an organized and coherent summary of what the client had to say. Most of this client's comments have to do with transfers.

S: *Client told OT she has really bad arthritis in her right shoulder and Ⓛ knee.*
Client rates pain at the site of her Ⓡ BKA as 8 out of 10.
Client said, "It hurts to stand on my left leg."
Client stated, "It [sliding board] needs to be moved further up on the seat."
When asked if she was okay after the transfer, she said, "I'm just tired."
Client stated, "I'm through," and requested help to get closer to the bed.
When client transferred to the bed for dressing tasks, she said, "This is the hardest part."
Client stated she prefers to transfer toward the Ⓡ side so she can push off with her Ⓛ LE and avoid bumping her Ⓡ BKA on the tire-rim of the w/c.

Write a more concise version of this "S," remembering to leave yourself out:

S:

WORKSHEET 11-5

"O"—Writing Good Opening Lines

Rewrite the following opening statements to show how your skill as an occupational therapist is important in each situation and to indicate the primary deficits addressed in the session.

1. *Client seen in room for 45 minutes for self-care activities.*

    Additional information: Client is on total hip precautions, which raises safety concerns during mobility, especially during toilet transfer. Adaptive equipment is available if needed. Client has underlying memory deficits.

2. *Client seen at workshop for 1 hr. to work on job skills.*

    Additional information: Client has deficits in sequencing tasks, which ↓ his ability to work ①. Ⓑ coordination problems interfere with client completing essential job function of opening/closing boxes. Sensory registration deficits contribute to client's high distractibility during task completion.

3. *Client seen bedside for 30 minutes for morning dressing.*

    Additional information: Deficits include ↓ balance and ↓ Ⓑ motor control of UEs that ↓ ability to safely complete ADL activities and use a manual w/c for mobility during ADLs.

4. *Client seen in kitchen for 1 hr. to work on ① in cooking.*

    Additional information: Client's problems include decreased dynamic standing balance and inattention of affected Ⓛ UE, which raise safety concerns.

WORKSHEET 11-6

"O"—Being Specific About Assist Levels

Do each of the following statements include the **specific part of the task** requiring assistance?

_____ *Client required max Ⓐ x 2 bed → bedside commode and bed → w/c; Ⓓ for pericare.*

_____ *Child required HOH Ⓐ to stay in the lines when following path with crayon.*

_____ *Client needed mod verbal cues to participate in discussion during life skills group.*

_____ *Resident needed min Ⓐ to don sock due to pain.*

WORKSHEET 11-7

Revising the "O"

Rather than rewriting this note to improve it, just write down your suggestions for what it needs to make it better.

O: **Toilet transfers:** *max Ⓐ*
　　Toileting: *max Ⓐ 2° inability to support self c̄ Ⓛ arm and to dress*
　　UE dressing: *min Ⓐ, verbal cues, set-up, Ⓘ in pulling shirt over head*
　　LE dressing: *min Ⓐ pants to hips; max Ⓐ pants to waist*
　　　modified Ⓘ to don Ⓛ shoe (elastic laces); modified Ⓘ to don Ⓡ shoe
　　Ⓡ hand status: *Ⓡ fingers: small spasticity (index finger greatest amount)*
　　　Thumb: CMC joint painful in abd & flex
　　　Ⓡ wrist: flaccid

◆

◆

◆

◆

◆

Worksheet 11-8

Differentiating Between Observations and Assessments

Identify which of these statements are **observations** and which are **assessments**. Remember that an observation tells you what the client did. An assessment will tell you how the contributing factor that is a problem affects an area of occupation.

_____ Client is unable to don AFO and shoe Ⓘ for ambulation.

_____ Inability to don AFO and shoe Ⓘ prevent client from ambulating safely around the house for IADL performance to live alone.

_____ Decreased sensory tolerance limits the client's attention to task in the classroom.

_____ Client required verbal cues to stay on task due to decreased sensory tolerance.

_____ Client was unable to incorporate breathing and energy conservation techniques, requiring several prompts to complete task.

_____ Inability to incorporate breathing techniques and energy conservation techniques into basic ADL tasks $\bar{s}$ verbal prompts limits her ability to live alone Ⓘ $\bar{p}$ discharge.

The following statements are **observations** of something the occupational therapist saw the client do. Reword them so that they become **assessments**.

1. Client demonstrated difficulty with laundry and cooking tasks due to memory and sequencing deficits.

2. Client unable to complete homemaking tasks or basic self-care activities independently due to decreased endurance and not following hip precautions.

3. After the use of behavioral modification techniques, client displayed courteous behavior for the remainder of the treatment session.

WORKSHEET 11-9

Problems, Progress, and Rehab Potential

Mr. Y is a 68-year-old man who had a Ⓛ CVA 1 week ago. His Ⓡ UE is getting some return, and occupational therapy was ordered yesterday. Your colleague who assessed Mr. Y yesterday is out sick today, and you are beginning treatment with him. Her initial note stated that his activity tolerance was less than 1 minute and she was not sure how much aphasia was present.

O: *Client participated in 30-minute session in OT clinic to work on functional use of Ⓡ UE in prep for ADL activities. Client deficits include Ⓡ UE hemiparesis, decreased sitting balance, and decreased cognition. Client needed mod Ⓐ in shifting weight to get to edge of w/c and max verbal cues to use correct posture and shift feet during stand pivot transfer w/c → mat. Client required max verbal cues to initiate grasp of small beanbag. Client needed mod Ⓐ in reaching with Ⓡ UE. Client able to complete Ⓡ UE shoulder flexion required to toss beanbag ~2 ft. with max verbal cues. Client demonstrated cognitive understanding of activity with mod verbal cues by stating desired goal to be achieved by accurate aim. Client tolerated up to 3 minutes of activity before requiring rest break.*

Now assess the meaning of these data. Note the problems, progress, and rehab potential that you see for this client.

Problems:

Progress/Rehab Potential:

Now write an "A" that assesses how engagement in occupation is affected. Include what the client would benefit from. Then write a "P" that describes your plan for this client.

A:

P:

WORKSHEET 11-10

Writing the "A" and "P"—The School Note

Now you will assess and plan for a school-age child. Remember that treatment in public school always relates to the child's educational performance. Cody is a second grader who is receiving occupational therapy in the public schools. He has several problems, including low muscle tone, which contributes to his upper body weakness and decreased proximal stability. At the time of the last note, he was able to achieve 70% accuracy in letter formation with verbal cues.

S: *Child stated, "This is hard!" during a bilateral coordination exercise requiring UE strength and stability.*

O: *Child participated in 30-minute session in school therapy room to address skills related to handwriting and other visual motor classroom tasks. Child presents with deficits in oculomotor movements, fine motor skills, and upper body strength and stability necessary for dynamic UE function in the classroom.*
***Visual tracking:** Child visually tracked a moving object 4 times ⓇⓇ → Ⓛ @ 40% accuracy and Ⓛ → Ⓡ @ 20% accuracy. Child demonstrated 20% accuracy of eye convergence 4x staring 12" from nose and breaking at ~6" from nose.*
***UE coordination:** Child performed Ⓑ UE coordination activity (Zoom ball) at 80% accuracy with hyperextended knees and trunk movement to compensate for upper body weakness.*
***Handwriting:** Child able to write letters P, E, F, D, M, N, R from memory with 90% accuracy and 75% accuracy for staying in line boundaries with min verbal cues.*

What problems, progress, and/or rehab potential do you see for Cody?

Write your assessment and plan below.

A:

P:

WORKSHEET 11-11

Writing the "A" and "P"— Mr. S's Communication Skills

Mr. S is a 35-year-old male who is in a maximum security unit in a state psychiatric facility. He has criminal charges against him for a violent crime but was sent to the state mental institution rather than to prison. His current diagnosis is schizophrenia, r/o personality disorder. Today he participated in assertion group.

S: *Mr. S stated he knows what assertion is, but reports, "Manipulation and aggression have always worked better for me." When asked to explain assertion, Mr. S stated, "The problem with that is the sugar and fruit in the cake."*

O: *Mr. S attended 1-hr. assertion group this date for skilled instruction and role play activities to improve assertion and effective self-expression skills. Mr. S was on time to the group, neatly dressed with hair combed. He was unable to correctly define assertion and did not respond to any of the three role-play activities, either by taking a role or by offering suggestions to others. During the role-play, Mr. S placed his head down and closed his eyes. Following the session, Mr. S quickly left the room.*

What problems, progress, and/or rehab potential do you see for Mr. S?

Write your assessment and plan below.

A:

P:

WORKSHEET 11-12

Revising the "Almost" Note

This note is **almost** good enough. In fact, it is quite good on the surface, but has major flaws in organization and clinical reasoning. Mrs. B is a 78-year-old female who has had a Ⓛ CVA and has Ⓡ hemiparesis. You do not have to rewrite this note, but as you read through it, keep track of suggestions that you have for improving it:

S: *Client reports stiffness in her Ⓡ hip, but improvement from previous pain. She states a preference for transferring to her left side. Client states she is willing to do "whatever it takes to get out of the hospital."*

O: *Client participated in 45-minute session in room to work on dressing and functional mobility during ADLs. Pt. deficits include decreased balance and limited Ⓡ ROM.*
__Transfer:__ Stand pivot transfer bed → w/c to left side SBA. Min Ⓐ with transfers w/c → toilet using grab bar.
__Mobility:__ Client rolled supine to Ⓡ side SBA with VCs to flex trunk. Client supine → sit SBA; sit → stand min Ⓐ; Ⓘ with w/c mobility.
__Dressing:__ Client donned shirt Ⓘ.
   Client donned bra min Ⓐ with VCs while standing.
   Client donned socks and shoes Ⓘ.
   Client donned underwear and pants with min Ⓐ and VCs to stand with walker.
   Client needs set-up for dressing activities.
   UE ROM: Ⓛ UE: WFL; Ⓡ UE: ↓ range in shoulder flexion.
__Static standing:__ Client used walker for Ⓑ UE support with CGA.
__Dynamic standing:__ SBA with walker for balance.

A: *Deficits noted in Ⓡ UE coordination, Ⓑ UE strength, and dynamic standing balance. Client Ⓘ in dressing EOB, but is min Ⓐ in dressing when standing with a walker. Ⓛ UE AROM is WFL, but Ⓡ UE has deficits noted in shoulder flexion. Client needs SBA in bed mobility when rolling to unaffected side and min Ⓐ in sit → stand 2° ↓ UE strength. Client needs SBA for transfer to unaffected side in pivot transfer bed → w/c and min Ⓐ w/c → toilet. Client would benefit from skilled OT to continue UE strengthening and coordination exercise and to ↑ dynamic standing balance using walker to ↑ Ⓘ in ADLs.*

P: *Client to be seen 30 minutes bid for 2 weeks to continue work on dynamic standing balance during ADLs.*

What suggestions do you have for improving this note?

Chapter 12

Intervention Planning

Now that you know the basics of writing a SOAP note, we will back up a little and give some attention to the intervention planning on which your notes are based. You may recall from Chapter 1 that the *OTPF-III* (American Occupational Therapy Association [AOTA], 2014b) describes both the domain and the process of occupational therapy. The first part of the occupational therapy process involves a thorough evaluation, including development of an occupational profile as well as analysis of occupational performance. Through the evaluation process, problems are identified, client priorities are determined, and targeted outcomes are developed.

The next step in the occupational therapy process is documenting the intervention plan, "a plan that will guide actions taken and that is developed in collaboration with the client. It is based on selected theories, frames of reference, and evidence" (AOTA, 2014b, p. S10). A frame of reference guides practice by delineating evaluation and intervention strategies for a specific domain of practice (Cole, 2014). The intervention strategies selected and the terminology used to describe those interventions will vary depending on the frames of reference used for a particular setting or client.

The *OTPF-III* explains that interventions may be developed for a person, a group, or a population. For purposes of learning, this manual will focus only on interventions targeted at individuals. However, the techniques described in this manual can be adapted for occupational therapists who serve groups and populations.

As explained in Chapter 10, the intervention plan is part of the "P" section of an evaluation SOAP note. We will discuss additional requirements related to evaluation documentation in Chapter 13. In this chapter, we will focus specifically on the goals, objectives, and intervention strategies contained in the intervention plan.

THE INTERVENTION PLANNING PROCESS

From the moment a referral is received, intervention planning begins in the mind of the therapist. A name, age, and reason for referral should stimulate an occupational therapist to begin reviewing in his or her mind the areas of occupation likely to be assessed, the areas of deficit that might be found, and the possible interventions that will benefit the client. Each individual is different, and there will be many variations, as well as some surprises as the assessment begins. The mental preparation for "*Clyde C, age 68, Ⓛ CVA, evaluate and treat*" takes a therapist on a mental journey along one road of thought, whereas "*Brooke J, age 4, ADHD, evaluate and treat*" takes the therapist mentally down a different pathway. From day one, a good therapist also begins discharge planning based on the client's occupational profile, prior level of performance, and probable discharge placement.

The *Guidelines for Documentation of Occupational Therapy* (AOTA, 2014b, P. S35) identify the components that should be included in an intervention plan:

- Client name and demographic information
- Measurable, occupation-based goals and objectives

Gateley CA, Borcherding S. *Documentation Manual for Occupational Therapy: Writing SOAP Notes, Fourth Edition (pp 153-168).* © 2017 SLACK Incorporated

- Intervention approaches and types of interventions to be used
- Service delivery mechanisms including provider, location, and frequency/duration
- Plan for discharge including discharge setting, follow-up care, and discontinuation criteria
- Outcome measures such as standardized and nonstandardized assessments
- Professionals responsible for plan and date of plan development, review, or modification

The initial evaluation and intervention plan are written in whatever format the facility uses, and this will vary depending on practice setting. In earlier chapters, you learned how to write functional problem statements and how to address those problems by writing long-term (LTGs) and short-term goals (STGs), or objectives. Now we will discuss how to select intervention approaches and specific strategies to address the identified problems and to assist the client in meeting the established goals.

The *OTPF-III* (AOTA, 2014b) outlines five categories of intervention approaches that may be used in occupational therapy:

1. **Health promotion** to create activities, enrich contexts, and enhance performance
2. **Establishment** of skills not yet developed or **remediation/restoration** of impaired skills
3. **Maintenance** of performance capabilities, assuming that performance would decrease without intervention (Note: The word *maintain* is a red-flag word for reviewers; when documenting this approach, it is essential to elaborate on how the lack of occupational therapy services would lead to a significant decrease in occupational performance for the client. Examples include interventions for individuals with progressive disorders, such as Parkinson's disease or macular degeneration, that help the individuals continue to function as independently as possible in the least restrictive environment.)
4. **Modification** of context or activity through **compensatory** techniques or **adaptation**
5. **Prevention** of occupational performance problems for clients with or without a disability

The intervention approaches listed here are closely tied to the client's targeted outcomes. These approaches describe **what** you hope to accomplish through occupational therapy intervention. The *OTPF-III* also lists the specific types of occupational therapy interventions that may be implemented:

- Therapeutic use of occupations and activities
- Preparatory methods and preparatory tasks
- Education and training
- Advocacy
- Group interventions

The types of occupational therapy interventions described here explain **how** you will help the client meet the targeted outcomes. Let's take a closer look at each of these interventions.

THERAPEUTIC USE OF OCCUPATIONS AND ACTIVITIES

These types of interventions involve selecting specific occupations and activities as interventions to meet the client's goals. "To use occupations and activities therapeutically, the practitioner considers activity demands and client factors in relation to the client's therapeutic goals, contexts, and environments" (AOTA, 2014b, p. S29).

- *Occupations*: Occupations are "client centered daily life activities that match and support or address identified participation goals" (AOTA, 2014b, p. S29). Examples include completing morning activities of daily living (ADL) routine using adaptive equipment, playing on a playground, and using public transportation to go grocery shopping.
- *Activities*: Activities are components of occupations that **hold meaning or relevance** for the client. Examples include practicing tub and toilet transfers to determine best equipment options for home, creating a simulated monthly budget in preparation for transitional housing, and practicing making change to improve money management skills.

PREPARATORY METHODS AND PREPARATORY TASKS

Preparatory methods and tasks help prepare the client for performance of occupations. These intervention approaches may be "used as part of a treatment session in preparation for or concurrently with occupations and activities or provided to a client as a home-based engagement to support daily occupational performance" (AOTA, 2014b, p. S29).

- *Preparatory Methods*: Preparatory methods are "modalities, devices, and techniques to prepare the client for occupational performance. Often, preparatory methods are '**done to**' the client without the client's active participation" (AOTA, 2014b, P. S29). Examples include physical agent modalities, manual lymphatic draining, splinting, wound care techniques, identification of assistive technology, recommendations for environmental modifications, and recommendation of products and technology for seating, positioning, and mobility.
- *Preparatory Tasks*: Preparatory tasks are "actions selected and provided to the client to target specific client factors or performance skills. Tasks involve **active participation of the client** and sometimes comprise engagements that use various materials to simulate activities or components of occupations" (AOTA, 2014b, p. S30). Examples include participating in a fabricated sensory environment, performing a home exercise program, strengthening exercises with therapy putty or exercise bands, and removing and replacing clothes on hangers in a therapy gym closet for purposes of addressing shoulder ROM.
  - Students often have difficulty understanding the difference between activities and preparatory tasks. Activities hold meaning for the client. "**Preparatory tasks themselves may not hold inherent meaning, relevance, or perceived utility as stand-alone entities**" (AOTA, 2014b, p. S30). If you ask a client to refold clean towels taken from a linen cart because she hopes to return to her job as a housekeeper, that intervention would be classified as an activity because it involves practice of a component of an occupation that holds meaning for the client. In contrast, imagine a different client who has no history in housekeeping employment. If you ask that client to refold towels taken from a clean linen cart because you identified that task as another way to address shoulder ROM instead of exercises, that intervention would be classified as preparatory task because it holds no inherent meaning for the client. It is simply another form of exercise.

One error that students and new therapists sometimes make is getting stuck on preparatory methods and tasks while failing to move toward meaningful activities and occupations. If you keep your client's occupation-based goals in mind, you should be able to develop a comprehensive intervention plan that includes multiple types of intervention.

EDUCATION AND TRAINING

In addition to the hands-on intervention approaches described previously, occupational therapy practitioners often engage in education and training with their clients. The *OTPF-III* (AOTA, 2014b) distinguishes between these two types of intervention:

1. *Education*: Education is defined as the "imparting of knowledge and information about occupation, health, well-being, and participation that enables the client to acquire helpful behaviors, habits, and routines that may or may not require application at the time of the intervention session" (AOTA, 2014b, p. S30). Examples include educating family members about home safety modifications for a client with dementia, educating a client's family member or friend about the slope guidelines for building a wheelchair ramp at the home, and educating a client and family about stroke warning signs and when to seek medical attention. **The goal of education is enhanced understanding**.

2. *Training*: Training is the "facilitation of the acquisition of concrete skills for meeting specific goals in a real-life applied situation….Skills refers to measurable components of function that enable mastery" (AOTA, 2014b, p. S30). Examples include instructing a client in self-ROM exercises to prevent contracture, training a client and caregivers on the features of a new wheelchair, and training a paraprofessional how to implement proprioceptive strategies with a child to reduce behavioral outbursts during transitions. **The goal of training is enhanced performance**.

ADVOCACY

Advocacy involves "efforts directed toward promoting occupational justice and empowering clients to seek and obtain resources to fully participate in daily life occupations" (AOTA, 2014b, p. S30). Advocacy efforts may be undertaken by the occupational therapy practitioner or by the client. Examples of advocacy include collaborating with a client to procure reasonable work accommodations and serving on a community board to encourage universal design of parks and recreational facilities. Examples of self-advocacy include a college student with a learning disability making an appointment with the Office of Disability Services to procure reasonable educational accommodations and a group of individuals with disabilities attending a City Council meeting to address availability of public transportation for wheelchair users.

GROUP INTERVENTIONS

Group interventions involve the use of the occupational therapy practitioner's leadership to facilitate learning and skill acquisition through the dynamics of group and social interaction (AOTA, 2014b). Examples include a social skills group for adolescents on the autism spectrum, a cooking skills group for adults with developmental disabilities, an anger management group for individuals with mental health conditions, and an upper extremity (UE) exercise group for patients in a rehabilitation facility. Please note that there are specific billing guidelines that must be followed when billing for group interventions. Even in the context of high productivity expectations, "occupational therapy practitioners have an ethical and legal duty to be vigilant in knowing and following the standards and regulations related to clinical documentation to accurately report 'treatment time' and bill for their services" (AOTA, 2014a, p. 1).

OTHER CONSIDERATIONS

In addition to being aware of the different intervention approaches and techniques, there are other factors that must be considered when setting goals and selecting interventions to meet those goals.

ESTIMATING REHAB POTENTIAL

Rehab potential should always be stated as good or excellent for the goals you and the client have selected. If your client's rehab potential is not good or excellent for the stated goals, you may need to select smaller, more incremental goals. It is not as helpful to set and work toward goals that the client does not have a good chance of accomplishing. Estimating rehab potential as *poor, fair,* or *guarded* is a red flag to reviewers, and they may be reluctant to set aside health care dollars for someone who is unlikely to benefit from your intervention.

> Note: "Rehab potential" does not mean "independence." It means "potential to reach the goals you have set or potential for the client to make significant change."

SELECTING MEANINGFUL INTERVENTION STRATEGIES

Since selecting strategies and treatment media is a daily task for an occupational therapist, to an inexperienced therapist, it can seem like reinventing the wheel to select different strategies for each individual client. One of the striking differences between occupational therapy and other disciplines is the way in which strategies and media are selected to meet the client's goals. Occupational therapy is a client-centered profession and the selected interventions should be meaningful to the individual client (Gillen & Boyt Schell, 2014). Occupational therapy is a process of creative problem solving with each client in each area of occupation. What is meaningful to one client may not be meaningful to another.

Even the most basic task such as dressing may not seem meaningful to some clients. A person with tetraplegia who has a personal attendant, for example, may never need to dress himself and may consider it an enormous waste of time to be required to learn to do so. However, he may be very motivated to learn how to use a power wheelchair operated with head controls to be independent with mobility needed to re-engage in social participation with his friends. Some clients will never need to balance a checkbook, while others may not be able to return to living independently without this skill. The difference between competent and exceptional occupational therapy may lie in the ability to find meaningful activities, and design these into intervention strategies.

The occupational therapist asks questions such as the following:

- What do you want to be able to do?
- What keeps you from being able to do that?
- What are the possible options for making that happen?

The options for intervention strategies may include teaching new skills or patterns, working to increase client factors (ROM, strength, endurance), or modifying the environment (context) to improve occupational performance. Occupational therapists consider doing things in many different ways. The creativity of the individual therapist blossoms in intervention planning. How many ways are there to get light into a room if the client can no longer manage a light switch? How many activities that require wrist extension could be adapted to work toward a LTG of returning to an assembly line position that requires increased AROM of the wrist? Would any of these activities qualify as meaningful to this client?

The treatment media used in occupational therapy is also different from that used by other disciplines. Occupational therapists often use common household objects to accomplish tasks or activities related to occupational performance. For example, the client's own clothing is a common treatment media. The clothes may be used for dressing to teach the client to don clothing; for folding to have the client do a meaningful activity while increasing standing tolerance; or for hanging in a closet to help the client increase AROM at the shoulder. The approach would depend on what the client will need to do in the setting to which he or she will be discharged. An experienced occupational therapist can find many different uses for common household objects. The same mesh sponge that is used to wash dishes may be used for squeezing to develop grip strength or for throwing to develop AROM in the UEs.

CONSIDERATION OF "BOTTOM-UP" VERSUS "TOP-DOWN" APPROACHES

The concepts of "bottom-up" and "top-down" approaches for evaluation and intervention have received considerable attention in the recent occupational therapy literature (Brown & Chien, 2010; Giles & Morrison, 2014; Kennedy, Brown, & Stagnitti, 2013; Meriano & Latella, 2008). Bottom-up approaches use interventions that address foundational deficits related to occupations such as ROM, fine motor coordination, and attention skills. Top-down approaches involve the use of meaningful occupations and activities as a means of addressing underlying client deficits. Examples include engagement in dressing tasks, opening a toothpaste cap, opening a food package, and engagement in higher level cognitive processes such as self-awareness of stress levels during social interaction. Although both approaches have merit, top-down approaches are believed to result in better carryover and generalization of skills. Occupational therapy practitioners should ensure that they are not using only bottom-up approaches in their intervention plans. Effort should be made to focus on top-down approaches as well.

THEORETICAL BASIS OF INTERVENTION

Throughout your occupational therapy curriculum, you will be introduced to several theories, conceptual models, and frames of reference that guide occupational therapy practice. Cole and Tufano (2008) explained that these terms often are used interchangeably. However, they clarified that a frame of reference is "a system of compatible concepts from theory that guide a plan of action for assessment and intervention within specific OT domains" (Cole & Tufano, 2008, p. 62). As you are developing an intervention plan, you should be able to relate your planned interventions back to one or more frames of reference. It is common practice for occupational therapists to use a combination of approaches.

> Note: Students and new practitioners may need to be very intentional in connecting theoretical foundations to clinical decisions. Chapter 15 includes an example from an electronic documentation software package that gives the therapist an opportunity to specify one or more frames of reference. However, as occupational therapists gain experience, they rarely articulate or document the theoretical basis underlying specific strategies in their intervention plans. It is beyond the scope of this textbook to review the numerous frames of reference that guide occupational therapy intervention.

DETERMINING FREQUENCY AND DURATION OF TREATMENT

In Chapter 10, you learned that the frequency and duration of occupational therapy services vary greatly between settings and funding sources. It may seem impossible to a new therapist to estimate how much time will be needed to accomplish goals. With a little experience, you will find that you really can do it. Please remember that the intervention plan is made to be changed. If your original estimate does not turn out to be accurate, you change it as you find out how quickly your client progresses.

Clinical Pathways

A clinical pathway, also known as a *critical care pathway*, is a standardized interdisciplinary management plan involving a particular "sequence of clinical interventions, timeframes, milestones, and expected outcomes for a homogenous patient group" (Queensland Health, 2013, para. 1). The purpose of clinical pathways is to provide care in a cost-effective manner, essentially reducing the length of inpatient hospitalization. The clinical pathway includes a standardized intervention plan based on a predictable course of recovery.

In addition to standardizing intervention strategies and establishing check points along a timeline, the use of a standard intervention plan is also more efficient by avoiding unnecessary time rewriting the same plan for routine treatment approaches. The standardized plan does allow for adaptations to accommodate individual client differences such as comorbid diagnoses (e.g., knee replacement with a history of multiple sclerosis).

Some diagnoses, such as stroke, are too complex to use a clinical pathway, while others are very compatible with a standardized approach to treatment. Clinical pathways are most often used following orthopedic surgeries including hip and knee replacements and various spinal procedures (laminectomies, discectomies, fusions, etc.). See Table 12-1 for an example of a clinical pathway. Keep in mind that the clinical pathway lists the **interventions** that the therapist will use. The client's **goals still need to be written in occupation-based terms** as described in Chapter 6.

Table 12-1

Clinical Pathway—Total Hip Replacement

POSTOPERATIVE DAY 1

- Initial occupational therapist evaluation, including transfer bed ↔ w/c or bedside chair
- Skilled instruction of hip precautions; provide handout
- Have pt. verbalize and demonstrate precautions during ADLs, within activity tolerance
- Begin UE strengthening if needed; introduce home program and have client demonstrate

POSTOPERATIVE DAY 2*

- Reassess client's understanding of hip precautions and home exercise program
- Assess adaptive equipment needs for dressing, toileting, bathing
- Procure necessary equipment via hospital procedures
- Practice lower body dressing, toileting at bedside commode, grooming at sink in standing

POSTOPERATIVE DAY 3*

- Bathing assessment in tub or shower
- Practice toileting with riser or commode frame on toilet
- Practice car transfer in car simulator
- Provide home safety education (especially kitchen task if will be home alone) and have pt. practice as needed

---

* Note that in some settings, the occupational therapist may be expected to evaluate the patient on the day of surgery. Patient may be discharged postoperative day 2, 3, or 4 depending on progress. If discharge is planned for postoperative day 2, all interventions listed for postoperative day 3 should also be covered on postoperative day 2. A skilled nursing facility referral may be made for those patients requiring a longer recovery period.

SAMPLE INTERVENTION PLAN

Client Name: Norma H   *Age:* 83   *1° Dx:* Ⓛ CVA   *2° Dx:* DM
Frequency/Duration: 30 minutes 2x/day for 3 weeks
Occupational Profile: Mrs. H is a widow who lives with her daughter and grandson in a one-story house in a small town. Mrs. H was Ⓘ in all ADL and IADL tasks before her CVA. She has never worked outside her home. She raised 7 children in the town where she now resides and takes pride in her ability to do homemaking tasks such as cooking, sewing, and decorating. She drives in her own small town, but is not comfortable driving long distances. She intends to return to the home she shares with her daughter and grandson and hopes to return to her PLOF.
Problem: Client requires mod Ⓐ in self-care due to inability to spontaneously use Ⓡ UE 2° Ⓛ CVA.
LTG: Client will complete all ADL and IADL activities with modified Ⓘ within 3 weeks.

STG (Objective)	Intervention	Type of Intervention
STG #1: Client will complete grooming tasks with set-up using ⓡ UE spontaneously as a functional assist within 1 week.	1. Normalize tone through weightbearing on ⓡ UE while engaged in activities that require weight shifts (sorting laundry, playing a board game) 2. Therapy putty exercises to improve hand and finger strength 3. Neuromuscular electrical stimulation to strengthen ⓡ wrist extensors 4. Handling, joint approximation, and muscle stretch in preparation for facilitation of grasp/release for prehension 5. Provide activities that require use of ⓡ UE as an assist (stabilizing tablet or clipboard while writing) 6. Complete morning grooming routine involving stabilizing toothpaste while removing lid and applying body lotion	1. Preparatory task 2. Preparatory task 3. Preparatory method 4. Preparatory method 5. Activity 6. Occupation
STG #2: Client will dress self with min Ⓐ within 2 weeks using ⓡ UE as a functional assist.	1. UE exerciser ("arm bike") for increased ⓡ UE strengthening 2. Instruct in adaptive dressing techniques and adaptive equipment as needed: long shoehorn, elastic laces, reacher, button hook 3. Facilitate trunk control and balance in weight shifts forward and backward, side to side, and in rotational patterns while engaged in reaching for objects 4. Practice use of button hook to fasten buttons on shirt 5. Complete morning dressing routine using ⓡ UE to hold bra while hooking in front, assist in pulling up pants, and stabilize shirt while buttoning	1. Preparatory task 2. Preparatory method 3. Preparatory task 4. Activity 5. Occupation
STG #3: Client will complete light meal prep and clean-up using wheeled walker with SBA for safety within 3 weeks.	1. In collaboration with client and family, make recommendations for environmental modifications to adapt kitchen for safe accessibility and mobility 2. Select and instruct in use of adaptive equipment for one-handedness as needed to peel and chop vegetables, open cans and jars. 3. Remove/replace items from kitchen cabinet to improve ⓡ UE strength 4. Practice item transport in kitchen using a wheeled walker and rolling cart 5. Plan a meal with attention to money management, organization, and sequencing 6. Bake brownies in preparation for family visit	1. Preparatory method 2. Preparatory method 3. Preparatory task 4. Activity 5. Activity 6. Occupation

Note that the interventions planned for Mrs. H include a combination of preparatory methods, preparatory tasks, activities, and occupations. In an actual intervention plan, you would not need to specify the type of intervention. That column is included here to encourage you to think beyond preparatory methods and tasks and to move toward occupation-based goals and interventions. Note also that the planned interventions are based on multiple frames of reference including biomechanical, rehabilitative, and motor learning.

Common Errors in Writing Intervention Plans

Problem Identification

- Problems identified in the assessment are not addressed in the plan.
- Problems are not stated in terms of behavioral manifestations, areas of occupation, and contributing factors.
- The number of visits requested does not match the severity of the documented problems.

Goals

- Goals are not functional or do not focus on the reason for referral to occupational therapy.
- Intervention plan does not focus on specific rehabilitation goals that will increase a client's ability to engage in meaningful occupation in the probable discharge environment.
- Goals focus on the client participating in or cooperating with treatment (unless the client is in the habit of refusing treatment; more acceptable in mental health and behavioral health settings).
- Goals are not measurable or do not have a target date for completion.

Intervention Strategies

- Interventions do not focus on increasing functional behaviors to return the client to the least restrictive environment.
- Interventions do not take the age, sex, and interests of the client into account or are not meaningful to the client.
- Acquired skills are not transferred into more functional contexts in the client's life.
- Intervention strategies focus too heavily on preparatory methods without progression toward purposeful activities and occupation-based interventions.

Client Involvement

- The client is not involved in the treatment planning process. In many settings, you will be required to ask the client what his or her goal is and document that goal in your evaluation or intervention plan.
- Intervention plan does not reflect the client's strengths, desires, and preferences.

"Canned" Plans

- "Canned" intervention plans reflect the same goals, objectives, and interventions for each client based on the diagnosis and services available rather than on clients need (even clinical pathways need to be individualized to fit the client).

References

American Occupational Therapy Association. (2014a). Ethical considerations for productivity, billing, and reimbursement. Retrieved from http://www.aota.org/-/media/Corporate/Files/Practice/Ethics/Advisory/reimbursement-productivity.PDF.

American Occupational Therapy Association. (2014b). *Occupational therapy practice framework: Domain & process* (3rd ed.). Bethesda, MD: AOTA Press.

Brown, T., & Chien, C. (2010). Top-down or bottom-up occupational therapy assessment: Which way do we go? *British Journal of Occupational Therapy, 73*(3), 95.

Cole, M. (2014). Occupational therapy theory development and organization. In K. Jacobs, N. MacRae, & K. Sladyk (Eds.) *Occupational therapy essentials for clinical practice* (2nd ed., pp. 169-184). Thorofare, NJ: SLACK Incorporated.

Cole, M., & Tufano, R. (2008). *Applied theories in occupational therapy: A practical approach.* Thorofare, NJ: SLACK Incorporated.

Giles, G. M., & Morrison, T. (2014). Core concepts in neurocognition and stroke. In T. Wolf (Ed.) *Stroke: Interventions to support occupational performance.* Bethesda, MD: AOTA Press.

Gillen, G., & Boyt Schell, B. A. (2014). Introduction to evaluation, interventions, and outcomes for occupational therapists. In B. A. Boyt Schell, G. Gillen, & M. E. Scaffa (Eds.) *Willard & Spackman's occupational therapy* (12th ed., pp. 606-609). Philadelphia, PA: Lippincott Williams & Wilkins.

Kennedy, J., Brown, T., & Stagnitti, K. (2013). Top-down and bottom-up approaches to motor skill assessment of children; Are child-report and parent-report perceptions predictive of children's performance-based assessment results? *Scandinavian Journal of Occupational Therapy, 20,* 45-53. doi: 10.3109/11038128.2012.693944.

Meriano, C., & Latella, D. (2008). *Occupational therapy interventions: Function and occupations.* Thorofare, NJ: SLACK, Incorporated.

Queensland Health. (2013). Clinical access and redesign unit: Clinical pathways. Retrieved from https://www.health.qld.gov.au/caru/pathways/.

WORSHEET 12-1

Choosing Intervention Strategies

Intervention strategies do not stand alone. Strategies must be based on problems and LTGs, and they must be purposeful to the client to be useful. However, for purposes of learning to generate possible strategies, we will suspend that requirement and think of as many ways as possible to meet a treatment objective. Consider the following example:

STG (OBJECTIVE)	INTERVENTION	TYPE OF INTERVENTION
With SBA, client will complete ADL or IADL tasks while standing for 5-minute increments, taking rest breaks as needed, by discharge date of 1/10/17.	1. Have client complete 5 minutes on UE exercises ("arm bike") while standing.	1. Preparatory task
	2. Set-up task to make coffee while standing at counter in the ADL kitchen.	2. Activity
	3. Have client stand at the bathroom sink to complete face washing and tooth brushing.	3. Occupation
	4. Have client stand at a table to play a card game.	4. Activity
	5. Have client stand to retrieve clothing from closet when dressing in the am.	5. Occupation
	6. Have client stand to fill rehab unit bird feeder with birdseed.	6. Activity
	7. Instruct client to stand while watering plants in windowsill of rehab dining room.	7. Activity

Using the STG below, think of as many intervention strategies as possible that would help the client meet this goal. Try to use a mix of preparatory methods or tasks, activities, and occupations as described in the *OTPF-III*.

STG (OBJECTIVE)	INTERVENTION	TYPE OF INTERVENTION
Client will be independent in managing financial affairs within 3 weeks.		

WORKSHEET 12-2

Writing the Assessment and Intervention Plan—The Case of Georgia S

Name: *Georgia S*   **Age:** *87*   **Dx:** Ⓛ *SDH on 6/11/17; hx of HTN, hearing loss*
Date of Eval: *6/12/17*

Background data and beginning occupational profile: *Prior to her stroke, Georgia had been living for the past 10 years with her unmarried daughter, Janice, who is 60 years old and works full-time. They live in a two-story house with the only bathroom on the second floor. Georgia was in acute care and has just been transferred to a rehabilitation center. She expresses a desire to return to her daughter's home. Her daughter has concerns about being able to care for her mother at home. Georgia has Medicare as her only insurance coverage.*

S: *Client expressed frustration trying to brush her teeth with her affected dominant* Ⓡ *hand. Client c/o back pain 2/10 when standing for grooming. Client's daughter said that client was* Ⓘ *in self-care prior to her stroke but has not cooked or done housework for years; also stated that client has a hearing loss but no hearing aids.*

O: *Client participated in 45-minute OT session in room for initial evaluation. Pt. presents with* Ⓡ *UE weakness, decreased coordination, and decreased dynamic standing balance.*
   Dressing/Grooming: *Client stood with CGA for 5 min while brushing teeth after set-up and 2 verbal cues. Client modified* Ⓘ *in donning/doffing socks with extra time. Client attempted to don* Ⓡ *sock using same technique for several minutes before being successful. Client did not attempt an alternative technique. Client donned/doffed gown with mod* Ⓐ *pulling the robe around her back and threading the* Ⓡ *UE into the sleeve. Client required four 30-second rest breaks during dressing activity due to fatigue.*
   Functional Mobility: *Client sit → stand with SBA; mod* Ⓐ *needed for standing balance while managing clothing during bedside commode transfer. Client walked 3 ft. w/c → sink using walker with CGA.*
   UE ROM & Strength: *All UE AROM WNL except* Ⓑ *shoulder abduction and flexion which were WFL.* Ⓑ *UE strength 5/5 overall except 3/5 in* Ⓑ *shoulder flex. & abd.*
   Grip Strength: Ⓛ *37#,* Ⓡ *29#*   **Lateral Pinch:** Ⓛ *9#;* Ⓡ *7.5#*   **Tripod Pinch:** Ⓛ *7#;* Ⓡ *4#*
   Sensation: *Light touch and sharp/dull discrimination intact* Ⓑ. *Client correctly identified 1 of 4 objects in* Ⓡ *stereognosis test.*
   Coordination (9 Hole Peg Test):   *Placing pegs* Ⓛ *37 secs,* Ⓡ *52 secs*
                                              Removal Ⓛ *14 secs,* Ⓡ *26 secs*

Write the "A" and "P" as you learned in Chapters 9 and 10. Turn your problems into correctly worded problem statements. Identify the rehab potential you see for Ms. S. On the intervention plan, you will include some of these items as "strengths."

A:

P:

Strengths:

WORKSHEET 12-2 (CONTINUED)

Writing the Assessment and Intervention Plan—The Case of Georgia S

For space consideration, this worksheet does not include the column asking you to identify the type of intervention. However, be sure to include a mix of preparatory methods, preparatory tasks, activities, and occupations as you develop Georgia's intervention plan.

Functional Problem Statement #1:

LTG #1:

STG (OBJECTIVE)	INTERVENTION
STG #1:	
STG #2:	

Functional Problem Statement #2:

LTG #2:

STG (OBJECTIVE)	INTERVENTION
STG #1:	
STG #2:	

Discharge Plan:

WORKSHEET 12-3

Planning Interventions Using Groups—Heather's Suicide Attempt

In some practice settings, clients are seen primarily in groups rather than individually. This strategy has the advantage of using peer feedback and support as part of the treatment process. It also provides challenges for the therapist in finding ways to structure the group to meet the needs of all of the clients attending. Below is a description of a client who is being treated in a psychiatric unit where intervention strategies generally take place in groups. After you read about this client, choose intervention strategies to use for her in each of the groups she attends.

Heather S is a 40-year-old, unemployed woman with a psychiatric disability who recently separated from her husband. She has two children, a daughter age 22 and a son age 18. Heather was admitted through the emergency department after ingestion of an overdose of psychiatric medications. She was lavaged and admitted briefly to a medical unit, where she was stabilized in 8 hours and transferred to the psychiatric unit with a diagnosis of depression.

Heather was sexually abused from the ages of 10 to 13 years by an uncle who lived in the home where she was one of five children. Her estranged husband abuses alcohol and is emotionally abusive to Heather when he has been drinking. Heather married him when she was 18 years old and pregnant with her first child. They have been married 21 years.

Heather reports that she has trouble with expression of anger. She doesn't always know she is getting angry, and then "explodes" in ways that are destructive to herself, others, and property. She also says she is having a lot of trouble making decisions, and that her husband has traditionally made decisions for her. She says that she "just can't think" and has difficulty paying attention to anything for more than a few minutes. For example, she is unable to complete a magazine article she is reading. Her appearance is disheveled, her hair is uncombed, and she is wearing no makeup or jewelry. She picks at her clothing while she talks to you, looking at the floor and making little eye contact.

The problem areas identified by the treatment team include anger, decision making, and poor self-esteem with suicidal ideas. Heather's anticipated length of stay is 4 days. The psychiatric unit provides an array of individual and group treatment sessions. In addition to the medication group and the individual sessions with the psychiatrist, there is group therapy facilitated by the social worker, and an evening wrap-up group provided by nursing. Occupational therapist provides 3 groups per day:

- Goals group ½ hour each morning
- Stress management group 1 hour daily
- IADL group 1 hour daily

The IADL group covers topics such as money management, parenting, assertion skills, and other IADL skills depending on the needs and issues that are common to the current clients. For example, if several clients have difficulty expressing anger in useful ways, you could use IADL group time to address anger management.

In a psychiatric unit, the treatment plan is usually interdisciplinary, meaning that all team members work together to identify areas of concern, goals, and interventions. Because we are working with a 4-day length of stay and an interdisciplinary treatment plan, we will not write objectives for each of Heather's goals. Heather will be seen in occupational therapy groups every day while she is in the hospital. In this worksheet, you will decide how to use the group time to Heather's best advantage in meeting her established goals. Keep in mind that your interventions will include not only the activities you plan to use, but also your therapeutic use of self with Heather—the ways you might plan to interact with her and the behaviors you want to model.

Worksheet 12-3 (continued)

Planning Interventions Using Groups—Heather's Suicide Attempt

Problem #1: *Exacerbation of depressive symptoms resulting in a suicide attempt.*
LTG #1: *By anticipated discharge in 4 days, Heather will demonstrate improved self-esteem by verbally identifying strengths, caring for her appearance, making eye contact when interacting with others, and developing a plan for coping with suicidal thoughts.*

INTERVENTION	
Goals Group	
Stress Management Group	
IADL Group	

Problem #2: *Stress related to recent role changes results in Heather's inability to concentrate and make decisions for her daily life.*
LTG #2: *Heather will apply a decision-making strategy to her two most important current life decisions by discharge in 4 days.*

INTERVENTION	
Goals Group	
Stress Management Group	
IADL Group	

Problem #3: *Inability to manage anger constructively resulting in behaviors that damage self, relationships, and property.*
LTG #3: *By anticipated discharge in 4 days, Heather independently will identify potential anger triggers, identify her physical reactions to being angry, and develop a plan to prevent escalation and destructive behaviors.*

INTERVENTION	
Goals Group	
Stress Management Group	
IADL Group	

Chapter 13

Documenting Different Stages of Service Delivery

Different stages of the occupational therapy process require you to write different types of notes. The setting and a client's funding source may also impact the type of note required. As discussed in Chapter 1, the occupational therapy process of service delivery consists of evaluation, intervention, and outcomes. The *Guidelines for Documentation of Occupational Therapy* (American Occupational Therapy Association [AOTA], 2013, p. S33) outlines the reports for each part of the service delivery process:

- Screening
  - Screening report
- Evaluation
  - Evaluation report
  - Re-evaluation report
- Intervention
  - Intervention plan
  - Contact report note
  - Progress note/report
  - Transition plan
- Outcomes
  - Discharge summary/discontinuation report

In this chapter, we will review the specific content required for each type of note and provide examples for your reference. Please be aware that the information presented in this chapter is a summary of information found in the *Guidelines for Documentation of Occupational Therapy* (AOTA, 2013), reprinted with permission. This document, like all AOTA Official Documents, is updated approximately every 5 years. To be certain you are following current standards, you should refer to the most recent document published in the *American Journal of Occupational Therapy*. The document is also available at www.aota.org for AOTA members.

FUNDAMENTAL ELEMENTS OF ALL DOCUMENTATION

The *Guidelines for Documentation of Occupational Therapy* lists several elements that are essential to all types of documentation:

- Client's full name and case number (if applicable) on each page of documentation
- Date
- Identification of type of documentation (e.g., evaluation report, progress report/note)
- Occupational therapy practitioner's signature with a minimum of first name or initial, last name, and professional designation

Gateley CA, Borcherding S. *Documentation Manual for Occupational Therapy: Writing SOAP Notes, Fourth Edition (pp 169-181).*
© 2017 SLACK Incorporated

- When applicable, signature of the recorder directly after the documentation entry. If additional information is needed, a signed addendum must be added to the record.
- Co-signature of an occupational therapist or occupational therapy assistant on student documentation, as required by payer policy, governing laws and regulations, and/or employer
- Compliance with all laws, regulations, payer, and employer requirements
- Acceptable terminology defined within the boundaries of setting
- All errors noted and signed
- Adherence to professional standards of technology, when used to document occupational therapy services with electronic claims or records
- Disposal of records (electronic and traditionally written) within law or agency requirements
- Compliance with confidentiality standards
- Compliance with agency or legal requirements of storage of records
- Documentation should reflect professional clinical reasoning and expertise of an occupational therapy practitioner and the nature of the occupational therapy services delivered in a safe and effective manner. The client's diagnosis or prognosis should not be the sole rationale for occupational therapy services.

Reprinted with permission from *Guidelines for Documentation of Occupational Therapy* (AOTA, 2013).

> Note: In the next section, you will find a list of elements to be included in each type of occupational therapy note. While each **category** in the list must be present, the **specific elements** in each category will vary depending on facility requirements and your client's individual situation. These lists are intended to be a reference for you as you learn to write notes for different stages of treatment. Also note that for purposes of anonymity, sample notes in this chapter and the following chapters show only the therapist's first name and last initial. You should always sign your notes with first name (or initial), last name, and professional designation.

EVALUATION

SCREENING REPORT

An occupational therapy screening "consists of an initial brief assessment to determine [the] client's need for an occupational therapy evaluation or for referral to another service if not appropriate for occupational therapy services" (AOTA, 2013, p. S 33). A screening should include the following content:

- *Client information*: Name/agency; date of birth; sex; health status; and applicable medical/educational/developmental diagnoses, precautions, and contraindications.
- *Referral information*: Date and source of referral, services requested, reason for referral, funding source, and anticipated length of service.
- *Brief occupational profile*: Client's reason for seeking occupational therapy services, current areas of occupation that are successful and problematic, contexts and environments that support and hinder occupations, medical/education/work history, occupational history (e.g., patterns of living, interest, values), client's priorities, and targeted goals.
- *Assessments used and results*: Types of assessments used and results (e.g., interviews, record reviews, and observations)
- *Recommendation*: Professional judgments regarding appropriateness of need for complete occupational therapy evaluation.

Reprinted with permission from *Guidelines for Documentation of Occupational Therapy* (AOTA, 2013).

EVALUATION

After a referral for occupational therapy is received for a client, you begin gathering information about the client's occupational history as well as other factors that impact his or her engagement in occupation. This is the beginning of the occupational profile, which will tell you what the client needs and wants from occupational therapy. First you collect data from the client, the family, the chart, and any other pertinent sources. Then you select and administer any standardized tests or survey instruments that will help you determine more specifically what contributing factors support or hinder participation in occupations. You also use your clinical observation skills to analyze occupational performance. Finally, you compile all of your data into a comprehensive report. Suggested content with examples includes the following:

- *Client information*: Name, date of birth, sex, health status, medical history, and applicable medical/educational/developmental diagnoses, precautions, and contraindications
- *Referral information*: Date and source of referral, services requested, reason for referral, funding source, and anticipated length of service
- *Occupational profile*: Client's reason for seeking occupational therapy services, current areas of occupation that are successful and problematic, contexts and environments that support and hinder occupations, medical/educational/work history, occupational history (e.g., patterns of living, interest, values), client priorities, and targeted outcomes
- *Assessments used and results*: Types of assessments used and results (e.g., interviews, record reviews, observations, standardized and/or nonstandardized assessments)
- *Analysis of occupational performance*: Description of and judgment about performance skills, performance patterns, contexts and environments, activity demands, outcomes from standardized measures and/or nonstandardized assessments, client factors that will be targeted for intervention, and outcomes expected
- *Summary and analysis*: Interpretation and summary of data as related to occupational profile and referring concern
- *Recommendation*: Judgment regarding appropriateness of occupational therapy services or other services

Reprinted with permission from *Guidelines for Documentation of Occupational Therapy* (AOTA, 2013).

Most facilities still using paper documentation provide a form for an initial evaluation report, and evaluation results are recorded on the form along with comments and observations. Figure 13-1 shows an example of a form that can be used for evaluation in an inpatient rehabilitation setting. This form includes a combination of checklists, charts, and space for narrative documentation. Note that this form includes the intervention plan. The space allowed for the intervention plan is often larger than what is shown in this figure. However, for space considerations, this example was limited to a single page. Although the intervention plan represents a different stage in the occupational therapy process (intervention), it is often included along with the initial evaluation report since a plan must be in place before treatment is continued. Now we will present the guidelines for the intervention plan and the corresponding example in conjunction with the initial evaluation.

INTERVENTION PLAN

Chapter 12 provided a detailed discussion about the purpose and process of intervention planning, as well as several examples. The suggested content for an intervention plan includes the following:

- *Client information*: Name, date of birth, sex, precautions, and contraindications
- *Intervention goals*: Measurable and meaningful occupation-based long- and short-term objective goals directly related to the client's ability and need to engage in desired occupations
- *Intervention approaches and types of interventions to be used*: Intervention approaches that include create/promote, establish/restore, maintain, modify, and/or prevent; types of interventions that include consultation process, education process, advocacy, and/or therapeutic use of occupations or activities
- *Service delivery mechanisms*: Service provider, service location, and frequency and duration of services
- *Plan for discharge*: Discontinuation criteria, location of discharge, and follow-up care
- *Outcome measures*: Tools that assess occupational performance, adaptation, role competence, improved health and wellness, improved quality of life, self-advocacy, and occupational justice. Standardized and/or nonstandardized assessments used at evaluation should be readministered periodically to monitor measurable progress and report functional outcomes as required by client's payer source and/or facility requirements
- *Professionals responsible and date of plan*: Names and positions of persons overseeing plan, date plan was developed, and date when plan was modified or reviewed

Reprinted with permission from *Guidelines for Documentation of Occupational Therapy* (AOTA, 2013).

Client Name:		DOB:	Date of Eval:	Med Record #:

Diagnosis:

Medical Hx:

Prior Level of Function:

Prior Living Situation (Type of Home / Equipment / Steps / Caregiver Assistance):

Hearing: Vision / Visual Perception:

A&O: X1 X2 X3 X4   Memory / Attention / Cognition:

Follows Commands: Mini Mental Status Examination (MMSE) Score:

Self-Care Area	FIM Score	FIM Goal	Additional ADL / IADL Observations:	Current Transfer / Mobility Status:
Eating				
Grooming				
Bathing				
Upper Body Dressing				
Lower Body Dressing				
Toileting				
Toilet Transfer				
Shower Transfer				
Tub Transfer				

Hand Dominance   L   R

Left UE			Right UE		Other Observations:
ROM	MMT		ROM	MMT	
		Shoulder Elevation			
		Shoulder Flexion			
		Shoulder Extension			
		Shoulder Abduction			
		Horizontal Abduction			
		Horizontal Adduction			
		Internal Rotation			
		External Rotation			
		Elbow Flexion			
		Elbow Extension			
		Forearm Pronation			
		Forearm Supination			
		Wrist Flexion			
		Wrist Extension			

Left UE			Right UE	Initial Assessment of Problems / Strengths:
		Grip Strength		
		Lateral Pinch		
		Tripod Pinch		
		Tip Pinch		
		Light Touch		
		Sharp / Dull		
		Temperature		
		Proprioception		
		Stereognosis		
		9-Hole Peg Test		
		Edema		
		Pain		

Discharge Recommendation: Home   Home with Home Health   SNF   Outpatient   Other (Specify)

Equipment Needs:

Patient / Family / Caregiver Goals:

Estimated Length of Stay: Overall Long Term Goal:

Short Term Goals / Estimated Timeframe: Therapist Signature / Date:

Figure 13-1. Sample Rehabilitation Center Evaluation Form.

Occupational Therapy Initial Evaluation Report

Name: Rosa S   **Age:** 68   **Sex:** F   **Physician:** Dr. Grantham
Date of Onset: 2/1/17   **Date of Admission:** 2/2/17   **Insurance:** Medicare & supplement
Referral Data: Client referred by Dr. Grantham on 2/2/17 for evaluation and treatment.
1° Dx: Ⓡ CVA   **2° Dx:** Diabetes   **Date of Eval:** 2/3/17   **Time:** 10:00 am

Occupational Profile: Client was admitted after a fall resulting in confusion and left-sided weakness. Prior to admission, she was living alone in a one-story home and was Ⓘ in all ADLs. Client is a retired librarian and states she values her independence and fully intends to return to her own home. Hobbies include mostly sedentary activities such as sewing, reading, and playing cards with friends. Daughter works during the day, lives two blocks away, and is willing to visit daily and assist with transportation, but cannot provide 24-hr. supervision.

S: Client stated, "I'll work hard in rehab. I need to get home."

O: Client participated in 60-minute evaluation in room and shower room for Mini-Mental Status Examination (MMSE), and evaluation of ADLs, functional mobility, and contributing factors (MMT, AROM). Pt. presents with Ⓛ UE weakness, decreased balance, and limited activity tolerance.
   Bathing: Upper body: min Ⓐ to sequence task. Lower body: min Ⓐ except max Ⓐ to reach perineal area and feet.
   Dressing: Seated in chair with arms, min Ⓐ to maintain dynamic balance when bending, mod Ⓐ to initiate donning bra, and max Ⓐ to reach feet. Verbal cues needed for sequencing and environmental orientation.
   Toileting: Min Ⓐ to obtain tissue and manage clothing, verbal cues to flush.
   Transfers: CGA with verbal cues for safety/proper arm placement sit to stand; min Ⓐ from low surfaces.
   Bed Mobility: Rolls & supine ↔ sit with SBA for safety.
   Static Standing Balance: CGA
   Activity Tolerance: < 10 min tolerance for any activity with physical/mental challenges.
   Motor Planning/Perception: WFL
   Cognition: Score of 17/20 on MMSE. Sequencing problems during dressing tasks noted. Client unable to fasten bra in back; required verbal cues to fasten in front.
   UE AROM: WFL for all Ⓑ UE movements, except ¾ range Ⓛ shoulder flex/abd against gravity.
   MMT: Ⓡ UE 4+/5 throughout; Ⓛ UE 3+/5 throughout
   Strength: Grip: Ⓡ 42 lb, Ⓛ 21 lb   Lateral Pinch: Ⓡ 14 lb, Ⓛ 6 lb
   Tripod Pinch: Ⓡ 12 lb, Ⓛ 5 lb   Tip Pinch: Ⓡ 8 lb, Ⓛ 2 lb
   Sensation: Ⓡ UE intact; Ⓛ UE light touch, pain, temperature intact; stereognosis 3 of 5.

A: Client's poor problem-solving skills (needing cues to sequence activity and inability to initiate alternative way to don bra) and need for verbal cues to initiate some ADL tasks limit her ability to manage ADLs and IADLs Ⓘ. Decreased AROM and strength in Ⓛ UE along with slow response to cognitive tasks, decreased ability to sequence tasks, and decreased short-term memory raise safety concerns in returning to independent living. Client's motivation indicates good potential for returning to modified Ⓘ in ADL activities. Client would benefit from environmental cues to orient her to environment, facilitation of problem solving, sequencing activities, and activities to increase strength in Ⓛ UE.

P: Client will receive OT for 45-minute sessions 5x/wk for 2 wks to work toward increased independence with ADLs, with focus on improving sequencing, problem solving, Ⓛ UE strength, and activity tolerance. Calendar will be placed in client's room to increase orientation to month, day, and season. Client's ability to respond to emergency situations will be assessed during next session.

Shelby T., OTR/L

Intervention Plan

Functional Problem Statement #1: *Client needs min to max physical Ⓐ and verbal cues to dress self due to ↓ AROM, activity tolerance, and ability to sequence the task.*
Long-Term Goal #1: *Client will complete all dressing tasks with modified Ⓘ within 2 weeks.*

STG (Objective)	Intervention
STG #1: *Client will don bra with modified Ⓘ using adapted technique within 3 days*	1. *Teach adaptive techniques* 2. *Post picture of how to don bra by fastening in front* 3. *Reinforce correct responses* 4. *Teach strengthening program for Ⓛ UE*
STG #2: *Client will don shoes and socks with modified Ⓘ using adapted technique and long shoe-horn within 5 days*	1. *Provide long shoehorn and instruct in use* 2. *Instruct in adapted techniques for donning shoes and socks* 3. *Post picture of adapted technique using long shoehorn* 4. *Instruct in use of affected side as a functional assist in dressing* 5. *Expand exercise program to include AROM*
STG #3: *Client will complete dressing tasks without verbal cues for sequencing for 3 consecutive days within 10 days*	1. *Verbalize steps before beginning to dress* 2. *Verbalize steps while dressing* 3. *Post list of steps for client to follow* 4. *Take rest breaks as needed for activity tolerance*

Functional Problem Statement #2: *Lack of orientation to environment & inability to problem solve raise safety concerns with ADLs and home management.*
Long-Term Goal #2: *Client will correctly answer questions pertaining to time, date, schedule, and emergency situations using only environmental cues within 2 weeks.*

STG (Objective)	Intervention
STG #1: *Within 1 week, client will correctly identify time, date, and situation without verbal cues when asked on 3 of 3 attempts*	1. *Post calendar, schedule, and emergency information near clock in client's room* 2. *Instruct family, nursing staff, and other therapy staff to quiz client several times daily re: date, time, and situation and to reinforce correct responses*
STG #2: *Client will follow her daily printed schedule with <2 verbal cues within 1 week*	1. *Post daily schedule on wall near clock and review with client during ADL session each morning* 2. *Cue client to look at schedule to determine what she should be doing at any given time*
STG #3: *Client will correctly problem solve responses to emergency situations Ⓘ on 9 of 10 attempts within 2 weeks*	1. *Provide situations for client to problem solve, progressing from easy to more complex* 2. *Provide telephone directory or other props as needed for problem solving*

RE-EVALUATION REPORT

In some practice settings, clients must be re-evaluated at certain intervals, such as monthly or quarterly. In other settings, re-evaluation is done as needed. The frequency of re-evaluation depends on the setting, the funding source, and the progress of the client. The tests that were given initially are readministered, and the results are compared with the results of previous tests to determine the effectiveness of the treatment being provided. The goals and plans are revised at this time and new timelines are projected. Suggested content for this type of report includes the following:

- *Client information*: Name, date of birth, sex, applicable medical/educational/developmental diagnoses, precautions, and contraindications

- *Occupational profile*: Updates on current areas of occupation that are successful and problematic, contexts and environments that support or hinder occupations, summary of any new medical/educational/work information, and updates or changes to client's priorities and targeted outcomes
- *Re-evaluation results*: Focus of re-evaluation, specific types of outcome measures from standardized and/or nonstandardized assessments used, and client's performance and subjective responses
- *Analysis of occupational performance*: Description of and judgment about performance skills, performance patterns, contexts and environments, activity demands, outcomes from standardized measures and/or nonstandardized assessments, and client factors that will be targeted for intervention and outcomes expected
- *Summary and analysis*: Interpretation and summary of data as related to referring concern and comparison of results with previous evaluation results
- *Recommendations*: Changes to occupational therapy services, revision or continuation of interventions, goals and objectives, frequency of occupational therapy services, and recommendation for referral to other professionals or agencies as applicable

Reprinted with permission from *Guidelines for Documentation of Occupational Therapy* (AOTA, 2013).

Hand Clinic Re-Evaluation Report

Name: *Leanna G*   **DOB:** *5/12/76*   **Sex:** *F*   **Physician:** *Dr. Oliver*
Primary Dx: *Osteoarthritis of* Ⓑ *CMC joints*   **Secondary Dx:** *None*
Precautions/Contraindications: *None*   **Date of Referral:** *6/27/2017*
Reason for Referral: *Client is 1 month post-surgery (LRTI) to the* Ⓛ *CMC joint and carpal tunnel release.*
Date of Initial Evaluation: *7/05/17*   **Date of Re-evaluation:** *8/04/17*
Funding Source: *University insurance*

Occupational Profile: *Leanna is a 41-year-old White female who works as an administrative assistant in the English department at the university. She lives alone in a small, two-story farmhouse 7 miles outside of town. The house is heated with wood that Leanna cuts and stacks in the summer. Leanna plants a large vegetable garden each year, in addition to holding both a full-time job at the university and a part-time job in a department store. She began experiencing pain in the CMC joints of both hands approximately 3 years ago. She intends to continue her present living arrangement and both of her jobs. She was originally admitted to the outpatient hand clinic on 7/05/17 at 1 month post-surgery for hand rehabilitation following a successful LRTI of the* Ⓛ *CMC joint and a* Ⓛ *carpal tunnel release. She is being re-evaluated this date (8/04/17) to determine whether further OT services are needed.*

S: *Client initially reported continuous pain at a level of 3/10 in* Ⓛ *hand and pain on overexertion at a level of 5/10 in* Ⓛ *hand, resulting in irritability and difficulty performing bilateral work and daily living tasks, as well as some tasks requiring left hand use. On this date, she reports no continuous pain and pain at a level of 1/10 when typing for more than 45 minutes without rest breaks.*

Initial ability to engage in work/ADL/IADL tasks (by client report):
- *Unable to use keyboard with all fingers of* Ⓛ *hand. Typed with one finger on standard keyboard.*
- *Unable to grasp cylindrical objects smaller than 1½ inches (broom handle, toothpaste tube) due to* ↓ *AROM.*
- *Unable to wear watch or rings on* Ⓛ *hand due to swelling.*
- *Unable to turn door knob with* Ⓛ *hand to enter house when* Ⓡ *hand is full.*
- *Unable to lift laundry basket and other items requiring* Ⓑ *UE use. Unable to lift purse or other items needed for IADL tasks with* Ⓛ *hand.*

Current ability to engage in work/ADL/IADL tasks (by client report):
- *Able to use new ergonomic keyboard for primary work task using all fingers.*
- *Able to sweep floors with a regular broom.*
- *Able to fold laundry using* Ⓑ *hands.*
- *Able to grasp small items needed for ADL and IADL tasks (toothpaste tube, key, lids) with* Ⓛ *hand, but not at PLOF.*
- *Able to turn doorknob with* Ⓛ *hand if door is unlocked.*
- *Able to hang clothes on clothesline, including carrying basket and holding garments with* Ⓛ *hand.*

O: *Client has participated in three 45-minute visits in outpatient hand clinic since admission on 7/05/17. Active and passive range of motion have been performed and taught to client, and home program has been modified as she progressed. Heat has been used, and the client has purchased a home paraffin unit. Electrical stimulation has been used to elicit specific motion and facilitate strengthening of the flexor pollicis longus. A strengthening program has been added to the HEP, and client is able to demonstrate all HEP exercises correctly. Client has received education on the structure and use of the hand, common features of CMC arthritis, ergonomics of the workstation, energy conservation, use of heat for pain relief, and adapted techniques for ADL activities. Client has been given written material covering the same content and reports implementing recommendations into both home and work activities.*

A: *Increase in Ⓛ grip strength of 7# shows good progress in strength needed to perform functional tasks. Improved thumb AROM (WFL) and wrist AROM (80% of average) now allow client to perform most work and ADL tasks Ⓘ in ways that do not damage the joint. Change to an ergonomic keyboard and understanding and correct self-administration of HEP indicate good potential to continue improvement without further OT services. Client would benefit from continuation of daily HEP.*

P: *Plan to discontinue OT services at this time as results of re-evaluation indicate no further need for OT services unless new problems arise. Client to call hand clinic if questions arise and follow the home program of heat, exercise, and adapted techniques.*

Brad E., OTR/L, CHT

Intervention

Occupational Therapy Service Contacts

Contact, visit, or treatment notes are used to document each visit or individual occupational therapy session. In some situations, contact notes are required in the health record each time a client is seen. In other cases, the occupational therapist keeps attendance records, logs, or informal contact notes, which will later be used for the purpose of writing a progress note. Contact notes are also written to document telephone or e-mail contacts and meetings with others regarding the client. Suggested content includes the following:

- *Client information*: Name, date of birth, sex, and diagnosis, precautions, and contraindications
- *Therapy log*: Date, type of type of contact, names/positions of persons involved, summary or significant information communicated during contacts, client attendance and participation in intervention, reason service is missed, types of interventions used, client's response, environmental or task modification, assistive or adaptive devices used or fabricated, statement of any training education or consultation provided, and the client's present level of performance
- *Intervention/procedure coding* (i.e., CPT code), if applicable

Reprinted with permission from *Guidelines for Documentation of Occupational Therapy* (AOTA, 2013).

Acute Care Unit Contact Note

Client: *Curt G*   **Sex:** *M*   **DOB:** *9/12/56*   **Health Record #:** *123456*
Dx: *Guillain-Barré syndrome*   **Physician:** *Dr. McDonald*
Date: *4/14/17*   **Time:** *8:30 AM*

S: *Pt. reports, "I want to get out of this bed. It's been a long night."*

O: *Client participated in bedside OT session in ICU for instruction in ADL tasks and AROM in Ⓑ UEs. Pt. presents with significant trunk and Ⓑ LE weakness, and moderate Ⓑ UE weakness. Client required mod Ⓐ supine → sit to roll to Ⓡ sidelying and push up through Ⓡ elbow. Upon sitting, O_2 saturation dropped to ~85%. Grooming, dressing, and UE AROM activities not completed due to low O_2 levels. Client returned to supine with min Ⓐ to bring Ⓑ LEs up onto bed. After ~2 minutes, O_2 levels returned to ~95%. Client washed face p̄ set-up in supine but declined further activity, citing fatigue. ICU nurse was notified of pt.'s change in O_2 saturation during activity.*

A: *Ability to transition supine to sit indicates improved activity tolerance from yesterday when pt. was unable to tolerate this. Expressed interest for out-of-bed activity is a good indication for improving strength and function. Decreased activity tolerance related to drop in O_2 saturation with exertion limits ability to participate in self-care tasks. Client would benefit from instruction in energy conservation as well as correct positioning to ↓ exertion and ↑ activity tolerance for ADL tasks. At this time, pt. does not have the ability to tolerate 3 hours daily therapy required for rehab unit stay; however, pt. would benefit from continued therapy at skilled nursing facility level once medically stable.*

P: *Continue skilled OT daily to ↑ activity tolerance and ① in ADL tasks for 5 days or until discharge from acute care.*
Billing: Total tx time 13 minutes. 1 unit Self Care

Evan D., OTR/L

Outpatient Clinic Contact Note

Client: *Molly T*	**Sex:** *F*	**DOB:** *6/16/13*	**Health Record #:** *123456*
Dx: *Spina bifida*	**Physician:** *Dr. Wright*		**Date:** *8/19/17*

Received phone call from child's mother canceling today's appointment due to schedule conflict. Mother was reminded of clinic attendance policy as child has now missed 3 of last 5 scheduled weekly appointments; mother voiced understanding that one more missed appointment may result in Molly being discharged from OT services. Offered to change OT appointment to a more convenient time for family, mother declined this offer. Also reminded mother of 6-month meeting with therapy team and service coordinator from county agency that is scheduled for 8/24/17; mother reports plan to attend that meeting and next OT visit on 8/26/17.

Nikki P., OTR/L

PROGRESS REPORT

Progress notes are written on a regularly scheduled basis (usually weekly or monthly), with the time frame determined by the facility. The facility policy is guided by accrediting agencies and funding sources in determining the time frame in which progress notes must be written. The progress note provides a **summary** of the intervention process and documents the client's progress toward goals. It also includes recommendations for continuation/discontinuation of services and referral to other health care professionals if appropriate. Suggested content includes the following:

- *Client information*: Name, date of birth, sex, diagnosis, precautions, and contraindications
- *Summary of services provided*: Brief statement about the frequency of services and length of time services have been provided; techniques and strategies used; measurable progress or lack thereof using age-appropriate current functional standardized and/or nonstandardized outcome measures; environmental or task modifications provided; adaptive equipment or orthotics provided; medical, education, or other pertinent client updates; client's response to occupational therapy services; and programs or training provided to the client or caregivers
- *Current client performance*: Client's progress toward the goals and client's performance in areas of occupation
- *Plan or recommendations*: Recommendations and rationale as well as client's input to changes or continuation of plan

Reprinted with permission from Guidelines for Documentation of Occupational Therapy (AOTA, 2013).

Behavioral Health Center Progress Note

Client: *Audrey I*	**Sex:** *F*	**DOB:** *10/12/76*	**Health Record #:** *123456*
Dx: *Depression*	**Physician:** *Dr. Abraham*		**Date:** *8/19/17*

S: *In assertion group on 8/17/17, client talked about how her life had taken a "downward spiral" since early July, and she had become more passive and less proactive in getting her needs met, although she had not been aware of it at the time. She reported having "no energy or desire" to engage in daily activities, but reports she feels "more like myself" in recent days.*

O: *This week, client attended assertion group 2/2 times, communication group 1/1 time, and IADL group 3/5 times. She was on time to 4/6 groups without reminders, wearing neatly pressed clothing, makeup, and hair ties. In assertion group on 8/17, she shared without prompting 2 stories about her usual way of dealing with retail situations. In communication group, she spontaneously answered one question addressed to the group as a whole, and in IADL group, she offered to assist another client with his checkbook.*

A: *Low energy level and lack of initiative limited client's participation in ADLs and IADLs at time of admission. Client's spontaneous actions in groups and willingness to share verbally indicate an improved mood this week. Group attendance for 6/8 groups is much improved this week as compared to 2/8 group attendance last week. Improved dress, hygiene, and makeup also indicate an improved mood from last week. Client would benefit from planning a structure for her days to prevent another "downward spiral" after discharge.*
Goals #1 (assertion) and #2 (communication) are met as of this date.
Goal #3 (leisure skills) is continued through discharge on 8/20/17 pending formulation of a plan.
Goal #4 (parenting skills) was discontinued on 8/15/17.

P: *Client to be seen in IADL group for 1 more day, with discharge anticipated tomorrow afternoon 8/20/17. IADL group will be used for preparing the structured plan for using her time. Will meet with client individually if needed to ensure that written plan is completed.*

Kayla R., OTR/L

Early Intervention Progress Note

Client: *Brooklyn M*   **Sex:** *F*   **DOB:** *5/30/15*   **Health Record #:** *123456*
Dx: *Shaken Baby Syndrome*   **Physician:** *Dr. Halbrook*   **Date:** *11/30/17*

Occupational Profile: *Brooklyn is a 2½-year-old girl with a history of shaken baby syndrome from abuse by her biological mother's boyfriend at age 3 months. Brooklyn has been in foster care since her diagnosis, and her foster family recently received approval for adoption, which will become official in December 2017. Brooklyn lives with her foster parents, and two teenage siblings (biological children of her foster parents). She is home with her foster mother the majority of the time, although she does occasionally receive respite care services from the local County Family Support Agency so her foster mother can run errands and attend her older children's school events.*

S: *Brooklyn's foster mother reports new skills in recent months including putting simple shapes into a puzzle and scribbling with a crayon. Brooklyn has begun saying more single words during therapy sessions and occasionally puts two words together such as "More bubbles."*

O: *Brooklyn has participated in weekly early intervention sessions June 2017 through November 2017 in her foster home with foster parent and/or respite care provider present during each session. 22 of 26 sessions occurred as scheduled; 2 visits cancelled due to client illness, 1 for family schedule conflict, and 1 for Thanksgiving holiday. For this 6-month progress report, Brooklyn was reassessed using the fine motor subtests of the Peabody Developmental Motor Scales—2nd edition. See chart below for comparison of performance May 2017 and November 2017:*

Parameter	5-30-2017			11-30-2017		
	Standard Score	Percentile Rank	Age Equivalent	Standard Score	Percentile Rank	Age Equivalent
Grasping	4	2nd	10 months	6	9th	13 months
Visual Motor Integration	3	1st	11 months	5	5th	19 months
	Total Fine Motor Quotient = 61 (< 1st %ile)			Total Fine Motor Quotient = 73 (3rd %ile)		

*Standard scores on the PDMS-2 have a mean of 10 and a standard deviation of 3. Total fine motor quotient scores have a mean of 100 and a standard deviation of 15.
New skills observed during OT sessions in recent weeks include turning pages in a thick-page book, stacking 2 to 3 blocks, scribbling using a pronated grasp on crayon, and placing large stacking pegs into a pegboard. She is also beginning to show interest in using a spoon to feed herself rather than relying on finger feeding.

A: *Delayed fine motor skills continue to impact Brooklyn's ability to participate in play and self-care activities. Improved standardized test scores indicate steady developmental progress. Brooklyn's recent increased interest in new fine motor activities indicates good potential for future improvements toward developmental milestones. Brooklyn would benefit from continued early intervention services once weekly for 6 months to address development of fine motor and self-skills in preparation for transition to early childhood special education (ECSE) services when she turns 3 years old.*

P: *Client to receive OT once weekly for 45-minute sessions in her home to address developmental deficits in play and self-care. Parent education in home program activities will be provided. Also, plan to coordinate transition services with local family county support agency and local public school district to ensure a smooth transition to ECSE services.*

Cara A., OTR/L

Transition Plan

A transition plan is written whenever a client transfers from one setting to another within a service delivery system. It is designed to provide client information to the new service provider so that care is uninterrupted. Transition plans summarize the client's current occupational status, specify what service setting the client is leaving, state what setting the client is entering, and tell how and when the transition will occur. Suggested content includes the following:

- *Client information*: Name, date of birth, sex, diagnosis, precautions, and contraindications
- *Client's current status*: Client's current performance in occupations
- *Transition plan*: Name of current setting and name of setting to which client will transition, reason for transition, time frame in which transition will occur, and outline of activities to be carried out during the transition plan
- *Recommendations*: Recommendations and rationale for occupational therapy services, modification or accommodations needed, and assistive technology and environmental modifications needed

Reprinted with permission from *Guidelines for Documentation of Occupational Therapy* (AOTA, 2013).

Transition Plan

Name: *Kanisha G*   **DOB:** *4/29/14*   **Sex:** *Female*
Date of Plan: *4/11/17*   **Expected Transition Date:** *May 2017*   **Diagnosis:** *TBI, s/p MVA*
Precautions: *Seizure disorder*

Occupational History: *Kanisha experienced head and multiple orthopedic injuries following a MVA at 9 days of age. Since that time, she has had multiple cranial, hip, and leg surgeries. She is currently under the management of a neurologist as well as an orthopedist. The mother carries out a home program daily, which is designed to stimulate development.*

S: *The mother reports that, although Kanisha's seizures, multiple surgeries, and illnesses have slowed her development, the family is hopeful that Kanisha will progress more rapidly through her developmental milestones now that the surgeries are finished and the seizures are under control.*

O: *Child received her first OT screening in the hospital 1 week post-injury. She received formal developmental assessments at 2, 4, 6, 12, and 24 months of age. Parents were given home program following the initial formal assessment. OT sessions were started twice weekly at 12 months of age and have continued to this date; Kanisha has also been followed every 3 months in the Birth-to-Three Developmental Clinic. She is now eligible for ECSE services through the local public school as she will be turning 3 years old later this month.*
Current occupational performance: Current problems being treated in OT include visual regard and visually directed reach, midline orientation, postural symmetry, and motor overflow. Current goals for Kanisha include functional reach, grasp and release, rolling, and ability to sustain antigravity positions for ADLs and developmental play activities. Kanisha requires an adaptive chair to maintain upright positioning. She is dependent in all self-care tasks, including feeding. She requires hand over hand assistance to initiate play with toys. Kanisha's current skills indicate functioning at approximately a 4-month level of development.

A: *Low vision, low proximal tone, and increased tone of all extremities limit Kanisha's performance in self-care and play activities. Attentive family members and stimulating home environment are good indications for future progress toward goals. Kanisha would benefit from continuation of regular OT, PT, and speech therapy services to facilitate her ongoing progress through the developmental sequence.*

P: *Kanisha will receive her first ECSE evaluation next month in May 2017. Parents have been given a home program, which has been updated as child has progressed in treatment. Home program will continue through the transition to early childhood services.*

Casey L., OTS
Claire U., OTR/L (co-signature of a student's note by the supervising therapist)

OUTCOMES

DISCHARGE REPORT—SUMMARY OF OCCUPATIONAL THERAPY SERVICES AND OUTCOMES

A discharge summary (also called a *discontinuation report*) is used to summarize the changes in the client's ability to engage in occupation and to make recommendations for referral or follow-up care if needed. Discharge notes often follow a format of their own, stating the date and purpose of the referral and giving a summary of the initial findings, the course of treatment, a summary of progress, and any recommendations for follow-up care. Discharge summaries may be done as SOAP or narrative notes, or the facility may have a particular form that is used. Some facilities use the same form for evaluation, re-evaluation, and discharge, making it quicker to prepare the discontinuation report. Suggested content includes the following:

- *Client information*: Name, date of birth, sex, diagnosis, precautions, and contraindications
- *Summary of intervention process*: Date of initial and final service; frequency, number of sessions, summary of interventions used; summary of progress toward goals; and occupational therapy outcomes—initial client status and ending status regarding engagement in occupations, and client's assessment of efficacy of occupational therapy services
- *Recommendations*: Recommendations pertaining to the client's future needs; specific follow-up plans, if applicable; and referrals to other professionals and agencies, if applicable

Reprinted with permission from *Guidelines for Documentation of Occupational Therapy* (AOTA, 2013).

Occupational Therapy Discharge Summary

Name: *Cindy C*   **DOB:** *4/10/46*   **Dx:** Ⓛ *SDH*
Physician: *Dr. Armin*   **Date:** *2/19/17*

S: *Client reports that she is very pleased with the outcome of her OT treatment, and with her ability to take care of herself at home. She reports no steps to the front entrance of a one-story home, and no architectural barriers inside the house. She reports that she owns the following adaptive equipment already: wheeled walker, reacher, dressing stick, sock aide, long shoehorn, tub bench, raised toilet seat, and grab bars near the toilet and in the tub/shower.*

O: *Client participated in 20/20 OT sessions bedside and in OT clinic from SOC on 2/06/17.*

ADL Status on 2/06/17	ADL Status on 2/19/17
• Mod Ⓐ in ADL transfers	• SBA in ADL transfers
• Mod Ⓐ in toileting	• SBA in toileting
• Mod Ⓐ in feeding	• SBA in feeding after set-up
• Mod Ⓐ in dressing	• Set-up and SBA for dressing from arm chair
• Max Ⓐ for safety in bathing	• Min Ⓐ for tub bench transfer; SBA for bathing

Client education provided in adaptive equipment techniques and HEP; client demonstrated ability to perform correctly. Home modifications were discussed with client and caregiver.

A: *Continued deficits in safety awareness limit client's independence in ADLs. Differences in admission and discharge abilities for ADLs show good progress. Since caregiver is available to provide SBA needed for safety in ADL tasks, all treatment goals have been met, and client is ready for discharge. Client would benefit from continued HEP for strengthening and endurance for functional tasks.*

P: *Client will be discharged home tomorrow. Client to continue home exercise program. Adaptive equipment recommended: walker basket and reacher holder for walker. Client and caregiver to decide how to implement home modifications. Client will continue with outpatient PT. No direct OT services are recommended at this time.*

Lydia E., OTR/L

Now let us consider the same note, written on a form provided by the rehabilitation facility:

Rehabilitation Center—Occupational Therapy Discharge Note

Name: *Cindy C*   **DOB:** *4/10/46*   **Dx:** Ⓛ *SDH*
Physician: *Dr. Armin*   **Date:** *2/19/17*

Course of Rehabilitation: *Client participated in 20/20 session from SOC on 2/06/17. Skilled instruction in adaptive techniques for ADLs provided. Client progress was good and she met all tx goals. Client now requires SBA in all transfers, lower body ADLs, upper body ADLs, grooming/hygiene. She is Ⓘ in toileting. Client also requires SBA in feeding after set-up. Client completes dressing from arm chair with wheeled walker, set-up, and SBA for standing to pull pants over hips. Bathing is SBA with min Ⓐ w/c ↔ shower using tub bench.*

Client Education: *Recommendations for additional adaptive equipment and modifications to home discussed with client and caregiver. Client and caregiver were instructed in HEP of theraband, free weights, wands, and other activities to choose from for Ⓑ UE strengthening. Client demonstrated ability to perform exercises correctly.*

Discharge Recommendations/Referrals: *Discharge home with caregiver. Continue home exercise program. Adaptive equipment recommended: walker basket and reacher holder for walker. Client already has wheeled walker, reacher, dressing stick, sock aid, long shoehorn, and functional bathroom equipment and has demonstrated ability to use these correctly and safely. Client will be seen in outpatient PT. No direct OT services are recommended at this time.*

Lydia E., OTR/L

REFERENCE

American Occupational Therapy Association. (2013). Guidelines for documentation of occupational therapy. *American Journal of Occupational Therapy, 67,* S32-S38. doi: 10.5014/ajot.2013.67S32 .

Documentation in Different Practice Settings

In this chapter, we will examine documentation in several different practice situations. Each of these practice settings has some requirements that are specific to the setting or the primary payment source. Documentation in these settings is different in some ways from the examples you have learned so far.

DOCUMENTATION IN MENTAL HEALTH

Although the occupational therapy profession has historical roots in mental health (Christiansen & Haertl, 2014), fewer than 3% of all occupational therapists report working primarily in a mental health setting (American Occupational Therapy Association [AOTA], 2015a). However, AOTA has identified mental health practice as an "emerging niche" of practice, explaining that "one in four U.S. adults have a diagnosable mental health condition in any given year" and occupational therapy can "assist people to restructure their daily lives" (AOTA, 2016, para. 1). Mental health occupational therapy is on the rise for military veterans to address home and community reintegration with combat-related post-traumatic stress disorder (AOTA, 2011a, 2015b).

Psychosocial interventions are at the very root of occupational therapy and are still fundamental to occupational therapist practice as a whole (AOTA, 2014b). From its inception to the present, occupational therapy has been holistic and client-centered. Occupational therapy in mental health is based on the belief that meaningful occupation has therapeutic value in establishing and restoring balance in daily life routines. Whether in a rehabilitation center or in a mental health setting, the attention to psychosocial aspects of a client's life is critical to the ability to resume engagement in meaningful areas of occupation. Client-centered occupational therapy means collaborating with the client throughout the process to maximize engagement in meaningful areas of occupation (Boyt Schell, Scaffa, Gillen, & Cohn, 2014). This is most important in psychosocial practice settings, where clients come to us with serious disruptions in their ability to engage in meaningful occupations.

If you go from a job in a rehabilitation center to one in a mental health setting, you might think that nothing you have learned about documentation applies. Problems, goals, and interventions are often interdisciplinary or transdisciplinary in nature and may be written in a different format from what you have learned. The language used in the documentation may seem less specific. Some mental health issues, such as suicide risk or past sexual abuse, may not fit very neatly into the OTPF-III (AOTA, 2014c). Intervention is often provided in groups or within a therapeutic environment or milieu. Occupational therapy services may be included in a treatment service designated as adjunctive therapy, activity therapy, or expressive therapy, which may include therapeutic recreation specialists, music therapists, art therapists, and dance therapists. Professional roles often overlap and there is often a blurring of professional identities. Reimbursement may not be discipline-specific and therapy services may be included in the room rate for the facility.

One of the exceptions is geriatric psychiatric mental health units or partial hospitalization units where services are reimbursed through Medicare. With Medicare reimbursement, documentation is similar to inpatient Medicare requirements, but the types of intervention covered include psychiatric occupational therapy services as well as self-care interventions (Centers for Medicare & Medicaid Services [CMS], 2014).

Gateley CA, Borcherding S. *Documentation Manual for Occupational Therapy: Writing SOAP Notes, Fourth Edition (pp 183-196).* © 2017 SLACK Incorporated

INITIAL EVALUATION REPORTS

While you may be contributing to an interdisciplinary initial evaluation, it is essential to obtain a comprehensive occupational profile from which to plan interventions. This may be achieved through an informal interview or by using one of the many standardized occupational performance measures that are available (Mental Health 4 Occupational Therapy [MH4OT], 2016). The occupational profile will highlight the areas of occupation that are dysfunctional or interrupted and provide information about the context(s) to which the client will return.

FUNCTIONAL PROBLEM STATEMENTS

Functional problem statements in a mental health practice setting are traditionally divided into two parts. The problem itself is stated in one or two words, such as *chemical dependence, noncompliant behavior,* or *suicide risk.* The behavioral manifestations that follow define the areas of occupation and the contributing factors involved.

Problem: *Chemical dependence*
Behavioral Manifestations: *Mark has been using alcohol since age 12, with increasing frequency over the past year, and also admits to using cocaine, crystal meth, opium, and marijuana, resulting in a failed marriage, loss of two jobs, and involvement with the criminal justice system.*

Problem: *Noncompliant behavior*
Behavioral Manifestations: *Client disobeys foster parents by running away, refusing to follow rules or requests, and engaging in sexual activity, resulting in six foster home placements in the past 4 years.*

Problem: *Suicide risk*
Behavioral Manifestations: *During the week prior to admission, the client verbalized suicidal ideation, stating that life was no longer worth living. On the day of admission, he purchased a handgun.*

Problem: *Increased auditory hallucinations*
Behavioral Manifestations: *For 2 weeks prior to admission, client reported that he was hearing more voices, frequently telling him to hurt himself because he is "no good." Client reports that the voices made it difficult for him to concentrate, and staff at his group home described him as becoming more irritable and less attentive or responsive when approached or asked to participate in a task or activity.*

INTERVENTION PLANS

Intervention plans in mental health are usually interdisciplinary. The "therapeutic milieu," or the total environment of the setting, is often considered to be critical in caring for clients who have mental health disorders. The individualized treatment plan (ITP) in a mental health setting is a contract for change between the client and the treatment team. Ideally, after the client's needs and strengths have been assessed by the team, each individual discipline suggests goals, objectives, and interventions for treatment within that discipline. All goals, objectives, and interventions for each discipline involved in the client's care are then written into one comprehensive plan. Major problems or concerns identified in the evaluation are documented on the ITP. The client is a collaborative participant in the intervention process and signs the treatment plan to show agreement with it. These plans are similar to those developed by teams in a rehabilitation or school setting but differ in that all clinicians work toward the same goals through different interventions.

Success in writing an interdisciplinary treatment plan depends on the following:

- The involvement of the client (and family, if they are currently involved in the client's life)
- The willingness of each member of the treatment team to cooperate in a coordinated effort to effect change
- Regular evaluation of the effectiveness of the plan and changes in direction in interventions that have not been effective

In actual practice, however, the length of stay is sometimes so brief that a client may be discharged before a comprehensive intervention plan can be formalized.

INTERVENTION STRATEGIES

Occupational therapists use a wide variety of interventions in psychosocial settings to promote empowerment and facilitate personal change, including the following:

- Modification of the environment

- Reintegration into the community
- Motivational interviewing
- Cognitive behavioral approaches

While the goal of occupational therapy in mental health is improved engagement in areas of occupation, the interventions often target specific performance skills, such as the following:

- Assertiveness
- Problem solving
- Self-awareness
- Anger management
- Sequencing
- Prioritizing
- Role identification and development
- Communication and social skills (AOTA, 2014b)

Occupational therapy interventions focus on the occupations that are disrupted or that the client would like to pursue in the future. Ideally, the documentation of services provided in psychosocial programs reflects the occupation-based approach of our profession. This means that your documentation should be objective, measurable, and focused on the client's occupational profile and ability to engage in necessary and valued life activities.

Interventions may be specific to occupational therapy, or they may be broader and applicable to activity therapy. The choice of interventions may depend largely upon which treatment groups are being provided by the facility, with the ability to individualize intervention strategies within the groups themselves. Selecting meaningful treatment interventions can be an interesting challenge. For example, most clients may attend communication groups, but within those groups, you will customize the way you choose to increase communication skills for each individual client. With a little experience, you will learn to individualize goals for each client in the group, while still providing for the needs of the group as a whole.

When planning intervention strategies, the client's assets (good verbal skills, intelligence, etc.) will be the tools that the client has to use in overcoming his or her problems. A "strength" in this context is an ability, a skill, or an interest that the client has used in the past or has the potential for using. Assets can include the client's interests (enjoys playing music), abilities (writes well), relationship skills (has a good relationship with her father), and social support systems (minister keeps in contact). Assets may also be past abilities that the treatment team wants to encourage as treatment progresses (Jane was physically active before she became ill). Some interests (enjoys going to bars on weekends) may not be assets.

CONTACT AND PROGRESS NOTES

The use of contact and progress notes may vary by facility. Some of the exceptions are geriatric psychiatric inpatient and partial hospitalization units where the clients are insured through Medicare. In these settings, the documentation follows Medicare requirements.

If a client with a mental health diagnosis is seen in home health, the Medicare standards for home health apply, with a treatment note required for each visit. In long-term psychiatric facilities, where progress notes rather than treatment notes are used, the therapist keeps a log of attendance and makes notes about participation and behaviors that show progress each day, and then compiles that information into a progress note in the health record at regular intervals. In acute care psychiatric facilities, where length of stay may be just a few days, notes may be written for each group the client attends in order to reflect the client's progress from day to day.

When you begin thinking in the language of mental health, terms like *brightened affect, less delusional,* or *improved mood* begin to enter your vocabulary, and you may be tempted to write in less objective and measurable terms. However, there are observable behavioral manifestations that help you determine that the client's affect is brighter or his mood is improved. Perhaps you are seeing him smile more frequently, initiate conversation more often, or respond to your "hello" by making eye contact. Perhaps the client's comments had less delusional content and were directly related to the topic discussed in group. Perhaps she takes less time to get up and dress in the morning or is more easily persuaded to attend occupational therapy. These indicators are all measurable, and it is very helpful to the treatment team if you are able to report your observations in measurable and behavioral terms.

The trend toward role diffusion is making it more difficult to document occupational therapy as a service that offers value for the dollars spent in mental health care. As resources shrink and costs expand, we need to focus on documenting **functional changes** that are cost-effective and meaningful to both the payer and to the consumer. There are myriad factors present in the lives of people with serious mental illness and chemical dependency that hinder their ability to engage in meaningful occupations. In a situation where so much role diffusion is present, occupational therapists need to be clear and specific about the way our services facilitate "positive outcomes such as improvements in sensorimotor, cognitive, and psychosocial abilities, which all contribute to overall health, well-being, and life satisfaction" (Mathieson & Hahn, 2010, p. 10).

CRITICAL CARE PATHWAYS IN MENTAL HEALTH

As length of stay has shortened for psychiatric diagnoses, some mental health settings have begun using critical care pathways and computer-generated intervention plans for the most common problems seen in that setting. These are time savers and can be customized to the client by adding desired outcomes and treatment interventions specific to the individual client.

Critical care pathways in mental health are interdisciplinary and are conceptually the same as those in rehabilitation. The plan for the client's care each day for each discipline is preplanned in order to make the most efficient use of staff time during the short length of stay, while still making sure the client's needs are met.

COMPUTER-GENERATED PLANS

In an electronic "mix-and-match" program, the computer provides prompts from which the team or the individual therapist selects the problem statements, goals, objectives, and treatment interventions that will be used for the individual client. When using prepackaged treatment planning sheets, the problems are expressed briefly (e.g., *depressed mood*, *drug abuse*, *suicide risk*), and the behavioral manifestations that apply to the individual client are written in.

There is a list of long-term goals, or outcomes, such as the following:

- *Within 1 week, the client will identify 3 new coping strategies to use when he feels the urge to use drugs.*
- *Within 1 week, the client will identify 2 social or leisure activities that do not involve the use of drugs or alcohol.*

The treatment team chooses goals for each client who is admitted. All members of the interdisciplinary treatment team work on these goals during the client's hospital stay. On a computer-generated form, there is also a list of potential interventions that would be addressed by the treatment team. Interventions might include strategies such as the following:

- *Evaluate the client*
- *Encourage client to express emotions*
- *Teach new coping skills*
- *Encourage the client to verbalize alternatives to previous coping strategies*
- *Assist the client to develop a discharge plan that will prevent recurrence*

Interventions are chosen for use with each client. Each discipline implements the interventions in its own way. In relation to the five intervention strategies listed, you might do the following:

- Complete an occupational profile to determine specific problems in each area of occupation.
- Use occupational therapy media to encourage the client to express emotions.
- Facilitate occupational therapy groups to teach new coping skills and to help the client find alternatives to strategies that have not worked well in the past.
- Assist the client in making a plan for any areas of occupation that were part of the previous problem.

Social work adapts the same treatment interventions to individual and group therapy, and nursing implements the interventions on the unit. In this situation, there are sheets provided for each goal that is commonly used. The interventions are individualized to the client by stating behavioral manifestations of the problem and by adding and deleting outcomes and/or interventions. An example of a prepackaged treatment planning sheet for alcohol dependence can be found on the next page. It is provided only as an example of what might be seen in practice. Please note that the desired outcomes may not meet the COAST criteria you have learned since they are general outcomes to be addressed by the interdisciplinary treatment team.

In Chapter 12, we considered treatment interventions for Heather, a psychiatric client admitted after a suicide attempt. If a treatment team were using computer-generated planning for Heather's care, the first step would be to go to the computer and pull up interdisciplinary treatment planning sheets. For Heather, some of the choices might be as follows:

- Suicide attempt
- Poor concentration
- Anger
- Poor self-esteem

On each sheet, there would be a place to identify Heather's behavior in relation to the problem. Following that might be a list of interventions commonly used for that problem, starting with evaluation and ending with discharge planning. Interventions that really do not apply to Heather would be deleted, and any additional interventions that apply to her uniquely would be added. The groups provided by the facility would be listed as interventions and you would plan for ways to make occupational therapy groups offered daily meet Heather's needs. There would be a list of desired outcomes for each of Heather's identified problems, with a place to add outcomes specific to Heather's situation.

BEHAVIORAL HEALTH INTERDISCIPLINARY TREATMENT PLAN

Client Name: **Date:**
Problem #:   **Problem Name:** *Alcohol dependence*
Behavioral Manifestations:

DESIRED OUTCOMES	TARGET DATE	DATE ACHIEVED
1. Client will verbally acknowledge that alcohol use has been a problem and will state intent to abstain from alcohol use.		
2. Client will have developed at least three new ways to deal with stress and will have demonstrated use of these.		
3. Client will have an aftercare plan in place.		
4. Client will have established a 5-day period of sobriety and of attending AA meetings daily.		
5.		
6.		

TREATMENT INTERVENTIONS	STAFF RESPONSIBLE
1. Evaluation of the client's alcohol intake and use patterns	
2. Provide individual, group, and family therapy	
3. Education re: the disease model of chemical dependency	
4. Provide opportunities to express feelings	
5. Teach coping skills	
6. Assist client to restructure environmental situations	
7. Evaluate and teach relationship skills	
8. Facilitate peer confrontation and feedback	
9. Introduce social/leisure activities that do not include alcohol	
10. Develop plan with client on how to respond when experiencing cravings for alcohol	
11.	

I agree with this plan.

_____

Client's signature

DOCUMENTATION IN SCHOOL-BASED PRACTICE

AOTA (2011b) explains occupational therapy's role in the following performance areas in the school setting:

◆ *Academic*: Occupational therapists can provide consultation regarding accommodations for curricular processes, standardized testing, and transition planning.

◆ *Developmental*: Occupational therapists can "foster development of pre-academic skills, including prewriting and pre-scissor skills, toileting skills, eating and drinking skills, dressing and grooming tasks, communication skills, management of sensory needs, social skills" as they related to performance in the educational setting (AOTA, 2011b, p. S51).

◆ *Functional*: Occupational therapists can "facilitate use and management of school-related materials; daily routines/schedule; written school work; task/activity completion; transitions among activities and persons; adherence to rules; self-regulation; interactions with peers and adults; participation in leisure and recreational opportunities at home, school, and the community; use of adaptive and assistive technology to support participation and performance" (AOTA, 2011b, p. S51). Furthermore, occupational therapists may assist the school in planning for adaptive driver education training and developing positive behavioral support systems and positive mental health programs for students with disabilities.

If you provide occupational therapy services in a school setting, your documentation will be related to the child's individualized education program (IEP). The IEP is a written document that details a student's educational and functional needs (Bazyk & Cahill, 2015; U.S. Department of Education, 2016). In other occupational therapy practice settings, occupational therapists write a specific intervention plan. In school-based practice, the IEP serves as the intervention plan. The *Individuals with Disabilities Education Act* (IDEA), federal legislation that is scheduled for review and reauthorization approximately every 5 to 7 years, "requires that states and public educational agencies provide a free appropriate public education (FAPE) to children with disabilities in the least restrictive environment (LRE)" (Bazyk & Cahill, 2015, p. 665). Although the format of IEPs may vary between school districts, Bazyk and Cahill explained that all IEPs must contain the following information:

◆ A vision of the child's needs including a summary of current academic and functional performance and a description of how the child's disability affects his or her ability to participate in general education

◆ Measurable annual goals that are educationally relevant and a plan for measuring progress toward those goals

◆ A statement of the special education and related services to be provided to the child

◆ A statement of individual accommodations to measure the academic achievement and functional performance of the child on state and district assessments

◆ A statement of placement in the least restrictive environment, meaning that the child should be educated with students without disabilities to the maximum extent appropriate

◆ Beginning at age 16 years, a transition plan that identifies plans for services to prepare for employment, vocational training, independent living, and continued education as appropriate to the student

The U.S. Department of Education provides an example of a model IEP form at http://idea.ed.gov. Most states also have model forms that combine the federal requirements with specific state requirements. Regardless of the specific format used by a particular state or district, occupational therapy is considered a "related service" as described in the requirements listed previously (Bazyk & Cahill, 2015). The IEP is developed by a team consisting of the child's parents, regular education teacher(s), special education teacher(s), and related services personnel. Rather than writing separate occupational therapy goals, the occupational therapist should contribute to the development of the overall IEP. Since an IEP can be quite lengthy, the one provided here has been condensed to show only the aspects that are most pertinent to occupational therapy.

INDIVIDUALIZED EDUCATION PROGRAM

Name: *Truman T*   **Age:** *5 yr., 11 mo*   **Grade Level:** *Kindergarten*
Present Level of Academic Achievement and Functional Performance
Truman will be 6 years old in just a few days. He was diagnosed with pervasive developmental disorder (PDD) at age 2 years. He attended the Early Childhood Special Education program for 2 years and is currently enrolled in a full-day kindergarten. The decision has been made by the IEP team to retain Truman in kindergarten for the upcoming school year. Truman's parents are in agreement with this decision and hope that another year in kindergarten will allow him

to improve his academic performance and social skills prior to advancing to first grade. Truman does not qualify for Extended School Year services at this time.

Truman spends the majority of his day in the general education classroom with a paraprofessional present for support with classroom participation. He spends 60 minutes daily in the special education classroom for additional 1:1 and small group instruction in reading and writing skills. He also participates in adaptive physical education twice weekly for 45 minutes.

Truman's verbal skills are delayed in comparison to same-age peers, although he has demonstrated considerable improvement over the past year. He is now able to communicate in three- to five-word sentences consistently. He also uses a Picture Exchange Communication System (PECS) to supplement his verbal communication.

Truman is easily distracted by auditory and visual stimuli in and near the classroom and has difficulty remaining in his seat for more than 5 minutes at a time. He has difficulty with transitions between activities and locations, but this has improved following implementation of a visual schedule. Truman sometimes responds with negative behaviors (yelling, hitting, pinching) when classmates inadvertently touch or bump into him during classroom activities.

Truman is hesitant to engage in play activities with his peers. He prefers to play alone and does not initiate interactions with peers. Toward the end of last school year, he was beginning to participate in some simple ball activities with others during recess with significant support from his paraprofessional. He will continue participation in a weekly after-school peer communication group led by the elementary school counselor.

Truman is able to recognize all letters of the alphabet, but he does not yet read any words. He can copy the letters of his name when provided with a visual model, but legibility is inconsistent. His ability to copy other letters of the alphabet remains very inconsistent. Truman has difficulty achieving a tripod grasp on writing utensils and staying on the lines of standard writing paper. He also has difficulty with consistent letter size and spacing. His writing performance improves with the use of adaptive writing paper and rubber pencil grip. He does consistently copy basic shapes including circle, square, triangle, and cross.

Truman requires assistance to obtain and carry his tray in the lunchroom. He is easily upset by the noise in the lunchroom and often needs to be taken to a quieter room to finish lunch. Truman consistently indicates when he needs to use the restroom, but continues to have difficulty managing the button and zipper on his jeans. He needs hand-over-hand assistance to complete hand washing because he prefers to play in the water. Truman is now able to take his coat on and off independently. He can also manage Velcro tennis shoes independently.

Type of Service	Anticipated Frequency	Amount of Time	Location of Service
Special Education *Special education teacher will provide intensive reading and writing instruction in both 1:1 and small group formats.*	*Daily*	*60 minutes*	*Special Education Classroom*
Supplementary Aids & Services *Truman will have a paraprofessional present throughout the school day except when with the special education teacher.*	*Daily*	*340 minutes*	*General Education Classroom & Across Settings*
Program Modifications *Adaptive P.E.*	*Weekly*	*90 minutes*	*Indoor/Outdoor P.E. Settings*
Accommodations for Assessments *Truman will be allowed additional time for completion of classroom and state assessments.*	*Weekly*	*60 minutes*	*General and Special Education Classrooms*
Related Services *Occupational Therapy*	*Weekly*	*30 minutes*	*General and Special Education Classrooms & Across Settings*
Related Services *Speech Language Pathology*	*Weekly*	*90 minutes*	*General and Special Education Classrooms & Across Settings*

Annual Goal #1: *Using compensatory strategies, Truman will demonstrate legible handwriting in the classroom with appropriate baseline orientation, letter size, and spacing with 80% accuracy.*

Evaluation Methods:	Primary Implementers:
☐ Curriculum-Based Assessment ☐ State Assessments ☑ Data Collection Chart ☑ Work Samples ☐ Other:	☑ General Education Teacher ☑ Special Education Teacher ☐ Physical Therapy ☑ Occupational Therapy ☐ Speech Language Pathology ☐ Other:

Measurable Benchmarks/Objectives:	Date of Mastery:
1. Truman will demonstrate tripod grasp on writing utensils using adaptive pencil grip with 80% accuracy.	1.
2. Truman will write his first name on adaptive paper without a visual model, demonstrating appropriate letter formation, size, and line orientation on 4 of 5 consecutive days.	2.
3. Truman will copy 22/26 lowercase letters onto adaptive paper using a visual model, demonstrating appropriate letter formation, size, and line orientation on 4 of 5 consecutive days.	3.

Annual Goal #2: *Truman will demonstrate improved attention and work behaviors during classroom activities with no more than three sensory breaks per hour throughout the day on 4 of 5 consecutive days.*

Evaluation Methods:	Primary Implementers:
☐ Curriculum-Based Assessment ☐ State Assessments ☑ Data Collection Chart ☐ Work Samples ☐ Other:	☑ General Education Teacher ☑ Special Education Teacher ☐ Physical Therapy ☑ Occupational Therapy ☐ Speech Language Pathology ☐ Other:

Measurable Benchmarks/Objectives:	Date of Mastery:
1. Truman will remain seated at his desk or during circle time for 15 minutes with minimal verbal cues and no more than one sensory break.	1.
2. Truman will transition between classroom activities with minimal verbal cues using a visual schedule and without demonstrating negative behaviors (yelling, hitting, etc.) toward peers and staff on 4 of 5 consecutive days.	2.
3. Truman will tolerate unexpected touch from classmates without demonstrating negative behaviors (yelling, hitting, etc.) on 4 of 5 consecutive days.	3.

Annual Goal #3: *Truman will demonstrate school-related self-care skills using adaptive strategies with no more than minimal assistance on 4 of 5 consecutive days.*

Evaluation Methods:	Primary Implementers:
☐ Curriculum-Based Assessment ☐ State Assessments ☑ Data Collection Chart ☐ Work Samples ☐ Other:	☐ General Education Teacher ☐ Special Education Teacher ☐ Physical Therapy ☑ Occupational Therapy ☐ Speech Language Pathology ☑ Other: Paraprofessional

Measurable Benchmarks/Objectives:	Date of Mastery:
1. Truman will complete toileting without assistance to manage clothing fasteners on 4 of 5 consecutive days.	1.
2. Truman will wash hands following a visual schedule with minimal verbal cues on 4 of 5 consecutive days.	2.
3. Truman will obtain/transport his lunch tray and remain seated in the cafeteria for the duration of the lunch period with minimal verbal cues on 4 of 5 consecutive days.	3.

DOCUMENTATION IN SKILLED NURSING FACILITIES IN LONG-TERM CARE

Most clients who receive therapy services in skilled nursing facilities in long-term settings are covered by Medicare, and documentation may be done using written or electronic forms to gather information required by Medicare. When a client is first admitted, an interdisciplinary evaluation called the *Minimum Data Set* (MDS) is used to determine the specific level of care needed and is part of the overall Resident Assessment Instrument (RAI). The MDS is part of the federally mandated process for clinical assessment of residents in Medicare and Medicaid certified long-term care facilities (CMS, 2016). CMS provides instructions for completing the MDS at https://www.cms.gov. For ease and efficiency, each discipline may be assigned a specific part of the MDS to complete. Facilities may vary in how activities of daily living, cognitive, or other sections are divided between occupational therapy, nursing, or other disciplines. Facilities will also vary in terms of other formats for occupational therapy-specific documentation.

DOCUMENTATION IN OUTPATIENT SETTINGS

Documentation requirements in outpatient settings will depend on the facility requirements, accrediting agencies, and funding sources. Managed care insurance may require a special form that outlines the client's evaluation results and plan of care before additional visits will be approved. This form is in addition to the facility evaluation form that must be completed. Outpatient occupational therapy services are typically billed using CPT codes, as described in Chapter 3. Your documentation must support the billing codes that were used for each occupational therapy session. In other words, you need to describe in detail the interventions that you implemented as well as the time spent on each intervention. If your client has Medicare as a funding source, you will also need to report G-codes, which identify the primary issue being addressed by therapy. Refer back to Chapter 3 for a list of G-codes and further explanation regarding their use.

DOCUMENTATION IN AN INPATIENT REHABILITATION FACILITY

Clients admitted to an inpatient rehabilitation facility will have an interdisciplinary evaluation documented on a tool called the Inpatient Rehabilitation Facility Patient Assessment Instrument (IRF-PAI), available at www.cms.gov. Although it is likely there will be separate supporting documentation required in a specific facility format, the occupational therapist contributes to the IRF-PAI by providing information about the client's Functional Independence Measure (FIM) scores. As explained in Chapter 3, the FIM instrument measures the client's level of independence in 18 functional activities in the categories of self-care, sphincter control, transfers, locomotion, communication, and social cognition (Uniform Data System for Medical Rehabilitation [UDSMR], 2016). There are very detailed scoring criteria for each of the 18 functional activities, and scores are assigned based on the 7-point scale summarized as follows (Rehab Measures, 2016):

- 7—Complete independence
- 6—Modified independence (Extra time, use of equipment or modified technique, safety concern)
- 5—Supervision, set-up, and stand-by assistance
- 4—Minimal assistance (Client performs 75% or more of the task)
- 3—Moderate assistance (Client performs 50% to 74% of the task)
- 2—Maximal assistance (Client performs 25% to 49% of the task)
- 1—Total assistance (Client performs less than 25% of the task or requires more than one person to assist)

FIM scores for each area are documented at admission. FIM score goals are then set and tracked at regular intervals (typically weekly), and FIM scores are recorded again at the time of discharge. Documentation in the occupational therapy initial evaluation, contact/progress notes, and discharge summary should include information specific to the functional activities scored by the FIM instrument. If you work in a facility where FIM scores are used, you will be required to complete annual training and certification in administering the FIM. The training is provided by UDSMR and your employer will facilitate the training process (UDSMR, 2016). Additional FIM information and scoring examples are available at https://www.cms.gov.

Documentation in Early Intervention

As recently as a few decades ago, early intervention services were typically provided in an outpatient therapy clinic with a medical orientation (Myers, Case-Smith, & Cason, 2015). Amendments to the IDEA in 1997 required early intervention services to be provided in natural environments such as the home and community settings in which typically developing peers of a comparable age would participate (AOTA, 2011b, 2014a).

Children receiving occupational therapy as part of federally mandated early intervention services will have a document called the Individualized Family Service Plan (IFSP). Although each state will have a specific format for the IFSP, there are certain elements that must be contained in the document, such as the following:

- Present level of performance in the areas of motor, cognitive, communication, social-emotional, and adaptive development
- Family's resources, priorities, and concerns for the child
- Expected outcomes for the child and family
- Specific early intervention services needed
- Natural environments in which services will be provided
- Dates of initiation and anticipated duration of services
- Name of service coordinator
- Plan for transition to preschool or other services at age 3 years (Myers et al., 2015, p. 642)

A unique feature of early intervention services is that all documentation is written in plain language that is understandable to parents rather than in professional jargon. Although the SOAP note format is not used, you can see that all of the SOAP elements are still included:

Kiara participated in a 30-minute OT session in her home with her mother and grandmother present. Focus this date was on self-feeding. Mother reports that Kiara has been feeding herself finger foods from the highchair tray but is not showing much interest in using a spoon. With Kiara seated in the highchair, mother showed how she helps her hold the spoon to scoop yogurt out of the container, but Kiara became fussy and threw the spoon down. Suggestion was made to place yogurt in small bowl to make scooping easier, and Kiara was then able to scoop 4 bites without help, and needed only a little help from her mother to scoop 5 more bites. Recommendation also made for use of rubber mat (such as shelf liner) under bowl to keep it in place, and grandmother reports she will bring some from her house. Improved ability to feed herself with a spoon shows good progress toward expected outcome of Kiara feeding herself all meals without help. Plan to address drinking from sippy cup next session as mother has stated goal to "get her off the bottle."

Consultation

Consulting work is another area of occupational therapy practice that may use a slightly different method or language for documentation. Occupational therapists may consult on a wide variety of questions about which they have special expertise. For example, a psychiatric unit that relies on recreational therapists and activity aides for its activity therapy program might ask for an occupational therapy consult on a client who has both physical and psychiatric disabilities. A newborn nursery might ask for an occupational therapy consult on a high-risk infant. An occupational therapist may be asked to evaluate a work, home, or school setting to make recommendations regarding safety, adaptations for work simplification, ergonomics, energy conservation, or compliance with the Americans with Disabilities Act (ADA) standards. An occupational therapy consultant might be used to peer review charts for quality improvement monitoring or for reimbursement issues.

A consultant gives a professional assessment of what needs to be done, rather than actually doing it. Two of the most common requests for occupational therapy consultations are for consultation on individual consumers, or for consultation on the context in which the consumer works or resides.

Individual Consumers

A consult on an individual consumer is written in the consumer's health record, just as any occupational therapy note would be. In a problem-oriented medical record, the note is written in chronological order in the progress note section in a SOAP format. In a source-oriented record, the consult would more likely be written in a different format, and would be found in the section of the record marked "consults." It might be in the form of a letter or memo, or it might be written on some kind of form that the consulting occupational therapist uses routinely. The following note documents a consultation provided for a psychiatric client who had positioning needs, and is written in SOAP format so that you can see how that would be done. In Chapter 16, there is an example of a consultation on an individual client done in a different format.

Occupational Therapy—Positioning Consultation

S: *Consumer reports that he is not able to find a comfortable position in his wheelchair, and that he is not able to propel it in a straight line around his home or in the community due to a drag on one of the wheels.*

O: *At the request of Dr. Carter, consumer participated in consultation at community mental health center to assess his positioning needs. Consumer noted to be leaning to the Ⓡ with increased pressure on the Ⓡ elbow. Back of wheelchair noted to be hammocking badly. Arm rests do not provide a good position for functional use of arms. Gel cushion in chair seems to be working well as an anti-pressure device but transfers cold sensation to consumer. Upon inspection, wheel found to have hairs wound around the axle, and also in need of oiling.*

A: *Ill-fitting w/c limits client's independence with functional mobility and performance of ADLs and IADLs. Several changes in the wheelchair are needed to increase comfort and functional use. Client would benefit from the following:*
  - *Add an anti-sling insert to the back of the chair to provide a more upright posture.*
  - *Add a pad to the gel cushion to prevent cold transfer of gel to consumer and also for ease of cleaning in case of incontinence.*
  - *Ⓑ arm bolsters are needed for w/c arm rests to bring consumer's arms closer to midline for ↑ functional use.*
  - *Clean and oil wheels at axle.*

P: *The adaptations listed above have been ordered. Consumer to be re-evaluated after the wheelchair is repaired and adapted.*

Marisa B., OTR/L

SETTINGS IN WHICH THE CONSUMER WORKS OR RESIDES

In evaluating a client's home or workplace prior to discharge, a SOAP note might also be used. For an example of a home evaluation, see Chapter 16. However, if a work setting were evaluated for ergonomic correctness or for ADA compliance as a whole rather than in relation to one specific client, a letter or standardized evaluation form would be more appropriate. The following letter documents a work site evaluation that was done on a consulting basis.

MEMO
To: *Earl Y, R.Ph.*
From: *Charlet Q, OTR/L*
Re: *Computer ergonomics in the pharmacy*

A visit was made to the 2nd floor pharmacy in response to your request to perform an ergonomic evaluation of the computer work stations located there. This is in response to complaints of carpal tunnel pain and neck and shoulder discomfort. The following are my recommendations:

1. *Computer keyboards must be positioned low enough so that the shoulders can be relaxed during sustained usage and so that wrists can be maintained in neutral position rather than in extension or flexion. When the wrist is in extension or flexion, there is more stress on the median nerve that is compressed in the carpal tunnel and may cause pain.*
    The best position may be achieved by lowering some of the keyboards and/or angling them so the wrists can be kept neutral. Sometimes keeping the keyboards flat or even inclining them with the far end slightly down may help keep the wrists in neutral position. A wrist rest used in conjunction with the keyboard is helpful to some users. If an ergonomic keyboard is used to avoid wrist deviations, it still must be positioned so the wrists are not either flexed or extended. The correct position for each person will be slightly different since all body builds are different. It will be important for each user to know the correct body mechanics and be able to make some adjustments in the workstation to meet his/her needs.

2. *The chair should support the back while maintaining the trunk in an upright position (not leaning back or forward). Thighs should be supported and the entire foot should be supported while sitting in a chair at a computer station. Foot support may be either the floor or a footrest (flat or angled) as needed to support the feet. The rungs attached to the high stools do not allow adequate foot support and may tend to disrupt back alignment. Adjustable-height chairs are recommended to meet individual needs.*

3. *The monitor needs to be placed directly in front of the viewer, so it is not necessary to maintain a rotated position of the neck and trunk. Several monitors were angled to the side, requiring the user to maintain asymmetrical posture, causing neck and back strain. The height of the monitor should be adjusted so the eyes of the viewer look directly forward onto the upper one-third of the screen. This prevents neck strain, which can occur if the viewer has to look up for sustained periods of time.*

4. *If the mouse is to be used with any frequency, it should be positioned near the keyboard rather than requiring a forward reach. A wrist rest attached to the mouse pad is preferred to remove stress from the heel of the hand.*

5. *Ideally, it seems that the computer workstations should be lowered from high counters to normal table or desk work-height. Table-top should ideally be 26" from floor and the distance eye to screen should be 26" to 30". However, it is possible to manage the existing problems with the correct chairs, footrests, monitor positioning, and keyboard/mouse positioning.*

6. *Taking a break every 30 minutes to do some active movement and stretching exercises is recommended. A copy of sample exercises was left in the pharmacy.*

If you plan to purchase chairs, footrests, etc., it would be best to actually go to an office supply vendor to try out specific pieces of furniture, or arrange to have the items on loan so the potential users can check the fit. I hope this is helpful. Please let me know if I can be of further assistance.

Charlet Q., OTR/L

Documentation in Palliative Care

Occupational therapists who work in hospice settings or in other practice settings where clients have terminal illnesses often provide palliative care rather than rehabilitation. Palliative care provides comfort, relief from symptoms, and quality of life as clients prepare for death. In this situation, there is no expectation that the client will make progress in physical functioning. Goals often center around pain control, energy conservation, maintaining independence in areas of occupation that are meaningful to the client, obtaining adaptive equipment, and family/caregiver education. Relaxation, active listening, and complementary and alternative therapies are often used with hospice clients. The following note shows one of the complementary/alternative therapies (Tai Chi) being used to increase relaxation and social participation and to maintain activity tolerance, balance, functional mobility, and satisfaction with quality of life.

Jean is a 48-year-old woman whose throat cancer was diagnosed late and has now metastasized to the brain. She is a single woman who has devoted her life to her career in one of the health professions. She understands her prognosis and has entered a home-based hospice program where she receives occupational therapy as a part of her care. Jean wants to maintain her social participation and her independence in basic and IADLs as long as possible. She has always been physically active, but many of the physical activities she has enjoyed doing with friends are too strenuous for her limited energy.

S: *Client states, "I feel so much better after doing Tai Chi with you ladies, even on days when I think I'm too tired or just don't feel like I'm able to do anything."*

O: *Client participated in 45-minute session in her home with 2 friends present to increase social participation, decrease risk of falling, and incorporate energy conservation techniques taught last week into everyday tasks. Five minutes of warm-up exercises focused on breath-awareness and relaxation were followed by 15 minutes of modified therapeutic Tai Chi with one 5-minute rest period. Client touched chair back as needed for stability during movements requiring weight shift and balance on one foot. Gentle push hands activity was used to challenge balance and to provide physical contact and social engagement during movement activities. Friends remained for short visit and refreshments on the deck, and plans were made to repeat the activity as tolerated in 1 week. Home instruction sheets and a Tai Chi video with relaxation music were provided for use as desired over the next week.*

A: *Client's home bound status, decreased balance, and variable energy levels limit her social participation and IADLs. Her perception of increased energy and activity tolerance following the Tai Chi activity allows her to continue to engage in occupation she values. Using furniture as props allows client to practice weight shifting and balance in a safe environment. Physical contact and social exchange during push hands reduced social isolation and distress of "not being able to do anything." Client would benefit from continued Tai Chi activities to address energy conservation, balance, and safety concerns through breathing and relaxation activities done in a social setting.*

P: *Client to be seen in her home weekly for 45 minutes or as tolerated for 3 more weeks for instruction in mobility, balance, energy conservation techniques to maintain functional mobility, IADL tasks, and valued role as a friend in a modified home exercise energy conservation program.*

Sandy M., PhD, OTR/L

DIFFERENT FORMATS FOR NOTES

Remember that SOAP is just a format—an organizational structure that may be used for any type of note. An initial evaluation can be written in a SOAP format, as can a treatment or progress note. There are other styles of notes that may be used instead.

Checklists, flow sheets, and standardized forms created by the facility are often used instead of SOAP notes to save time. Forms are an especially popular way to document an initial assessment because they allow quite a lot of information to be communicated with little time spent writing. The evaluation form presented in Chapter 13 is a good example because it covers a lot of areas in a small space without sacrificing the ability to individualize the information. It also documents the areas of occupation before the underlying factors so that no time is wasted documenting underlying factors that do not impact function. There is ample space for comments so that the form can easily be individualized.

Narrative notes are not formally organized into sections the way SOAP notes are. Narrative notes may present any information in any order desired. Good narrative notes usually contain the "A" data of the SOAP note. Narrative notes reporting primarily the "A" data are becoming more popular due to time and space constraints.

DAP notes are an adaptation of the SOAP format used in some facilities. In this format, the "D" (data) section contains both the "S" and the "O" information.

BIRP, PIRP, or **SIRP notes** are sometimes used in mental health practice settings. Information in this format is distributed as follows:

- *B*: The behavior exhibited by the client
- *I*: The treatment intervention provided by the therapist
- *R*: The client's response to the intervention provided
- *P*: The therapist's plan for continued treatment, based on the client's response

- *P*: The problem/purpose of the treatment
- *IRP* for intervention, response, and plan, as stated previously

- *S*: The situation
- *IRP* for intervention, response, and plan, as stated previously

If you work in a facility that uses one of these formats, you categorize your information slightly differently than you do when you are writing a SOAP note.

REFERENCES

American Occupational Therapy Association. (2011a). AOTA fact sheet: Occupational therapy and community reintegration of persons with brain injury. Retrieved from www.aota.org.

American Occupational Therapy Association. (2011b). Occupational therapy services in early childhood and school-based settings. *American Journal of Occupational Therapy, 65*(6), S46-S54.

American Occupational Therapy Association. (2014a). Frequently asked questions: What is the role of occupational therapy in early intervention? Retrieved from www.aota.org.

American Occupational Therapy Association. (2014b). Focus on mental health. Retrieved from www.aota.org.

American Occupational Therapy Association. (2014c). *Occupational therapy practice framework: Domain & process* (3rd ed.). Bethesda, MD: AOTA Press.

American Occupational Therapy Association. (2015a). 2015 American Occupational Therapy Association salary and workforce survey: Executive summary. Retrieved from www.aota.org.

American Occupational Therapy Association. (2015b). AOTA fact sheet: Occupational therapy's role with post-traumatic stress disorder. Retrieved from www.aota.org.

American Occupational Therapy Association. (2016). Emerging niche: Depression. Retrieved from www.aota.org/Practice/Mental-Health/Emerging-Niche/Depression.aspx.

Bazyk, S., & Cahill, S. (2015). School-based occupational therapy. In J. Case-Smith & J. C. Clifford O'Brien (Eds.) *Occupational therapy for children and adolescents* (7th ed., pp. 664-703). St. Louis, MO: Elsevier.

Boyt Schell, B. A., Scaffa, M. E., Gillen, G., & Cohn, E. S. (2014). Contemporary occupational therapy practice. In B. A. Boyt Schell, G. Gillen, & M. E. Scaffa (Eds.) *Willard & Spackman's occupational therapy* (12th ed., pp. 47-58.) Philadelphia, PA: Lippincott Williams & Wilkins.

Centers for Medicare & Medicaid Services. (2014). Medicare & your mental health benefits. Retrieved from https:www.medicare.gov

Centers for Medicare & Medicaird Services. (2016). MDS 3.0 RAI manual. Retrieved from https://www.cms.gov.

Christiansen, C. H., & Haertl, K. (2014). A contextual history of occupational therapy. In B.A. Boyt Schell, G. Gillen, & M. E. Scaffa (Eds.) *Willard & Spackman's occupational therapy* (12th ed., pp. 9-34). Baltimore, MD: Lippincott Williams & Wilkins.

Mathieson, K., & Hahn, C. (2010). Qualified mental health professions. *ADVANCE for Occupational Therapy Practitioners, 26*(11), 10.

Mental Health 4 Occupational Therapy [MH4OT]. (2016). OT assessment index. Retrieved from http://mh4ot.com/resources/ot-assessment-index.

Myers, C. T., Case-Smith, J., & Cason, J. (2015). Early intervention. In J. Case-Smith & J. C. Clifford O'Brien (Eds.) *Occupational therapy for children and adolescents* (7th ed., pp. 636-663). St. Louis, MO: Elsevier.

Rehab Measures. (2016). FIM® instrument (FIM). Retrieved from http://www.rehabmeasures.org.

United Data System for Medical Rehabilitation. (2016). UDSMR services. Retrieved from http://www.udsmr.org.

United States Department of Education. (2016). A guide to the Individualized Education Program. Retrieved from http://www2.ed.gov.

Chapter 15

Electronic Documentation

In the past several years, electronic health records (EHRs) have become the norm rather than the exception, and they are used in numerous health care settings (Scott, 2013). There are packages available to schedule our days as well as to send and receive mail, to compile our occupational profiles and intervention plans, to write our notes, and to remind us when everything is due. Software packages for electronic systems offer us a menu from which to choose the initial evaluations we want to use and for recording the data. Other packages offer us choices of problems, goals, objectives, and possible intervention strategies rather than requiring us to compose these for individual clients. Such software can make our job simpler and save valuable health care dollars. However, there are some critical issues to be aware of when using electronic documentation systems (Waite, 2012).

First, there is so much information available in an EHR that it is often difficult to locate the particular piece of information or form that you are looking for. Rather than being able to scan quickly through the sections of a paper health record, EHRs may require a user to click through multiple lists and menus to locate the desired item.

Second, it is tempting to copy and paste information from one record to another if the clients have similar issues. This can result in problems ranging from small errors (saying "her" instead of "his") to major errors in accuracy regarding the client's status. Best practice is to enter the information for each client without use of a copy and paste method.

EHRs have also reduced the amount of face-to-face and phone communication between members of the health care team. While electronic documentation is a time saver, you should always remember the importance of collaborating directly with other members of the client's health care team to optimize the quality of your occupational therapy services and to maximize your client's outcomes.

Perhaps the most important issue when using EHRs is to remember the importance of developing a rapport with your client and including him or her throughout the occupational therapy process. There is a temptation to interact solely with the computer in selecting goals, objectives, and treatment strategies, particularly if you are using a computer in the treatment room. This practice should be avoided, regardless of the extra time involved in setting goals and choosing intervention strategies **with** the client rather than **for** the client. Effective treatment requires the teamwork of the client and therapist working toward mutually selected and agreed-upon goals.

Finally, there needs to be a way to individualize each section of the treatment plan or note. A good program will allow editing options or places for comments so that the documentation can be individualized to the client. One way to make an effective compromise between selecting from a menu and individualizing the statements is to use a "mix-and-match" system in which the menu offers components of the statement and allows the therapist to choose the components appropriate to the individual client. For example, in Chapter 12, we looked at critical care pathways for clients who have many of the same needs, and in Chapter 13, we examined mix-and-match treatment intervention

Gateley CA, Borcherding S. *Documentation Manual for Occupational Therapy: Writing SOAP Notes, Fourth Edition (pp 197-210).* © 2017 SLACK Incorporated

plans in mental health. In some situations, it is also possible to standardize contact or progress notes. In summary, we need to make certain that the client is our main focus, fitting the software to the client needs rather than fitting the client into the capabilities of the software package.

In the following note, the computer supplies the words in bold, and the therapist completes the sentences:

S: *When asked, client able to state 2/3 hip precautions correctly.*

O: *Pt. participated in 30 minute OT session bedside for skilled instruction in following hip precautions during personal ADL tasks.*

ADLs: Client able to dress upper body ① and lower body SBA using adaptive equipment with 2 verbal cues to remember hip precautions.

Functional Mobility: Client supine → sit mod ①, able to walk to bathroom using wheel walker c̄ verbal cues to avoid external rotation when turning.

Contributing Factors: Strength/endurance: Client able to lift 4 pounds using Ⓑ UEs. Rest break needed after 5 minutes of light activity.

Home Program:

A: *Contributing Factors: Overall deconditioning has resulted in weakness and lack of activity tolerance needed to complete ADL routine without several rest breaks. Client continues to make steady gains in strength and activity tolerance and has good potential to meet goal of modified ① in ADL tasks after discharge.*

ADLs: Ability to remember 2 out of 3 hip precautions when asked and to incorporate 2 of the 3 successfully into his ADL routine shows good progress and good potential to follow hip precautions after discharge.

Functional Mobility: Need for verbal cues to follow hip precautions during bathroom tasks results in continued safety concerns.

Client would benefit from continued instruction in incorporating hip precautions into daily activities and from a schedule that increases activity tolerance and overall conditioning.

P: *Client to be seen twice daily for 1 more day to complete skilled instruction using adaptive equipment for dressing; to teach tub, shower, and car transfers; and to instruct caregiver in home program.*

Shea S., OTR/L

This program cues the therapist to remember areas that need to be covered in the note and provides the words that must be repeated in every note. There is still opportunity for maximum flexibility in individualizing the documentation. You will note that she did not fill in the blank for home program since she has not yet taught that program. She could omit that section when saving/printing her note, or she could put "*Not yet taught.*"

Figure 15-1 shows an example of electronic documentation that allows the occupational therapist to document the initial evaluation, the plan of care, and the discharge summary all in the same report. You will see that this form includes several tables for entering data common to a work hardening setting as well as the option to include a standardized description of the tests that were performed. You will also note some abbreviations not covered in this manual that are specific to the work hardening setting:

- *PRE*: Progressive resistive exercise
- *CV*: Coefficients of variance
- *PILE*: Progressive isoinertial lifting evaluation
- *PDC*: Physical demand characteristics

With the trend toward electronic documentation software, students often question the relevance of learning the SOAP note format. We strongly believe that learning the SOAP format teaches students and entry level practitioners to use clinical reasoning in documenting a client's performance and response to therapeutic interventions. Furthermore, electronic documentation software typically contains all of the elements found in a SOAP note, although they may be presented in a different order or format. Some software programs specifically use a SOAP note format. Take a look at Figure 15-2 to familiarize yourself with some of the features of a comprehensive billing and documentation software program based on the SOAP note format:

BIO-ERGONOMICS, INC.
AN INDUSTRIAL REHABILITATION CONSULTING COMPANY
VICTOR J. ZUCCARELLO, OTR/L, C.E.E.S., ABDA

WORK HARDENING EVALUATION – SUMMARY REPORT
Initial Evaluation Date: 4/1/17
Exit Evaluation Date: 4/28/17

Name	Chet D.
Age	40
Height (inches) - 72	Weight (lbs) - 250 Dominance (L/R handed) – R
Physician: Dr. Lance Sawbones	Follow-up Physician Appointment: 4/30/17
Diagnosis	s/p L4-5 Fusion
Date of Injury	1/2/17
Mechanism of Injury/Medical Tx (as reported by patient)	"Lifted a box at work and felt a pull in my back". Conservative tx for 2 weeks including PT, medications, and time off w/o relief. MRI (+) for large HNP. Fusion 2/1/17 & PT 2/22 to 3/15/17. Attempted return to work on 3/18/17 but unable to tolerate. Rx for Work Hardening written 3/25/17.
Employer & Job Title	XYZ Corporation – Order Filler
Insurance Carrier/Adjuster	Coverall Insurance/Sue Payer
Case Manager	Nancy Nurse, RN, CCM

Work Hardening Program Attendance
Attended 18/18 visits for up to 7 hour days. No tardies.

Work Hardening Treatment Program:
Aerobic exercise, stretching/stabilization, PRE, functional tasks, and body mechanics education.

Work Hardening Exit Evaluation Performance Criteria Profile:
Consistency of Effort – CVs low. Cross validation in PILE v. Occasional lifts acceptable.
Quality of Effort – HR during evaluation >/= 25% variance. Acceptable kinesiophysical signs.
Non-Organic Signs – Subjective reports consistent with test behavior. Complaints specific.

Work Hardening Exit Evaluation Assessment:
Significant progress noted in program. He is currently meeting all return to work goals. See the work requirements/goals v. demonstrated physical tolerances on the following page. Feasibility for success at return to work is **GOOD** at this time.

Work Hardening Exit Evaluation Recommendation/Plan:
Pending physician f/u and exam, I recommend return to work at full duty at this time.

Vic Zuccarello, OTR/L, C.E.A.S. II, ABDA

Chet D.

Page 1

BIO-ERGONOMICS, INC.

Figure 15-1. (Reprinted with permission of Vic Zuccarello, OTR/L, C.E.A.S. II, ABDA Owner - BIO-ERGONOMICS, INC.) *(continued)*

Work Hardening Evaluation		Chet D.		Page Two
Demonstrated Physical Tolerances				
Task	Initial Eval – 4/1/17	Exit Eval – 4/28/17	Job Description	Met? (yes/no)
Pain Level (0-10)	6/10	**3/10**	*Job Description Information (Goals to be Met) Provided By: Employer & Employee*	
Chief Complaints	Midline lumbar aching into R hip.	**Midline lumbar aching.**		
Material Handling Lifting in pounds unless stated otherwise/Push/Pull in Pounds of Force (Occ. = 0-33% of day, Freq. = 34-66%, Const. = > 66%) or (Occ. = 1-12/hr, Freq. = 13-60/hr, Const. = > 60/hr)				
Floor to Waist Lift	25# occasional	**75# occasional, 35# frequent**	**70# occasional, 25# frequent**	**MET**
Waist to Shoulder Lift	"	"	"	**MET**
Overhead Lift	"	**50# occasional, 25# frequent**	**40# occasional, 20# frequent**	**MET**
Carrying (50 feet)	"	**75# occasional, 35# frequent**	**70# occasional, 25# frequent**	**MET**
Pushing (Force)	55#	**100#**	**Pallet jack, dolly**	**MET**
Pulling (Force)	43#	**97#**	"	**MET**
Non-Material Handling Positions and movements in activities and associated tasks (Occ. = 0-33% of day, Freq. = 34-66%, Const. = > 66%) or (Occ. = 1-12/hr, Freq. = 13-60/hr, Const. = > 60/hr)				
Standing	Occasional	**Frequent**	**Frequent**	**MET**
Walking	"	"	"	**MET**
Squatting/Bending	"	"	"	**MET**
Kneeling/Crawling	"	**Occasional**	**Occasional**	**MET**
Reaching/Grasping	Frequent	**Constant**	**Constant**	**MET**
PDC Level (S,L,M,H,VH)	**MEDIUM**	**HEAVY**	**HEAVY**	**MET**
Perceived Disability	Oswestry – 44%	**Oswestry – 22%**		

Physical Demand Levels of Work *Dictionary of Occupational Titles (US Dept. of Labor, Fourth Edition, Revised 1991)*

PDC Level	Occasional (0-33% of day)	Frequent (34-66% of day)	Constant (>66% of day)
Sedentary	*1# to 10#* / Stand & Walk	*Negligible/* Sitting	*Negligible/* Sitting
Light	*11# to 20#*	*Up to 10#* / Stand & Walk *and/or* Standing pushing/pulling controls	*Negligible and/or* Seated & pushing/pulling arm/leg controls
Medium	*21# to 50#*	*11# to 25#*	*Up to 10#*
Heavy	*51# to 100#*	*26# to 50#*	*11# to 20#*
V-Heavy	*Over 100#*	*Over 50#*	*Over 20#*

END OF SUMMARY

Chet D.   Page 2

Figure 15-1 (continued). (Reprinted with permission of Vic Zuccarello, OTR/L, C.E.A.S. II, ABDA Owner - BIO-ERGONOMICS, INC.) *(continued)*

Example of Work Hardening Evaluation Data Pages (from Chet's Initial Evaluation)	Page Three

LUMBAR MUSCULOSKELETAL SCREEN

Resting HR	84 (min acceptable increase = 105)	Resting BP	124/66
Pre Pain Level	5/10	Description	Midline lumbar and R hip
Posture	increased lumbar lordosis, protruding abdomen, PSIS even, no shift.		
Gait	mild R antalgia	Palpation	increased muscle density lumbar PVM's

NEUROLOGICAL

	L	R	Comments
Knee Reflex (L4)	2+	2+	symmetrical
Ankle Reflex (S1)	"	"	"

WADDELL SIGNS
(+) = abnormal response to examination, or possible non-organic sign

TENDERNESS		SIMULATION		DISTRACTION		REGIONAL		OVER-REACTION
Superficial	-	Axial loading	-	L SLR +	R SLR -	Cogwheel	-	-
Non-anatomic	-	Simulated rotation	-	Sit 75	Sit 75	Numb	-	
				Supine 30	Supine 55	Weak	-	

RANGE OF MOTION
(Pre test AROM take 3 trials and calculate coefficient of variance; CV >15% = Inconsistent Test)

MOTION	PRE TEST (°)			AVERAGE (°)	CV%	POST TEST (°)	NORM
Lumbar flexion	35	30	35	33	7.1	30	60
Lumbar extension	10	10	12	11	8.8	15	25
L lateral flexion	20	22	22	21	4.4	15	25
R lateral flexion	20	25	25	23	10.1	25	25

STATIC STRENGTH

MOTION	TRIALS			AVERAGE	CV%	Manual Muscle Test
R knee flexion	34.4	36	40.1	36.8	6.5	4
L knee flexion	26	25	22	24.3	7.0	5
R knee extension	77.3	88	80.2	81.8	5.5	4
L knee extension	33	31	25	29.7	11.5	5
R plantarflexion	33.3	30	34	32.4	5.4	4
L plantarflexion	36.2	36	32	34.7	5.6	5
R dorsiflexion	22	24.4	18.6	21.7	11.0	4
L dorsiflexion	20	22.6	20.6	21.1	5.3	5

QUALITY OF MOVEMENT (Non-Material Handling) SCREEN (5x each)

Squatting	full, UE assist required	Overhead Reach	full, fluid, unguarded
Bending	50%	Finger Flexion	as above
Kneeling	full, UE assist	Opposition	as above
Crawling	symmetrical, guarded	Climbing	step to step, decreased RLE WB.
Comments	Guarding in lower level postures.		
Post-Pain Level (0-10)	6/10 – no change in location of symptoms. Denies need for break, "let's go".		

Chet D.   Page 3

Figure 15-1 (continued). (Reprinted with permission of Vic Zuccarello, OTR/L, C.E.A.S. II, ABDA Owner - BIO-ERGONOMICS, INC.) (continued)

Work Hardening Evaluation	Chet D.	Page Four

Material Handling Test

Description of lift/carry test: This test format is based on other commercial lifting tests and utilizes a lifting box and weights. The worker is instructed in proper body mechanics, the therapist demonstrates proper procedure, and the worker is then allowed to perform a preferred number of practice trials. After each successful lift, weight is added in progressive fashion and the worker is asked if the load is "light, medium, or heavy". The worker is also asked if they feel safe to perform the lift with heavier weight. If the worker answers with a "yes" response and the form on the previous load was safe, weight is added (5-10# for a 'heavy' response, 10-15# for a 'medium' response, and 15-20# for a 'light' response) until one of three termination criteria are met: physiological (ie heart rate, perspiration, flushed complexion); kinesiophysical (ie recruitment of surrounding body parts, substitution, counterbalancing, muscle tremor)); or psychophysical (ie desire to stop because of 'heaviness' of load, perceived pain, or perceived cardiopulmonary exertion). During the test, these aspects of performance are observed and utilized to determine if the worker provided acceptable effort, and if the worker's subjective reports are in proportion with test behavior. Maximum safe effort is solicited and encouraged. The worker is never forced to perform a task they feel is unsafe.

- 50-foot Carrying is assessed by first testing with the max load achieved in the waist to shoulder lift and progressing as in the above procedure.
- Upon reaching the end-point, the load is decreased by 50% and 10 repetitions are performed to determine the frequent carrying load.

Description of push/pull test: Static testing is performed to assess for level of participation in testing as well as to elicit a measure of pushing/pulling strength. The worker is instructed in safe technique (including by not limited to avoidance of jerking or holding the breath, etc.), the therapist demonstrates proper procedure, and a preferred number of practice trials are performed. The worker then performs 6-second trails at their own preferred safe-maximum force. A maximum rest period of 15 seconds is given between 3 trials. Therapist observes for physiological (heart rate, flushed complexion, perspiration); kinesiophysical (substitution, recruitment, tremor, counterbalancing); and psychophysical (pain level, heart rate v. rate of perceived exertion) indicators. Maximum safe effort is solicited/encouraged, but subject is not coerced into providing higher force than they feel is safe.

Pre-test Heart Rate	90	Pre-test Pain Level	5/10

Test	Load (#)	Heart Rate	Rate of Perceived Exertion (6-20)	Pain Level (0-10+)	Kinesiophysical Indicators
Floor to waist lift	25	114	14-15/20	6	Counterbalance and recruitment
Waist to shoulder	25	114	13-14/20	6	"
Overhead Lift		110	14-15/20	6	"
* Carrying Max	25	110	15-16/20	6	"
Pushing (force)	55	115	11-12/20	6	"
Pulling (force)	43	122	"	6	"

Comments: Body mechanics were safe and steady. HR and kinesiophysical signs suggest acceptable effort.

END OF EVALUATION

Figure 15-1 (continued). (Reprinted with permission of Vic Zuccarello, OTR/L, C.E.A.S. II, ABDA Owner - BIO-ERGONOMICS, INC.)

Figure 15-2. (Reprinted with permission of PT Practice Pro.)

- This software is structured much like common office software programs, presenting a dashboard with various tabs and windows that enable the user to move efficiently through different screens such as scheduling, notes, charges, goals, and patient demographic information.

- To the left, you can see the Subjective, Objective, Assessment, and Plan of Care sections of the SOAP note format, each with a drop-down menu for easy access to additional tools for reporting patient data.

- In this example, the occupational therapist has the ability to enter narrative data in the Subjective portion of the note. The occupational therapist can also can easily enter data regarding range of motion and manual muscle testing into pre-formatted tables in the Objective section of the note.

- Note that in the center of the screen, there are tabs for "Show All" and for each section of the SOAP note, so the occupational therapist has options regarding how to view and enter data.

- At the top of the screen, you will see that this software has integrated ICD diagnosis coding, as discussed in Chapter 3. Health care entities were required to switch to the use of ICD-10 codes in October 2015, but patients that were in your documentation system prior to that may have information in the older ICD-9 coding system.

- On the far right is a "Patient Information" pop-up window showing pertinent information about the patient's diagnosis, insurance, and number of authorized visits. By clicking "Dock" in the top right corner, this window would be minimized to allow the occupational therapist to view more of the SOAP note section of the screen.

- The "Snippets" tab at the top of the screen allows the occupational therapist to establish word prediction or shortcuts for commonly used words and phrases. For example, you could type "FL" and the software would automatically change that to "functional limitations."

- In addition to customized patient documentation and billing, this software also has a "Reports" tab that allows managers to track therapist productivity, use of procedures codes, patient cancellation rate, and other clinical measures of interest to employers, funding sources, and accrediting agencies.

- The "Sign" tab at the top of the screen takes the occupational therapist to a page where a password is required to electronically sign the note once documentation has been completed.

Figure 15-3. (Reprinted with permission of AOTA PERFORM developed by Cedaron Medical, Davis, CA, in conjunction with the AOTA.)

Some software systems, like the example in Figure 15-2, can be customized for different rehabilitation disciplines while still retaining a general overall structure. Other software systems are very specific to the occupational therapy profession. For example, AOTA PERFORM software was developed by Cedaron Medical in conjunction with the American Occupational Therapy Association and is based on the *OTPF-III* (AOTA, 2014). See Figures 15-3 through 15-9 for examples of how a software program can be customized to address the specific domain and process of the occupational therapy profession:

- *Figure 15-3*: Similar to the example in Figure 15-2, this screen presents the "Patient Dashboard" which allows the occupational therapist to navigate through a variety of screens to see and edit information related to the patient.
  - To the far left, there is a folder for each date of service, with a drop-down menu to access various documentation forms.
  - Note the box at the top right which alerts the occupational therapist to important information about authorized visits and billing. This box and the "Medicare Fee Schedule" at the bottom of the screen let the occupational therapist know where the patient's billing to date falls in regard to the Medicare Fee Cap, which was discussed in detail in Chapter 3. If the patient requires additional therapy beyond the cap, the occupational therapist must use specialized billing codes or payment will be denied.

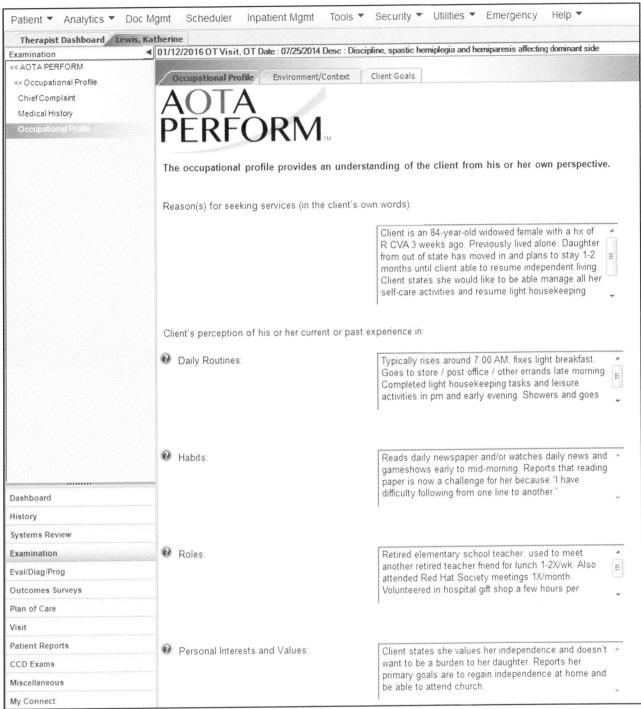

Figure 15-4. (Reprinted with permission of AOTA PERFORM developed by Cedaron Medical, Davis, CA, in conjunction with the AOTA.)

- *Figure 15-4*: Using terminology straight out of the *OTPF-III*, this Occupational Profile tab allows the occupational therapist to enter narrative data about the client's history, routines, habits, roles, and personal interests and values.

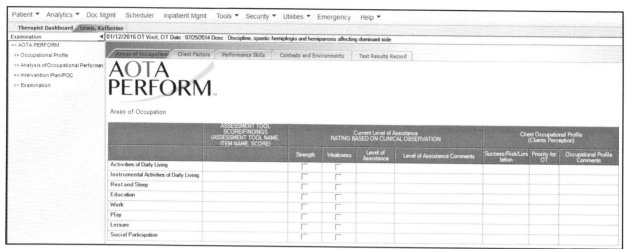

Figure 15-5. (Reprinted with permission of AOTA PERFORM developed by Cedaron Medical, Davis, CA, in conjunction with the AOTA.)

- *Figure 15-5*: This screen lists the eight Areas of Occupation identified in the *OTPF-III* and allows the occupational therapist to enter specific information about any or all of those areas including specific assessment tools used and whether the client considers each area a priority for occupational therapy intervention.

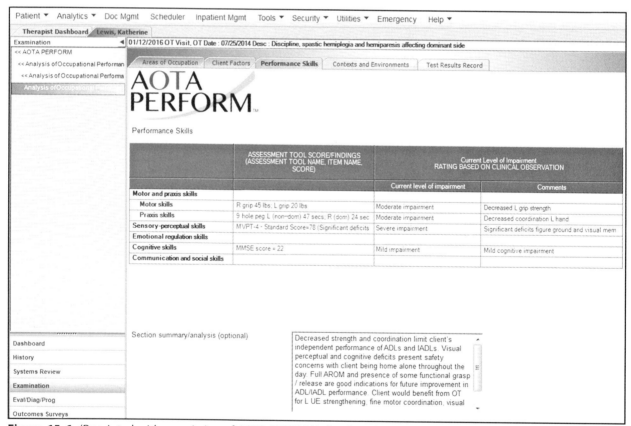

Figure 15-6. (Reprinted with permission of AOTA PERFORM developed by Cedaron Medical, Davis, CA, in conjunction with the AOTA.)

- *Figure 15-6*: This screen allow the occupational therapist to enter specific assessment scores for each Performance Skill identified in the *OTPF-III*. The current level of impairment can be selected from a drop-down menu and narrative comments can also be added in the far right column.

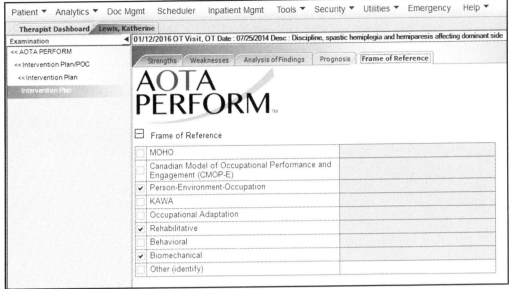

Figure 15-7. (Reprinted with permission of AOTA PERFORM developed by Cedaron Medical, Davis, CA, in conjunction with the AOTA.)

♦ *Figure 15-7*: As discussed in Chapter 12, your approach to client intervention should always be guided by an underlying theoretical framework. This screen allows you to select from many of the commonly used occupational therapy models and frames of reference or to select "Other" and specify a different frame of reference.

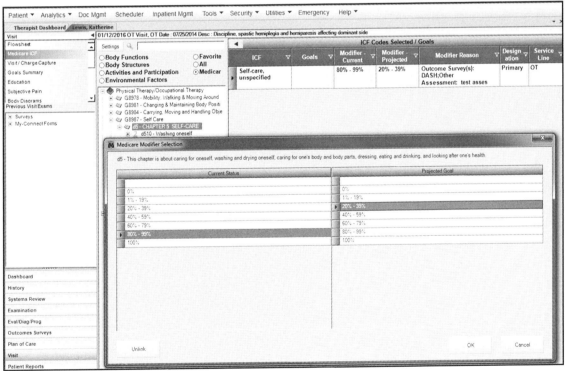

Figure 15-8. (Reprinted with permission of AOTA PERFORM developed by Cedaron Medical, Davis, CA, in conjunction with the AOTA.)

♦ *Figure 15-8*: In Chapter 3, we introduced G-codes that are used for outpatient Medicare billing. This screen shows how the G-codes are integrated into the AOTA PERFORM software. From the left side of the screen, the occupational therapist selects the specific code on which to report and a pop-up screen allows the occupational therapist to select the current status of impairment and projected goal.

Goal Type	#	Goal	Note	Time	Period	Term	Status	Status Date
Occupational Therapy	1	Client will complete bathing task with modified independence using tub transfer bench and hand held- shower		3	Weeks	Long Term	New	12/08/2015
Occupational Therapy	2	Client will complete 3-step cooking activity with modified independence using wheeled walker and rolling cart for item transport		3	Weeks	Long Term	New	12/08/2015
Occupational Therapy	3	Client will complete entire laundry task (washer/dryer/fold & hang-up) with modified independence using wheeled walker, reacher, and rolling cart in 3 weeks		3	Weeks	Long Term	New	12/08/2015
Occupational Therapy	4	Client independently will demo ability to schedule senior transport service via telephone for community outings		3	Weeks	Long Term	New	12/08/2015

Figure 15-9. (Reprinted with permission of AOTA PERFORM developed by Cedaron Medical, Davis, CA, in conjunction with the AOTA.)

- *Figure 15-9:* This Goals Summary screen allows you to select and modify pre-established template goals or to enter free text to create new goals in any format. Note that this therapist has used a COAST format. These goals contain the Client, Occupation, Assist Level, and Specific Condition in the text box, and the Timeline is documented in a separate column.

The examples of electronic documentation discussed thus far in this chapter have focused on adult clients. There are also software programs that are specific to pediatric practice. For example, school therapy doc developed an electronic documentation software for school-based occupational therapy practice. See Figures 15-10 through 15-13 for examples for examples of school-based occupational therapy documentation:

Figure 15-10. (Reprinted with permission of school therapy doc – electronic therapy documentation.)

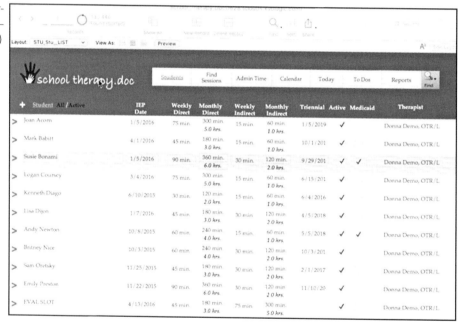

- *Figure 15-10:* This screen allows the occupational therapy practitioner to see a list of children currently on his or her caseload along with the amount of time that should be spent with each student on a weekly or monthly basis according to the student's Individualized Education Program, or IEP. Additionally, this screen provides reminders for the therapist about upcoming IEP dates. In school-based practice, students must receive a formal re-evaluation at least every 3 years. This screen lists the due date of each student's triennial evaluation and also indicates whether a student has Medicaid as a funding source, a situation which may require additional documentation.

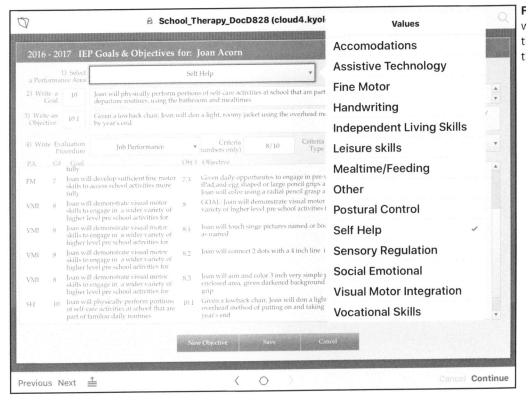

Figure 15-11. (Reprinted with permission of school therapy doc – electronic therapy documentation.)

- *Figure 15-11*: This screen shows an example of IEP goals and objectives. Most electronic software programs have a "bank" of goals that can be customized to fit the needs of each student. Note that with this software program, the therapist can choose a particular performance area to address such as fine motor, feeding, independent living skills, visual motor integration, or several other educationally relevant areas.

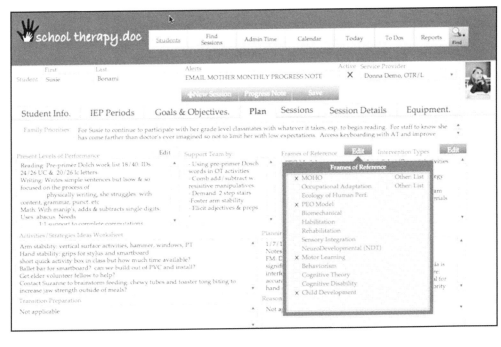

Figure 15-12. (Reprinted with permission of school therapy doc – electronic therapy documentation.)

- *Figure 15-12*: In Chapter 12, you learned how frames of reference guide evaluation and intervention across all areas of occupational therapy practice. This screen gives the documenting therapist an opportunity to identify the frames of reference used to guide each child's IEP goals and interventions.

Figure 15-13. (Reprinted with permission of school therapy doc – electronic therapy documentation.)

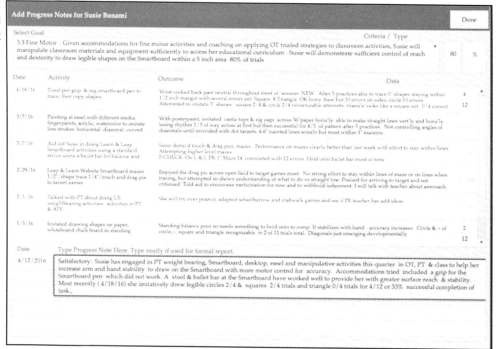

- *Figure 15-13*: IEP goals are often measured by a particular number of repetitions or percentage of correctly performed trials. Since IEP goals are set for 1 year, therapists must collect ongoing data on student performance that can be referenced when writing progress notes. This screen allows the therapist to describe interventions used to address particular goals and to record data and outcomes relating to those interventions. Additionally, this screen allows the therapist to enter a brief progress summary at periodic intervals.

The screenshots presented in this chapter are just a few examples of the dozens of software products available for use in different occupational therapy practice settings. Students often voice concerns that they do not get enough exposure to electronic documentation during their professional education. Some software programs have educational packages that allow instructors and students to practice use of an electronic documentation system. However, you likely will encounter a different software program in every practice setting. Anyone with basic computer skills can learn to use any electronic documentation system with a little bit of practice.

> Please note that the documentation samples contained in the software screenshots in this chapter may not follow the guidelines of this textbook precisely. Additionally, any client names included in the screenshots are fictional and provided only for purposes of demonstrating the features of the software.

REFERENCES

American Occupational Therapy Association. (2014). *Occupational therapy practice framework: Domain & process* (3rd ed.). Bethesda, MD: AOTA Press.

Scott, R. W. (2013). *Legal, ethical, and practical aspects of patient care documentation* (4th ed.). Burlignton, MA: Jones & Bartlett Learning.

Waite, A. (2012). Record time: Point-of-service documentation strategies help practitioners beat the time crunch. *OT Practice*, *17*(1), 9-12.

Chapter 16

Examples of
Different Kinds of Notes

This chapter provides examples of notes from all stages of treatment and from a variety of practice settings. The first group of notes illustrates different stages of treatment and the second set provides examples of single treatment sessions in different practice settings and with various patient populations. The specific format and wording of some notes may differ from the guidelines provided in earlier chapters of this textbook. They are provided here as examples of the wide variety of documentation that you may encounter across occupational therapy practice settings.

CHAPTER CONTENTS

EXAMPLES OF NOTES FOR DIFFERENT STAGES OF TREATMENT

EXAMPLES OF NOTES FOR DIFFERENT PRACTICE SETTINGS AND POPULATIONS

Gateley CA, Borcherding S. *Documentation Manual for
Occupational Therapy: Writing SOAP Notes, Fourth Edition (pp 211-234).*
© 2017 SLACK Incorporated

The notes in this chapter were written by students, faculty, and practicing therapists. The signatures were selected to make the notes anonymous. Required demographic and referral information is limited due to space considerations.

Screening: Neonatal Intensive Care Unit Follow-Up Outpatient Clinic

Name: *Peyton D*   **Age:** *11 months*   **Primary Dx:** *r/o developmental delay*

Pertinent History: *Peyton is an 11-month, 11-day-old male child whose adjusted age is 9 months, 27 days. He was initially discharged from hospital at chronological age 1 month, 2 weeks; adjusted age 2 weeks. Since discharge, Peyton has been seen twice for medical evaluation at the hospital at 3 months adjusted age and 6 months adjusted age. He is being seen today for his first OT developmental screening as a part of the Outpatient Neonatal Follow-Up Program. His mother is present at the evaluation.*

S: *Child is not yet old enough to use language to communicate, but makes sounds ("ba, da, ma," etc.) WFL for adjusted age. Client also makes frequent eye contact with parents and points/reaches toward desired items.*

O: *Today's screening reveals:*
- *Atypical patterns of posture and movement (persistent primitive reflexes, presence of tonic reflexes, moderate increase in muscle tone, limited repertoire of movement, and postural asymmetry).*
- *Possible visual difficulties (immature visual tracking and intermittent malalignment (one/both eyes drift inward).*
- *Delayed milestones (child exhibits skills clustering around the 4- to 6-month developmental level).*
- *Raw score of 24 on the Alberta Infant Motor Scale indicating motor performance below the 5th percentile in comparison to peers of the same adjusted age.*

A: *The findings of this screening indicate that Peyton is experiencing developmental delay, deviance in the pattern of development, and possible visual difficulties, all of which limit his success in play and emerging self-care skills. Peyton would benefit from referral to the state early intervention program to initiate comprehensive evaluation for occupational therapy and other therapy services.*

P: *The mother has been informed of the results of the evaluation, and is in agreement with the following plan:*
- *OT will contact the neonatal follow-up clinic physician regarding vision concerns.*
- *Referral made to state early intervention program to initiate OT services.*
- *Peyton scheduled to return to neonatal follow-up clinic in 3 months.*

Christy N., PhD, OTR/L

SCREENING: PRIMARY CARE CLINIC

Name: Emily S   **Age:** 83   **Primary Dx:** R/O dementia

Pertinent History: Client is an 83-year-old female with an unremarkable medical history. She has had no significant medical concerns up to this point and her only medication is a daily multi-vitamin. After living independently in a very rural area for several years after her husband's death, her family convinced her 3 years ago to move to a small house in town just two doors down from her daughter and son-in-law, who now check on her daily. She has been independent in completing her basic self-care and IADLs, including financial management and driving. Family members requested visit with primary care physician today due to concerns of recent decline in memory function and inability to figure out bank and credit card statements. They also note concerns about patient's safety with driving. Physician requested OT to complete a brief cognitive screen to determine need for more comprehensive evaluation.

S: Pt. reports, "I'm fine. I don't know what all this fuss is about." Pt. noted to have difficulty coming up with family member's names when OT asked pt. to introduce them.

O: Pt. participated in brief screening as part of primary care visit to determine present cognitive level and ability to complete IADL tasks.
Short Blessed Test: Pt.'s performance resulted in a score of 15, which suggests impairment consistent with dementia.
Check Writing Task: Pt. required max verbal cues to fill out a sample check to pay a bill. Handwriting was only minimally legible, and daughter reports this is a recent change.
Road Sign Test: Pt. correctly identified 2 of 8 road signs presented and was dismissive of her errors, claiming that her small town does not have those signs.

A: Cognitive deficits including decreased STM, inability to write checks, and difficulty identifying common road signs result in significant concern for pt. to be driving and managing her financial affairs. Family's awareness of deficits and willingness to provide additional support with financial management and transportation are good indications that pt. may be able to remain in independent living situation for the immediate future. Client would benefit from thorough evaluation by a neuropsychologist to determine extent of cognitive deficits. Client would also benefit from outpatient OT services to establish compensatory measures to maintain independent living status as long as possible. Finally, client would benefit from a thorough driving skills evaluation by an OT Driving Rehabilitation Specialist.

P: Reviewed results of screening and recommendations with patient, family members, and primary care physician. Provided written and online resources for patient and family in dealing with cognitive deficits. Also provided contact information for OT Driving Rehabilitation Specialists within a 2-hour radius of pt.'s hometown. This OT will follow up only if requested by physician during future primary care visits.

Kayleen B., OTR/L

INITIAL EVALUATION REPORT: HIP FRACTURE

Name: Rebecca S   **Age:** 80   **1° Dx:** Ⓛ hip fx   **2° Dx:** HTN

Brief Occupational Profile: Ms. S reports living alone and being Ⓘ in all ADLs prior to admission. She had gone upstairs to use the bathroom since there was none on the first floor. She became lightheaded, fell down the stairs, and broke her hip. She was admitted for a total hip replacement yesterday. Her family lives out of town and cannot stay with her. She wants to return home. Ms. S has supportive neighbors and lives in a small town where she is retired from her position as a second grade teacher. She lives across the street from the elementary school and is in the habit of visiting with the children and some of their families when school is out each day. She is also active in her church.

S: Client stated that she would like to "get this leg well" and go home to "live a regular life." Client rates current pain at surgical site as 6 out of 10.

O: Client participated in 45-minute ADL eval in room to assess capabilities following Ⓛ THR. Client supine in bed upon therapist's arrival; required min Ⓐ for supine to sit to move Ⓛ UE to side of bed while adhering to hip precautions. Client educated on use of ADL equipment for self-care tasks and adherence to hip precautions.

Client demonstrated ability to repeat 2/3 precautions. During ADL evaluation, client was observed flexing 8° to 10° beyond 90° and required 4 verbal cues to remain at or below 90° during the 45-minute session. Other 2 hip precautions were followed. Client performed sponge bath at sink p̄ set-up for upper body, and used dressing stick with washcloth and verbal cues for lower body. Client partial wt. bearing on Ⓛ leg; required min Ⓐ for balance with sit ↔ stand to bathe back peri area. Client able to complete upper body dressing after set-up. Client donned underwear and pants over hips using a dressing stick with min Ⓐ. Client donned socks using sock aid with min Ⓐ. Client completed grooming tasks and oral care Ⓘ from w/c level. Following verbal cues, client demonstrated good problem solving by trying different body positions to perform ADLs while adhering to hip precautions and demonstrated understanding of adaptive aids by utilizing reacher and dressing stick correctly after instruction. Client demonstrated ↓ activity tolerance as she required four 2-minute rest breaks during dressing tasks. Client then taken to OT clinic for evaluation of client factors:

Ⓑ *UE AROM: WFL* Ⓑ *UE strength: WFL*

UE sensation: Intact *Grip strength:* Ⓡ *47#,* Ⓛ *43# (*Ⓡ *hand dominant)*

Tripod pinch: Ⓡ *10#,* Ⓛ *5#* *Lateral pinch:* Ⓡ *10#,* Ⓛ *5#*

A: *↓ endurance, ↓ balance, and inconsistent compliance with hip precautions present safety concerns during lower body dressing and bathing. These problem areas negatively affect client's ability to be safe and Ⓘ with ADLs. Client's motivation, problem-solving skills, and understanding of equipment use indicate excellent rehab potential. Upper body strength and AROM WFL are beneficial to learning adaptive techniques for self-care and functional mobility. Client would benefit from skilled instruction on hip precautions and use of adaptive equipment with ADL performance, therapeutic activities that facilitate dynamic standing balance, and ↑ ADL activity tolerance. Exploration of interim living arrangement or possible continued home visits and home equipment procurement will be needed if progress warrants discharge to home.*

P: *Client to be seen bid for 1 hour the next 3 days to ↑ independence in self-care tasks through instruction on hip precautions and use of adaptive equipment, with tasks to ↑ activity tolerance, and dynamic standing activities.*

LTG: *By anticipated discharge in 4 days, client will:*

- *Safely complete lower body dressing and bathing modified Ⓘ utilizing adaptive equipment with 100% adherence to hip precautions.*
- *Safely complete toileting mod Ⓘ using adaptive equipment (walker & bedside commode).*

STG:

- *By next tx session, client will complete toileting with SBA for sit ↔ stand from bedside commode and manage clothing with no more than 2 verbal cues.*
- *By 2nd session, client will don shoes and socks with modified Ⓘ, utilizing adapted techniques and devices with 100% adherence to hip precautions.*
- *By 3rd session, client will complete all lower body dressing tasks with SBA using adaptive equipment with no more than one 30-second rest break.*
- *By 3rd session, client will complete toileting with SBA using wheeled walker and commode frame over toilet.*
- *By 4th session, client will safely bathe her peri area modified Ⓘ utilizing adaptive techniques and devices with 100% adherence to hip precautions.*

Tiffany B., OTR/L

INTERVENTION PLAN: HIP FRACTURE

Strengths: *UE strength & AROM WFL; intact cognition and motivation to return home*

Functional Problem Statement #1: *↑ fatigue, ↓ endurance for ADLs, and inconsistent compliance with hip precautions makes client unsafe in ADL tasks.*

Long-Term Goal #1: *By anticipated discharge in 4 days, client will safely complete lower body dressing and bathing modified Ⓘ utilizing adaptive equipment with 100% adherence to hip precautions.*

STG (Objective)	Intervention
STG #1: *By 2nd session, client will don shoes & socks with modified ①, using adapted techniques & devices with 100% adherence to hip precautions.*	1. *Instruct & have client verbalize 3/3 hip precautions.* 2. *Provide written handout of hip precautions.* 3. *Instruct in use of adaptive techniques/devices followed by demonstration of use in dressing activities.*
STG #2: *By 3rd session, client will complete all lower body dressing tasks with SBA using adaptive equipment with no more than one 30-second rest break.*	1. *Continue instruction in use of adaptive techniques/devices followed by demonstration of use in dressing activities.* 2. *Educate client and provide written instructions on energy conservation techniques. Evaluate understanding by her application during ADL task; ask about how she performs ADL tasks at home.*
STG #3: *By 4th session, client will safely bathe her peri area modified ① using adaptive techniques and devices with 100% adherence to hip precautions.*	1. *Instruct in use of adaptive techniques/devices followed by demonstration of use in bathing activities.* 2. *Instruct in manipulation of clothing and bathing items while standing in walker at sink s̄ violating hip precautions.* 3. *Assess for home equipment needs and continued home services if progress warrants discharge to home.*

Functional Problem Statement #2: ↓ *dynamic standing balance makes client unsafe during ADL tasks.*
Long-Term Goal #2: *By anticipated discharge in 4 days, client will safely complete toileting mod ① using adaptive equipment (walker & bedside commode).*

STG (Objective)	Intervention
STG #1: *By next tx session, client will complete toileting with SBA for sit ↔ stand from bedside commode and manage clothing with no more than 2 verbal cues.*	1. *Instruct client in safe transfer techniques; reinforce compliance with total hip precautions.* 2. *Provide UE strengthening through reaching and wt. bearing activities at sink and closet for grooming and dressing items and pushing up from chair and bedside commode.*
STG #2: *By 3rd session, client will complete toileting with SBA using wheeled walker and commode frame over toilet.*	1. *Continue instruction in safe transfer techniques; reinforce compliance with total hip precautions.* 2. *Interview client regarding home environment; explore and discuss interim living arrangements or possible equipment use & placement in home; discuss support services needed if discharge home is warranted.*

Initial Evaluation: Seating and Mobility

Name: *Breanna C*   **Age:** *17*
Primary Dx: *Incomplete C6 SCI due to motor vehicle accident (MVA)*   **Secondary Dx:** *Depression*
Medical History & Occupational Profile: *Breanna is a 17-year-old young woman with a diagnosis of incomplete C6 SCI resulting from an MVA on her prom night. Her boyfriend was killed in the MVA, and Breanna continues to deal with depression related to that event and her residual functional deficits. Breanna had no significant medical history prior to the MVA. She will be a senior in high school this fall and enjoys photography and playing piano. She lives at home with her parents and 15-year-old brother. Breanna has undergone 6 weeks of intensive inpatient rehabilitation. She is being evaluated for a power wheelchair in preparation for discharge home. Breanna, her mother, and the rehab facility OT attended this evaluation.*
Current Seating/Mobility: *For the last 2 weeks of her rehabilitation stay, Breanna has utilized a loaner tilt-in-space power wheelchair on a trial basis. Per client, family, & staff report, Breanna has been independent with mobility in her hospital room and throughout the facility.*

Home Environment: *(based on report from rehab facility OT)* Home is a large one-level ranch with an open floor plan. Family has already made considerable modification to the home including installation of ramp to enter front door, widening of doorways, and renovation of bathroom for w/c accessibility. Breanna completed a home visit with the facility OT 1 week ago and reportedly was able to access the bedroom, living room, kitchen, dining room, bathroom, and patio using the power w/c. Mother reports that an anonymous member from their church has donated a van with a w/c lift.

Cognitive/Visual Status: Rehab OT, speech therapist, and neuropsychologist report Breanna's cognitive and visual perceptual function as WNL.

ADL Status: Breanna is able to complete upper body dressing and bathing with set-up. She requires moderate assistance with lower body dressing and bathing using adaptive equipment. She currently requires maximum assistance for bowel program and catheter management, although rehab team is addressing client and caregiver training this week to increase Breanna's independence with these tasks.

UE Function: Breanna has 4/5 strength throughout her dominant Ⓡ UE. She has 3+/5 strength in her Ⓛ UE shoulder and elbow, and no active movement in her Ⓛ wrist or hand.

Sensation: Sensation intact Ⓡ UE; absent in distal Ⓛ UE. Impaired Ⓡ trunk & LE; absent Ⓛ trunk & LE.

Transfers/Mobility: Breanna requires minimal assist for bed mobility with a rail, including supine → sit. Breanna completes a squat pivot transfer w/c ↔ bed/toilet with moderate assist. She is independent in maneuvering a power wheelchair using a standard joystick. She is also able to operate the tilt-in-space option independently for pressure relief.

Assessment: Breanna is non-ambulatory due to motor impairments resulting from incomplete C6 SCI. She is unable to propel a manual w/c independently due to significant impairments of Ⓛ UE AROM and strength as well as decreased strength in Ⓡ UE. Breanna is not a candidate for a scooter as she would not be able to transfer safely into a scooter seating system or operate the tiller driving system effectively. Therefore, the use of a power wheelchair is necessary to improve Breanna's ability to participate in mobility-related activities of daily living. Tilt-in-space and air cushion are necessary as Breanna sits in the w/c for 10+ hours daily and is therefore at high risk for development of pressure ulcers. Breanna is unable to perform a functional weight shift and unable to transfer independently to the bed for pressure relief.

Without this device, Breanna would be at risk for decreased ability to participate in mobility-related activities of daily living such as accessing the bathroom for bathing and toileting and accessing the dining room for family meals. She would have no independent, safe, or effective means of mobility or function within her home, school, or community. Additionally, she would be at significant risk for development of pressure sores, postural deformity, and pain.

Recommendation: Recommend purchase of the following to accommodate Breanna's body dimensions, postural alignment, and pressure relief needs:

- 18" x 16" power wheelchair with power tilt-in-space
- Push-button lap belt
- Desk-length flip-up height-adjustable armrests with standard joystick mounted on right armrest
- Removable headrest
- Rear anti-tippers for stability during tilt of wheelchair
- Ankle straps & heel loops to maintain feet on footplates
- Air cushion with incontinence cover to prevent pressure ulcers
- Lap board for UE support during feeding and school activities
- Standard tires & casters with flat free inserts

Plan: Breanna will discharge home using existing loaner wheelchair from this company. Upon insurance approval of the above recommendations, equipment will be delivered to Breanna's home for fitting and training in safe and effective use. Follow-up appointments will be conducted as needed for modification of equipment.

Matt C., OTR/L, ATP, RTS

INTERVENTION PLAN: CANCER

Name: Allison M   **Age:** 35   **Primary Dx:** Mastectomy 2° breast CA

Strengths: Prior to surgery, Allison was in good physical condition and employed full-time. She has some social support from her sister who lives in another state.

Functional Problem Statement: *Allison avoids social outings with friends due to ↓ self-esteem secondary to cosmetic alterations imposed by mastectomy procedure, which precludes her ability to return to work.*

Long-Term Goal: *Allison will ↑ social interactions and activity to 6 outings/month within the next month, in preparation for return to work.*

STG (Objective)	Intervention
STG #1: Allison will identify one support group of interest to her within 1 week to ↑ willingness to be out in public for work and social activities.	1. Educate Allison re: available support groups and peer visitation groups, their contact persons, telephone numbers, and social media information, and ask her whether she has made contact. 2. Ask if Allison would like to have her contact information given to a volunteer from the hospital's peer mentor group.
STG #2: Allison will attend 1 support group activity within 2 weeks to ↑ confidence in social and work situations.	1. E-mail and/or phone call to remind Allison of upcoming support group meetings. 2. Discuss with Allison her experiences with the support groups.
STG #3: Allison will initiate conversation with at least one other support group member during her first visit to the group to ↓ negative impact of cosmetic alterations to body image.	1. Accompany Allison into the community the first time she goes out. 2. Encourage participation in group discussion.
STG #4: Allison will enroll in a women's exercise program to ↑ activity tolerance and positive body image.	1. Educate Allison re: area exercise groups for post-mastectomy clients. 2. Follow-up phone call/email to ask if she has enrolled in an exercise program.
STG #5: Allison will identify 5 assets she possesses other than physical to ↑ self-esteem and confidence in social and work situations.	1. Discuss Allison's assets with her, encouraging her to think of as many as she can. 2. Educate Allison regarding books and websites that address post-mastectomy concerns.

Functional Problem Statement: *Allison is unable to return to work 2° 3/4 AROM, 4-/5 muscle strength, ↓ activity tolerance (fatigues after 1 hr.), and sensory changes.*

Long-Term Goal: *Allison will return to work part-time within 4 weeks.*

STG (Objective)	Intervention
STG #1: Within 2 weeks, Allison will complete 2 hours of work tasks with no more than one 15-minute rest break.	1. Scar massage and myofascial release to incision area along with client education on self-massage. 2. PROM to Ⓛ shoulder—instruct in self-ranging program. 3. Work simulation tasks.
STG #2: Allison will retrieve 5 items from overhead shelf Ⓘ using Ⓛ UE in work simulation task within 3 weeks.	1. Active resistive ROM to Ⓛ UE. 2. Resistive strengthening with thera-tubing, weights, and graded functional activities. 3. Work simulation tasks.
STG #3: Within 3 weeks, Allison will transfer twenty 5# boxes from one table to another in < 10 minutes using Ⓑ UEs with reported pain level < 2/10.	1. Work simulation with client education on energy conservation principles. 2. Provide home exercise program and modify as client progresses.
STG #4: Within 3 weeks, Allison will complete seated and active work tasks using correct body mechanics Ⓘ to have pain level of < 2/10 while working.	1. Educate in ergonomics and posture to prevent pain. 2. Provide education on women's exercise groups.
STG #5: Allison will complete work and daily living tasks while Ⓘ demonstrating sensory precautions within 2 weeks.	1. Provide education on safety concerns with sensory loss. 2. IADL tasks and work simulation with sensory hazards to check application of safety techniques.

RE-EVALUATION: WORK HARDENING (FACILITY FORMAT)

Note: This example contains terminology and abbreviations specific to a work hardening setting that are not listed in Chapter 4.

Worker: *Joe Fireman*   **Age:** *33*   **Job Title:** *Firefighter/Paramedic*
Physician: *Dr. Pain*   **Dx:** *s/p Ⓛ shoulder reconstruction*   **Attendance:** *5/5 sessions*
Subjective Complaints: *Pain level was rated as 3-4/10 pre-test and post-test. He described sharp pain near the left acromioclavicular (AC) joint, with aching in the anterior/posterior deltoid and into the left upper trapezius musculature.*
Work Plan: *Return to his usual and customary job when able.*
Perceived Disability: *Worker scored 14/70 on the Pain Disability Index, which indicates a low level of self-perceived disability. This represents a moderate improvement from 39/70 upon initial evaluation.*
Musculoskeletal Screen
Musculoskeletal Deficit Changes Since Last Eval: *In comparison to the unaffected right shoulder, slight ROM gains are noted with the Ⓛ UE, while still remaining below expected AMA norms. Left shoulder strength is 5/5 within the given range (exception for external rotation 4+/5), while Ⓡ UE strength is 5/5 in all planes. Occasional sustained forward/overhead reaching task continues to be completed at an above competitive proficiency level*
Quality of Movement Changes: *Functional overhead reaching and internal/external rotation with the Ⓛ UE has improved, but remains decreased vs Ⓡ UE. Mild decreased control was noted with the Ⓛ UE with maximum load handling at all levels. Mild compensation patterns were observed with use of Ⓛ UE when crawling and climbing ladders.*

Summary of Demonstrated Abilities

MATERIAL HANDLING	MAX OCCASIONAL (LBS.)			EMPLOYER-REPORTED JOB REQUIREMENTS
	Entrance (5/03/17)	*Re-Eval (5/17/17)*	*Re-Eval (6/07/17)*	
Floor—Waist Lift	55	60	70	*May lift > 100 lbs from floor to chest or shoulder height in emergency scenarios (occas.); may handle tools up to 45 lbs lifting floor to overhead (up to frequent as needed).*
Waist—Shoulder Lift	20	45	55	
Shoulder—Overhead Lift	15	35	40	
Bilateral Carry	60	60	70	
Unilateral Lift/Carry (L/R)	30/55	55/55	55/55	
Pushing (force) (L/R)	73 (31/42)	57 (31/31)	89 (39/51)	*Up to 70 lbs (hands in front); up to 35 lbs overhead push/pull with pike pole.*
Pulling (force) (L/R)	70 (33/37)	57 (35/25)	80 (41/39)	
NON-MATERIAL HANDLING	FREQUENCY DISPLAYED			JOB REQUIREMENTS
Sitting	*Unrestricted*	*Unrestricted*	*Unrestricted*	*Occasional*
Standing	*Unrestricted*	*Unrestricted*	*Unrestricted*	*Frequent*
Walking	*Unrestricted*	*Unrestricted*	*Unrestricted*	*Frequent*
Climbing	*Limited*	*Improved*	*Frequent*	*Frequent*
Bending	*Unrestricted*	*Unrestricted*	*Unrestricted*	*Frequent*
Reaching (Forward/Overhead)	*Occasional/ Limited*	*Occasional/ Limited*	*Frequent*	*Frequent*
Squatting/Kneeling	*Unrestricted*	*Unrestricted*	*Unrestricted*	*Frequent*
Crawling	*Occasional*	*Occasional*	*Up to Frequent*	*Occasional*

Consistency and Quality of Effort

Client continues to provide good and consistent effort with testing, based upon positive HR response to activity, low coefficients of variation (CV) values with ROM/static strength tests, and the presence of external effort indicators. Please see chart below for description of criteria.

Global Effort Rating: Consistency and Quality of Effort Indicators

CRITERION	RESULT	COMMENTS
Pain Diagram: *Reports of circumferential pain, glove, or stocking presentation would in most cases be supported in the literature as inconsistent with the diagnosis.*	*Expected*	*No unusual markings for given diagnosis.*
Pain Behavior and Function: *High pain ratings should be consistent with altered movement patterns and range of motion. Alteration of movement patterns should be consistent in associated tasks/transitional movement patterns v. direct measurement. A patient's behavior should consistently reflect distress, and not only during performance of evaluation tasks.*	*Expected*	*Pain level was rated as 3-4/10 pre-test, up to 5/10 with testing, and as 3-4/10 post-test. Subjective reports were consistent with displayed function.*
Perceived Disability Score: *In the absence of organic findings, high-perceived disability may compromise recovery from injury.*	*Expected*	*Client's score on the Perceived Disability Inventory (14/70) indicates a low level of self-perceived disability at this time.*
Coefficients of Variation: *Repeated test trials must be low to indicate consistent effort.*	*Expected*	*Worker displayed high CV values during 0 of 10 ROM tests and 0 of 6 static strength tests.*
5-Position Grip (bell-curve): *Deviation from bell-curves may indicate submaximal effort, especially when performed on non-hand diagnoses.*	*Expected*	*Worker displayed modified bell-shaped distribution on right/left.*
Cross-Reference Validity Check: *Tests repeated at intervals with full volitional effort with >20% variation may be indicator of sub-maximal effort.*	*Expected*	*Variance between results for position 2 on standard grip test and Maximum Modified Voluntary Effort (MMVE) test was 12.1% to 18.8%.*
Static Force Curve Analysis: *Force curves during static trials should follow a predictable pattern. Delayed and/or erratic force curves may indicate that maximal effort was not achieved during that test.*	*Expected*	*During static strength testing, delayed peak contractions and erratic force curves were noted during 0 of 18 trials.*
HR and RPE Correlation: *A patient's report of physical exertion (RPE) should correlate with a corresponding increase in working HR.*	*Expected*	*Working HR and corresponding RPE values were proportionate in all instances.*

Impression

- *Client has provided high levels of effort while attending 5 scheduled sessions on the most recent prescription, resulting in additional gains with heavy load handling, pushing/pulling ability, and tolerance for sustained work-simulated activities. He continues to wear his turn-out gear during sessions to simulate completing essential job functions.*
- *Mr. Fireman has displayed safe function in at least the Medium work demand level, with some function into the heavy demand level, up to the above-listed tolerances. The abilities displayed with testing this date do not meet the employer-reported essential job demands. The main factors limiting return to work continue to be decreased tolerance for the required work demand level, decreased load handling ability, decreased push/pull tolerances, decreased tolerance for sustained work tasks involving the Ⓛ UE (reaching, tool use), decreased active ROM for overhead job tasks, and his subjective pain complaints at this time.*

Plan

Mr. Fireman has a follow-up appointment with physician 7/08/17. We will await your recommendations.

Shelia T., OTR/L, CHT, CEAS

RE-EVALUATION NOTE: DRIVER REHABILITATION

Name: *Alex L*   ***Age:*** *71*   ***Dx:*** *Multiple transient ischemic attacks*

S: Client reports successful completion of 6-week mature driver improvement course recommended during initial evaluation 2 months ago. "I do okay during the day, but I'm afraid to drive at night. I just don't see that well." Client declined opportunity to drive on 4-lane highway during on-road assessment, indicating that he only drives short distances in his small community and relies on family for longer distance transportation.

O: Client participated in driving re-evaluation this date to determine safety and independence with community mobility. Previous evaluation 2 months ago revealed minor hearing deficits, decreased reaction times, mild left inattention, and impaired ability to recognize and understand road signs.

In-Clinic Evaluation: Visual acuity WFL with bifocal lenses; depth perception WFL. No left inattention observed. Client scored WFL on brake reaction time test. Client correctly identified meaning of 29 of 30 road signs (missed side road intersection sign).

On-Road Evaluation: Client completed 20 minutes driving in car in residential and commercial areas of a suburban area. Results are as follow:

- Client demonstrated proper use of mirrors and over-the-shoulder checks; observed and responded to turn signals of other drivers by slowing down and obeyed all road signs and traffic control devices. Client demonstrated adequate visual scanning when entering the roadway and at all intersections.
- Client correctly used turn signals at appropriate times and activated horn, headlights, and emergency flashers when instructed to do so.
- Client observed posted speed limits and made appropriate adjustments to speed related to intersections, traffic flow, and roadway surfaces. Client demonstrated proper vehicle positioning while moving forward in traffic and before, during, and after all turns.
- Client demonstrated appropriate time and space judgment when changing lanes and negotiating intersections. Client demonstrated adequate brake, accelerator, and steering control when driving forward, backing up, merging, and parking.

A: Improvements noted in visual perception, reaction time, cognition (understanding road signs), and functional driving performance as compared to initial evaluation 2 months ago. Client's performance this date indicates ability to operate a motor vehicle safely in residential and commercial environments. Decreased night vision and comfort level with driving on busy highways pose safety concerns for driving in those situations. Client would benefit from continued family assistance for night-time or long-distance transportation.

P: It is recommended that client's driving be restricted to daylight hours in rural and small town areas. Client should not drive at night or on large, busy highways. Recommendations have been discussed with client and family. They voice understanding that the results of this evaluation are indicative only of the client's functional driving ability on this date. Any changes in health or cognition that would affect driving should be addressed through follow-up with client's physician for potential referral to a Certified Driving Rehabilitation Specialist (CDRS).

Travis L., OTR/L, CDRS

Adapted from content in *Documenting Driver Rehabilitation Services and Outcomes*, Shipp & Havard, 2006.

PROGRESS NOTE: INPATIENT MENTAL HEALTH

S: During the first 2 days of admission, Ms. J elected not to attend OT group sessions, stating that she was too "anxious and overwhelmed."

O: Client stayed in her room most of the time for first 2 days despite consistent invitations to attend groups and participate in recreational activities. On this day, the client attended a stress management group. Initially she was quiet, but gradually began entering into the activity. She was able to identify specific physical, emotional, and behavioral symptoms that she experiences when feeling overwhelmed or anxious. Ms. J stated that she previously had not been aware of these stress reactions.

A: *Anxiety related to social situations limits client's social interactions with others and participation in community and leisure activities. Initiation of group attendance and participation are good indications of progress. Additional progress indicated by recognizing specific symptoms of stress as opposed to relating only general feelings. Client would benefit from participation in daily OT groups focused on stress management.*

P: *Continue all goals as originally stated. Client to be seen daily for 3 days to provide opportunities for Ms. J to learn basic stress management techniques so that she may recognize and control stress reactions when she begins feeling overwhelmed or anxious.*

David L., OTR/L

PROGRESS NOTE: COMMUNITY MENTAL HEALTH

Transitional Housing Facility Monthly Progress Note

Name: *Marco*   **1° Dx:** *Schizophrenia*   **2° Dx:** *Substance abuse*

S: *Client reports feeling "very stressed" thinking about the upcoming holidays and "having to do what my family wants me to do. They think just because I have schizophrenia, I'm also stupid." Client also reports feeling "great" about his ability to maintain sobriety for 1 month.*

O: *Client completed first month at transitional housing facility. OT attendance, participation, and goals addressed are summarized below:*

GROUP PARTICIPATION		
Group Name	**# Attended**	**Full Participation**
Cooking Club	2 of 3	2
Procovery	2 of 4	2
House Meeting	4 of 4	4
Health Class	4 of 4	3
Substance Abuse	2 of 3	2
Grocery Shopping	3 of 4	3
Leisure Trips	3 of 4	3

INDIVIDUAL SERVICE PARTICIPATION	
1-on-1 Appointments	**#**
Completed	7
No Shows	0
Cancelled/Rescheduled	0
1-on-1 Hours	**#**
Total Spent with OT	6 hrs
Total Spent with OTS	2 hrs

Goals Addressed During Groups & Individualized Service Meetings

	Access/Linkage/ Transportation	X	Computer Skills		Hygiene/ Self-Care		Medical Health	X	Self-Esteem
X	Advocacy (Personal/Political)	X	Cooking		IADL Assessment	X	Mental Illness Education	X	Substance Use
X	Anger/Emotion/ Stress Mgmt		Discharge Planning	X	Interpersonal Skills		Non-Grocery Shopping	X	Symptom Mgmt
	BADL Assessment		Education/GED		Laundry/ Clothing Care	X	Nutrition/Meal Planning	X	Time Mgmt
X	Budgeting/Money Handling		Family Support/ Development	X	Leisure/Social		Problem Solving		Vocational/Work
	Bus Training	X	Goal Setting		Literacy	X	Routine/Schedule and Organization		Volunteering/ Productive Occupation
	Cleaning/Home Care	X	Grocery Shopping		Medication Mgmt		Safety		Others (specify below)

Family Interactions: Client set a plan for self-advocacy with family with max verbal cues. Following interpersonal skills training, client requested to contact family members to practice new skills. In two 30-minute visits, client demonstrated reciprocal conversation without outbursts, accusatory statements, or passive-aggressive behaviors.

Sobriety: Despite noted stressors, he independently was able to follow sobriety plan he created at admission.

Internet Use: Client able to access novel and routine websites of choice with min verbal cues (required moderate assist at admission) required for impulsivity and attention to task. Client has also established 2 social media accounts and posts thus far have been socially appropriate.

IADLs: Client completed grocery shopping with min verbal cues for item location and price comparison (required mod assist at admission). Client declined to work on budgeting/savings plan this month due to spending all his income on the upcoming holidays. Client indicated desire to budget next month with intent to save $50 toward a television set for his room.

A: Stress related to family perceptions and expectations results in ineffective interactions with family members. Ability to participate in reciprocal conversation without negative interactions demonstrates progress toward goals. Sobriety for 1 month indicates great progress toward client's goal of refraining from drug & alcohol use. Impulsivity and decreased attention to task limit client's independent Internet usage, but decreased need for verbal cues this month indicates progress. Continued need for assistance with budgeting and grocery shopping limit client's ability to transition to more independent living situation, but progress with grocery shopping indicates good potential for this goal. Client would benefit from continued group and individual service participation in this transitional housing facility to address limitations in social interaction, sobriety, Internet usage, and independent living skills.

P: Client to attend all scheduled weekly groups and twice-weekly individual OT sessions to address social participation, sobriety, Internet usage, and independent living skills. Plan to help client establish and follow monthly budget, increase social contact with family, maintain sobriety plan, and increase independence with Internet usage.

Stephanie S., OTR/L, QMHP

Progress Note: Balance and Vestibular Rehabilitation

Name: *Juanita S*   **Age:** *73*
1° Dx: Ⓛ *peripheral vestibulopathy*   **2° Dx:** *OA, CAD,* Ⓑ *cataracts*

S: Pt. reports continued feelings of spinning, blurred vision, and difficulty walking. She reports she has not completed the home exercises provided 2 weeks ago during evaluation because they make her feel dizzy and she gets scared. She also reports needing to hold onto the shower door for support when stepping in/out of the tub. No recent falls reported.

O: Client has participated in two 45-minute balance sessions in outpatient OT clinic to address balance deficits identified during initial eval. 2 weeks ago.

Current Status: Client is able to keep eyes forward on target and perform 10 reps of slow head turns with report of increased dizziness from 1 to 3 (0 = no symptoms, 10 = most extreme symptoms). Client is able to follow visual target up and down with report of dizziness from 1 to 3 (same scale). With min verbal cues, client able to increase speed of head movements without further increase in reported dizziness.

Client Education: Client was re-educated regarding the balance system, her dx, the reason for OT, and the importance of consistency with her home exercises for balance; client voiced understanding. HEP modified to accommodate client's comfort level with exercises, and she demonstrated ability to complete:

- Steady gaze with head turns
- Following visual target vertically, horizontally, diagonally during IADL task (putting away dishes)

Pt. also instructed to have family member present for safety when bathing; voiced understanding. Written recommendations provided to client and reviewed with daughter at end of session.

A: Continued report of dizziness and habit of holding onto shower door during shower transfer indicate safety concerns with ADL & IADL tasks. Decline in dizziness rating (3/10) this session shows progress from initial evaluation rating (6/10). With consistent performance of HEP and continued balance & vestibular rehabilitation, *client has potential to decrease dizziness and increase her safety in her independent living situation. Client would benefit from continued occupational therapy to address compensatory strategies during ADLs and IADLs.*

P: *Continue occupational therapy 1x/wk for 4 wks to address safety concerns related to symptoms of Ⓛ peripheral vestibulopathy. Sessions to focus on increasing client's tolerance of head movements without increased dizziness and client education regarding compensatory strategies for increased safety during ADLs and IADLs.*

Patricia D., OTR/L

TRANSITION PLAN: REHAB

S: *Client said, "I feel so much better than I did a while back. I feel like I've come a long way."*

O: *Client participated in 15/20 scheduled tx sessions from SOC, with last few sessions focused on transition planning from inpatient to skilled nursing setting. Client illness and medical testing prevented attending 5 sessions. OT sessions focused on ADL retraining, toileting, functional transfer training, ↑ AROM, and strength. Client level of function at transition is as follows:*

GOALS	INITIAL	TRANSITION
Dressing: UE mod Ⓘ LE mod Ⓘ	Min Ⓐ for balance Mod Ⓐ for balance	Set-up CGA when standing to don underwear & pants
Bathing: UE mod Ⓘ LE mod Ⓘ	Min Ⓐ Min Ⓐ	Mod Ⓘ seated on shower chair Mod Ⓘ using long-handled sponge
Transfers: • sit ↔ supine Ⓘ • stand ↔ w/c & toilet mod Ⓘ	SBA Min Ⓐ	SBA SBA
AROM – WFL Ⓡ	Shoulder abd 65° (strength 2) Shoulder flex 55° (strength 2) Elbow 0° to 125° (strength 3)	Shoulder abd 90° (strength 3) Shoulder flex 60° (strength 3) Elbow WFL (strength 4)

A: *Residual deficits in balance and strength limit client's independence with ADLs and functional transfers. Increased Ⓡ UE AROM and strength indicate progress. Client has met bathing and hygiene goals. Dressing and transfer goals partially met. Client continues to make progress and would benefit from further OT intervention to increase UE strength and activity tolerance to perform ADLs Ⓘ and meet all goals.*

P: *Discharged from inpatient occupational therapy 2° change of status from Medicare Part A → Medicare B. Request physician's orders to re-evaluate under Medicare B in SNF. Upon physician's orders, recommend skilled OT intervention 3x week to increase activity tolerance and strength to perform ADLs Ⓘ.*

Jessica T., OTR/L

DISCHARGE NOTE: SOAP FORMAT

S: *Client reports "doing a lot better" and being "less confused" than he was on admission.*

O: *Client initially presented with multiple trauma 2° to MVA. Occupational therapist evaluation 1 week ago indicated client had deficits in short-term memory, safety awareness, attention to task, and ADL status. Client participated in 5 OT sessions of ADL retraining for dressing and grooming and functional mobility. Client and family received skilled instruction in safety precautions in the home. Client's functional status on admit and discharge as follows:*

Goal #	Admit Status	Goal	Discharge Status
1	Min Ⓐ in grooming	Set-up/supervision	Set-up/supervision
2	CGA toilet transfers	SBA	SBA
3	Supine → sit c̄ min Ⓐ	SBA	SBA
4	Min Ⓐ UE dressing	Set-up/supervision	Set-up/supervision

A: All goals achieved due to improved cognitive status, awareness of safety precautions, and skilled instruction in ADLs. Residual attention and short-term memory deficits limit client's safety independence with higher level ADL and IADL tasks. Client would benefit from supervision at home 2° remaining cognitive deficits.

P: Client discharged to home. Recommend home health occupational therapist evaluation for safety in home environment and potential for necessary durable medical equipment. No home exercise program given. No other referrals at time of discharge. Occupational therapist will follow-up in 1 month by phone to check client's functional status in the home.

Kayleen B., OTR/L

Discharge Note: Facility Format

Name: Marjorie P   **Primary Dx:** CVA   **Secondary Dx:** Arthritis
_X_ Occupational Therapy   __ Physical Therapy   __ Communicative Disorders
Course of Treatment: Client participated in 30-minute sessions daily for 9 days following CVA to work on ↑ independence in self-care skills, functional mobility, UE strengthening, energy conservation, and activity tolerance.
Status at Discharge: Client reports feeling much better and is ready to go home.

Admit Status	Discharge Status
Self-care mod Ⓐ	Self-care Ⓘ and safe
Functional mobility mod Ⓐ	Functional mobility Ⓘ and safe
Activity tolerance 7 minutes for ADLs	Activity tolerance 10 minutes for ADLs

Goals Met: Client has met self-care and functional mobility goals using energy conservation techniques.
Goals Not Met: Activity tolerance goal not met due to client declining last 2 treatment sessions when she learned she was being discharged.
Client/Family Education: Client instructed in and demonstrates understanding of HEP. Handouts provided. Client reports having weights at home she can use for continued UE strengthening as instructed in her HEP.
Recommendations: Discharge client to her sister's home due to goals being met. HEP attached. No home health recommended at this time.

Hailey S., OTR/L

Consulting Note: Assistive Technology (Facility Format)

Occupational therapists are often members of an assistive technology team when assessing clients for augmentative and alternative communication (AAC) devices or other assistive technology equipment. The following note was co-written by an occupational therapist and a speech-language pathologist (SLP). It is not in SOAP format because it is being sent to a local agency for funding of recommended equipment.

Name: Micaela N   **Age:** 13   **Dx:** Muscular dystrophy   **Funding:** County Agency
Micaela participated in a consultative appointment at assistive technology clinic to determine effective hardware and software adaptations for independence in computer use.
Subjective: Micaela states, "I want to be able to use the computer for school stuff, e-mail, and Facebook without my mother helping me." Mother reports that client currently navigates the Internet by telling her mother what to click.
Hearing: WNL

Vision: *Micaela presented with decreased visual acuity but demonstrated compensation using high contrast, enlarged computer screen, and a large high-contrast cursor.*

Speech & Language: *The client's receptive skills were commensurate with her expressive language skills. She was able to process and follow complex verbal directions for her age. Due to decreased air volume, speaking becomes fatiguing after just a few minutes of conversation.*

Mobility: *Micaela uses a power wheelchair with a mini proportional joystick for mobility with modified independence in a familiar spacious environment.*

Neuromuscular Skills: *Micaela presents with progressive quadriparesis throughout her body. Due to the nature of her diagnosis, she fatigues very quickly.*

Visual Skills: *The client presents with good visual scanning skills to scan keys on a keyboard and good visual tracking to follow a cursor.*

Sensory Processing: *Micaela demonstrates good cause/effect understanding and functional attention to access a computer. She demonstrates high motivation to access a computer and the Internet.*

Results of Assistive Technology Assessment: *Micaela is physically unable to use a standard keyboard or mouse but likes to navigate the Internet by telling her mother what to click. Micaela was unable to use a joystick mouse, trackball mouse, or glide point. She demonstrated good use of a mini proportional joystick to drive her wheelchair. She does not have Bluetooth capabilities in the electronics of her wheelchair. After observing her use with the mini proportional joystick, Micaela was presented with an ABC joystick and an XYZ mini-joystick, ABC and XYZ onscreen keyboards, USB switch interface, and an ultralight switch. Micaela demonstrated the ability to move the highly sensitive ABC joystick and spell on both onscreen keyboards, but preferred the letter contrast and simplicity of XYZ keyboard using small movements of her right index finger and thumb. She clicked on choices using her left hand and the ultralight switch. She was highly successful with this combination and independent to navigate the Internet and spell out messages using a word processing document. She also demonstrated the ability to check her e-mail and social networking accounts with the above-mentioned adapted computer equipment. She was unable to move as accurately or quickly with the XYZ mini-joystick. Micaela also presents with low vision related to the above diagnosis. It was thought during the evaluation that Micaela would benefit from text enlargement software, which would provide screen reading as well as magnification as needed.*

Recommendations: *As a result of the assistive technology evaluation, it has been determined that Micaela is an excellent candidate for adaptive software/hardware to allow her improved access to her computer and Internet. It is recommended that she receive an ABC joystick USB, a USB switch interface, XYZ keyboard, text enlargement software, and an ultralight switch to increase her independence on the computer and Internet. It is also recommended that Micaela receive an updated computer system to increase her independence with written communication needs.*

Shawna D., MLS, OTR/L, ATP   Michelle W., MS, CCC-SLP

CONSULTING NOTE: OUTPATIENT PEDIATRIC CLINIC

This consulting note is not done in a SOAP format since it is designed to be sent to the school rather than written in the child's health record. This note also provides an example of a note that is done by a student co-signed by the supervising occupational therapist.

Hospital and Rehabilitation Center - Motor Skills Clinic
Name: *Kelsey Joy Sample*
Chronological Age: *5 years, 2 months*
Parents: *Russ and Jamie Sample*
Kelsey Joy Sample is a 5-year, 2-month-old girl who is being seen today upon request of her family and the UMC Kindergarten Program. Kelsey was an active, healthy child until April of this year, at which time she developed Haemophilus influenzae type-B meningitis. Kelsey was hospitalized for 10 days and had a "long recovery" by the family's report. Even though Mr. and Mrs. Sample feel that Kelsey has now made a full recovery, they are concerned that this illness slowed her previously fast progress and that she may not be ready for kindergarten this fall. The parents and the UMC Kindergarten Program are requesting an evaluation to assess her readiness for kindergarten.
Assessment Results: *Three subtests of the Peabody Developmental Motor Scales, 2nd edition (PDMS-2, 2000) were administered to Kelsey. The PDMS-2 is a standardized norm-referenced evaluation designed to assess fine and gross motor skills in children birth to 71 months of age. Today's evaluation of Kelsey (at chronological age 5 years, 2 months) reveals:*

Subtest	*Standard Score	Percentile Rank	Age Equivalent
Object Manipulation	11	63rd	5 years, 11 months
Grasping	10	50th	5 years, 3 months
Visual-Motor Integration	11	63rd	5 years, 8 months

*Standard scores are based on a mean of 10 and a standard deviation of 3.

Kelsey's combined performance on the grasping and visual motor integration subtests resulted in a Fine Motor Quotient of 103 (mean of 100, standard deviation of 15), placing her in the 58th percentile for overall fine motor skills.

Kelsey was alert and cooperative throughout the 25-minute evaluation. She exhibited a right hand dominance, utilizing the right upper extremity as the main initiator of activity and the left upper extremity as an assist and stabilizer. Posture, muscle tone, strength, and endurance all appeared to be WNL for chronological age. Response to auditory stimuli in the environment was appropriate. The parents do not report any hearing or vision concerns. During the evaluation, the child did not squint, rub eyes, nor exhibit any difficulties with visual regard/tracking.

Summary: Results of the three subtests of the PDMS-2 indicate that Kelsey is functioning slightly above the mean in the area of fine motor skills at chronological age 5 years, 2 months. Motor coordination and response to environmental stimuli appear to be WNL for chronological age. Even though Kelsey was recently hospitalized with a serious illness, she currently exhibits adequate fine motor abilities to perform kindergarten activities.

Actions Taken: Evaluation results were discussed with Kelsey's parents who attended the evaluation session today. A copy of this report will be sent to the family and to the UMC Kindergarten Program as requested by the family.

Plan: Re-evaluation upon request.

Bailey M., OTS   7-25-17   Christy N., PhD, OTR/L   7-25-17

CONSULTING NOTE: COMMUNITY LIVING

Background Information: Amber is a 20-year-old female with spastic quadriplegic cerebral palsy. Client has lived at home with her family her entire life, with her mother providing maximum to dependent assistance for all basic self-care tasks. Client's mother was recently diagnosed with multiple sclerosis and is no longer able to provide the level of physical assistance that Amber requires. Client will be transitioning into a group home for adults with developmental disabilities at the end of this month. County agency has requested an occupational therapy consult to determine adaptive equipment necessary for group home staff to provide care for Amber.

S: *Client is nonverbal but did communicate through facial gestures and by touching a yes/no response system mounted to her manual w/c. Client's parents provided information about how they had previously assisted Amber with ADLs at home.*

O: *Pt., family, and group home staff participated in a consultation at Amber's future group home to determine adaptive equipment necessary to provide care for Amber. Client presents in manual tilt-in-space w/c with lateral trunk supports, seatbelt, headrest, and footplate straps to maintain positioning. Per observation and family report, client has limited functional use of all extremities. Her parents have been completing total lift transfers between bed and w/c. The group home already has a ceiling track lift system installed in Amber's future bedroom. Group home staff demonstrated lift system transfer w/c ↔ bed with Amber, who smiled and vocalized throughout process. Concern was raised by group home staff regarding bathing. Amber's family previously lifted her into the bathtub but in recent months have been completing sponge baths at the bed level as it has become more difficult for Amber's mother to lift her. Group home has a zero-entry shower stall with hand held shower hose and a simple shower/commode transport chair. OT and group home staff attempted to transfer Amber bed → shower chair using the ceiling lift system. However, due to significant deficits in trunk control and spasticity in all extremities, Amber was not able to maintain upright positioning in the chair.*

A: *Limited trunk control and spasticity of Ⓑ UEs and Ⓑ LEs limits clients ability to maintain upright positioning and perform functional transfers during ADLs. Amber's positive response to use of ceiling track lift system is a good indication that she will transition well to her new home environment. Client would benefit from purchase of a reclining, rolling shower/commode with head support, lateral trunk supports, and straps for positioning pelvis, trunk, and LEs during transport and bathing.*

P: Reviewed equipment recommendations with Amber, group home staff, and family. Specifications for recommended shower chair sent to county agency who will coordinate funding and procurement. No further recommendations at this time. This OT is available for future consults as needed should new concerns arise with Amber's transition to her new home.

Ruchi S., OTR/L

CONTACT NOTE: ACUTE CARE

S: Client nonverbal and inconsistently made and maintained eye contact with occupational therapist and family members when spoken to.

O: Client participated in bedside OT session to work on initiating and attending to self-care tasks. Client presented with poor trunk control and limited attention span throughout session. Client demonstrated startle response $\bar{c}$ position change. When asked to point finger, client required multiple verbal cues and demonstrations, and demonstrated poor response time. Client required max Ⓐ supine → sit EOB. Client required multiple verbal cues and hand over hand Ⓐ 75% of the time to initiate holding on to washcloth. Client able to bring washcloth to water with 1 verbal cue but required hand over hand Ⓐ to bring washcloth to face. Client attended to looking at self in mirror for ~1 minute. Client required hand over hand Ⓐ to initiate brushing hair. Ⓡ shoulder AROM limited due to ↓ tone.

A: Deficits in motor planning, task initiation, and attention limit client's participation in ADL tasks. Ability to attend for 1 minute indicates progress toward participation in ADL tasks. Client would benefit from ranging activities to increase shoulder elevation, as well as further interventions focusing on the skills of initiating and attending to task to complete ADL activities.

P: Client to continue occupational therapy daily for 20-minute sessions until discharge in ~2 weeks to work on self-care activities and the underlying performance skills and client factors necessary to complete tasks Ⓘ.

Christina H., OTR/L

CONTACT NOTE: COGNITION

S: Veteran reports feeling fine, but says he does not remember the name of the occupational therapist with whom he has been working.

O: Veteran participated in OT session in clinic for cognitive tasks, Ⓡ UE AROM, strengthening, and fine motor coordination. Veteran oriented to person, month, year, and place after prompting. He followed two-step commands after max verbal cues and mod physical assist to complete basic self-care tasks. Veteran was unable to grasp and release items with Ⓡ hand. He required mod physical Ⓐ and verbal cues to complete UE AROM used in table top activities.

A: Decreased orientation to surroundings presents safety concerns. ↓ cognitive functioning leads to ↓ attention to completion of tasks, specifically dressing, feeding, and bathing. ↓ strength, coordination, and AROM in Ⓡ UE limits his ability to complete ADL activities. Orientation with prompting indicates good potential for successful use of environmental cues and visual schedules. He would benefit from instruction in using Ⓡ UE as an assist as well as from activities to ↑ Ⓡ UE strength, AROM, and coordination to perform self-care activities. Veteran would benefit from cognitive skills training and safety instruction.

P: Veteran will be seen daily for 3 weeks for 1 hour to improve cognitive skills, ↑ attention to task and safety awareness, and to ↑ Ⓡ UE strength, AROM, and coordination to complete self-care tasks.

Meredith A., OTR/L

Contact Note: Complementary/Alternative Therapy (Craniosacral)

As occupational therapists and occupational therapy assistants increase their skills in the use of complementary and alternative therapy techniques, questions arise about how to document interventions that may be focused on client factors and that use nontraditional components such as energy work or chakra balancing. Many of these visits are done on a private pay basis, since complementary therapy is often not reimbursable by either public or private insurance. It is best to report objectively on what was said, what was done, what impact the presenting problems have on the client's ability to engage in meaningful occupation, and what the plan is for continued services, just as you would for any service you might provide.

S: *Client reports ↓ in functional mobility and ↑ pain since hip replacement surgery. He has adaptive equipment and is able to state 3/3 hip precautions. He reports gains since last visit as follows:*
- *He was able to sleep 4/7 nights without medication and sleeps longer without waking.*
- *Headaches occur less often.*

O: *Client participated in 1-hour craniosacral session in clinic to decrease pain and increase functional mobility needed for work and both personal and instrumental ADL activities. He arrives using forearm crutches in place of the walker he used last week. On evaluation, the craniosacral rhythm is asymmetrical, as is the body, with the left side cephalad and the head tilting right. The major restrictions identified are in the pelvis, which is treated first with a series of diaphragm holds, and release of the sacrum in supine. With increased symmetry to the pelvis, the Upledger cranial series ending with a long still-point is used to facilitate homeostatic healing activity in the body.*

A: *Improvement in sleep (decreased need for pain medication and increase in time asleep from 1 to 1½ hours), decrease in headaches, and graduation from walker to forearm crutches all indicate good progress in treatment, as does visual and palpable increase in pelvic symmetry after today's session. Client would benefit from continued work to the pelvis to alleviate cumulative trauma and residual restrictions from recent hip surgery, followed by work to more subtle restrictions that have resulted from a series of previous serious accidents.*

P: *Client to return in 1 week, at which time reassessment will determine the frequency, duration, and direction of treatment. As soon as pelvic symmetry is improved sufficiently to allow mobility WFL for work and IADL tasks, regional tissue release can be included to increase the mobility of the head and neck, which is contributing to the headaches.*

Sharon B., OTR/L, CST

Contact Note: Hand Therapy Clinic

S: *Client reports pain @ the ulnar styloid with forearm supination. Client reports she is still unable to start her car c̄ her ⓇR hand but can now use it to turn a doorknob.*

O: *Client participated in 30-minute hand clinic visit for functional range of motion in UE. Moist heat applied to ⓇR hand and forearm for 10 minutes prior to beginning treatment.*
AROM/PROM measurements for ⓇR hand and forearm are:
Key: [Flexion/extension; ( ) passive range of motion; −extension lag; +hyperextension]

ⓇR Hand	Metacarpophalangeal Joint	Proximal Interphalangeal Joint	Distal Interphalangeal Joint
Index	0/90	0/105	0/75
Long	0/90	0/105	0/80
Ring	0/90	0/105	0/80
Small	0/90	-14/105 (0/105)	0/79

® wrist: +45/40 composite (+60/50) composite +45/50 noncomposite
® forearm: supination 62 (78); pronation 90
Client performed the following exercises c̄ ® UE: Isometric forearm supination x10, AAROM supination x5, AROM forearm supination x5. After exercise, client's supination ↑ to 77° AROM. HEP revised to include blue foam for flexion strengthening 2 to 3x day.

A: Decreased functional ROM and strength in dominant ® hand limit client's ability to complete ADL and IADL tasks. Client's gains in DIP joint flexion AROM since last week is due to ↑ strength of flexors. Active wrist extension ↑ 9° and extension ↑ 5° from last week. ↑ in active pronation is due to ↑ strength while client lost 14° of forearm supination since last week, which appears to be a result of muscle tightness. Client would benefit from continued skilled OT to regain functional ROM to complete IADLs and for general strengthening.

P: Client to be seen 2x/wk 30-minute sessions for 3 more weeks. Continue wrist exercises and modify treatment plan to include more supination stretching and strengthening.

Rachelle H., OTR/L, CHT

CONTACT NOTE: HOME ASSESSMENT

S: Client stated numerous times how nice it was to be home during this home assessment. Client verbalized more in this setting than at the facility.

O: Prior to admission, client lived at home alone with support from family, home health nurse, and housekeeping aide and was Ⓘ with all ADLs. Today, pt. participated in home assessment in preparation for discharge home next week. Pt. was transported by family in private vehicle, with OT meeting family at the home. Pt. demonstrated mobility with wheeled walker mod Ⓘ and adhered to all postsurgical hip precautions throughout home visit. The following are the results of the home evaluation:
- **Entry:** 2½" step, 4" door jam. Uneven grass to step. Concrete broken and no railings present.
- **Kitchen:** 26" area around table in center of kitchen, 27" between snack bar and fridge, 30"-high snack bar located on outskirt of kitchen. Little room to maneuver safely. Needs utensils and appliances within reach.
- **Hallway:** 22" wide from dining room → bedroom with bathroom between inaccessible for walker. Remainder of entries adequate to accommodate walker.
- **Bathroom:** 17" floor to tub top, 18" floor to toilet seat. Bathroom small, but can accommodate wheeled walker.
- **Other:** Throw rugs in all rooms. Chair blocks bedroom access with wheeled walker. End tables block access to living room from dining room with wheeled walker.

A: With the following modifications and recommendations, the home would be safe for client to return to after discharge:
- Remove all throw rugs to decrease falls; remove excess furniture to increase walking area and increase safety.
- Adaptive equipment needed:
  - Raised toilet seat with safety rails, shower chair with back support, grab bars, and hand-held shower.
  - Add railing to hallway to increase safety without walker.
  - Add railing and repair concrete to outside entry.
- Remove kitchen table and utilize snack bar or dining table to increase mobility in kitchen.
- Lower telephone by back door to improve reach.

P: Resident and family will implement the preceding recommendations and changes to allow discharge from facility to return home safely.

Carrie C., OTR/L

CONTACT NOTE: HOME HEALTH VISIT

S: *Client stated that he was "shaky" from his shower earlier in the AM. Client's daughter reported that client showered and dressed with min Ⓐ for balance and coordination to manage fasteners. Client reported that he has been following his HEP.*

O: *Client participated in home visit to assess current status in balance, coordination, level of compliance, and Ⓘ c̄ HEP and to introduce new hand strengthening exercises. OT and OTA both present for collaboration and update to intervention plan. Client presents with decreased balance related to recent CVA, and currently completes transfers and mobility during ADLs with CGA using grab bars and wheeled walker. Client required mod verbal cues to initiate and complete pre-existing HEP.*

New hand-strengthening exercises added—finger spread with rubber bands of various sizes; intrinsic muscle coordination worksheet (e.g., pen rolling, etc.).

Client and daughter participated in discussion about planning treatment activities to complement client's interests. Gun repair projects and small woodworking activities were suggested for coordination and strength in hands. Client demonstrated good static sitting balance throughout the session, but needed CGA for balance to stand safely from chair.

A: *Need for verbal cues to initiate HEP raises continued concerns about compliance. ↑ strength c̄ Theraband exercises since initial evaluation indicated through increased repetitions and decreased fatigue. Progress shown by ability to handle 1" items such as pajama buttons, although still has difficulty with smaller items. Rehab potential is excellent. Client would benefit from continued skilled OT to further instruct in energy conservation techniques, safety, and to modify HEP as client continues to progress.*

P: *Client to be seen 2x/wk for 1-hour sessions for 2 more weeks to continue work on increasing independence with self-care, with focus on showering and dressing.*

Bridget C., OTR/L

CONTACT NOTE: HOME HEALTH MENTAL HEALTH

Name: *John W*   **Length of Session:** *75 minutes*   **Goals Addressed:** *2, 4, and 5*

S: *John states that having a bank account instead of keeping all his money in cash in an envelope is very confusing to him, and he is never sure any more how much money he has. He also reported some continuing confusion regarding his medication.*

O: *John participated in home visit to review his grocery needs and for verbal cues to fill his medication organizer correctly. Skilled instruction provided in meal planning and calculating probable food costs. He was then taken to the bank to withdraw some money, and to a local grocery store to purchase food. At the bank, the teller figured John's account, which confused him. Skilled instruction provided in calculating a bank balance. At the grocery store, John purchased canned fruits and vegetables, ground beef, fresh lettuce, and a loaf of bread. Upon returning home he put the lettuce and meat in the refrigerator independently and consulted his weekly menu planner to determine what he had planned for lunch. John needed 2 verbal cues to fill his medication organizer with correct doses of all medications.*

A: *Limited understanding of bank account management results in need for supervision in managing finances. Decreased number of cues required to fill medication organizer correctly indicates progress from 4 cues required last week. Independent choice of canned fruits and vegetables and the addition of lettuce to his sandwiches indicates progress toward healthier eating habits. John would benefit from continued skilled instruction in ADL skills such as independent management of medication, food, and money to be able to live independently in the community without the support of a professional caregiver.*

P: *John will continue to be seen weekly in his home and community settings to work toward independence in meeting his daily needs.*

Alan T., OTR/L

CONTACT NOTE: MENTAL HEALTH (MULTIPLE GROUPS)

S: *Client reported she is currently not volunteering and has not worked for the past 4 years due to her disability status. Regarding volunteering, she says, "I need the structure," and further stated that she wants to be productive. Currently, client reports she sleeps "too much" and is having relationship problems.*

O: *Client was admitted yesterday and attended 4/4 group sessions today. During expressive therapy group, client participated in baking with the rest of the group, but did not eat anything. When each group member identified current emotions, client identified hers as miserable, angry, very anxious, overstimulated, frustrated, frightened, and alienated. During skills group, client identified a possible problem she may encounter upon discharge to be lack of organization, with her "red flags" being oversleeping and agitation. Client welcomed suggestions from others regarding restructuring her use of time.*

A: *Client is very perceptive of her emotions and limitations. Her refusal to eat with the group indicates continued appetite disturbance. Client would benefit from information about eating disorders. She would also benefit from continued group participation, with emphasis on increasing self-esteem and time management skills. Client's participation in all 4 group sessions today indicates good rehab potential.*

P: *Client will continue to attend all daily group sessions while on the acute unit to work on increasing self-esteem and ability to structure her time.*

Gabby H., OTR/L

CONTACT NOTE: MENTAL HEALTH (ONE GROUP)

The previous note summarized a client's participation in several groups on one day. Some mental health settings, particularly inpatient settings with short lengths of stay, require a note to be written for each group that the client attends. The following note illustrates this type of documentation.

S: *Client reports unhealthy self-esteem in the form of negative thoughts about herself. She describes feeling "stupid" and "ugly," particularly when she is under stress.*

O: *Client participated in 1-hr. self-esteem group in dayroom. Group session was designed to educate participants regarding healthy and unhealthy self-esteem and to instruct on goal setting and other ways to improve self-esteem. Client demonstrated active participation in all group discussion and activities. With encouragement from other group members and facilitator, client set goal for this week to decrease her negative thoughts and to plan for discharge. She independently identified a compensatory strategy to use when she recognizes negative thoughts; her plan is to replace negative thoughts with something more positive such as thinking about how much she enjoys being around her children. Client initiated discussion about setting up appointments for aftercare following discharge.*

A: *Focus on negative thoughts during periods of stress limits client's ability to complete IADL tasks, including caring for her children. Ability to set goals and identify steps to achieving those goals indicates excellent progress this date. Client has great potential to return to independent living. Client would benefit from continued practice in goal setting and assistance with identifying and replacing negative thoughts.*

P: *Client to attend self-esteem group daily for 3 days to address self-esteem issues that inhibit IADL performance. Sessions to include group discussions, role-play, and written discharge plan development, as well as facilitation of setting up aftercare appointments.*

David M., OTR/L

CONTACT NOTE: PEDIATRIC (PRESCHOOL AGE)

S: *McKenna said she wanted to play, but when the task was difficult for her, she said, "You do it. You fix it."*

O: *McKenna participated in an OT home visit to work on use of Ⓑ UEs to ↑ spontaneous use of hand as a functional assist, sitting balance while tailor sitting unsupported, and functional mobility, as a prerequisite to self-care and play skills. McKenna was engaged during ~90% of the session.*
*   **Bilateral UE Use:** McKenna required max Ⓐ to pull shirt over stuffed animal's arms with Ⓡ UE while holding it with Ⓛ UE. She spontaneously used Ⓛ hand to assist with stabilizing animal while pulling sleeve over its arm and shoulder c̄ Ⓡ hand. McKenna initiated snapping shirt, but needed max Ⓐ to use Ⓛ hand to stabilize shirt while fastening snaps. Spontaneously used Ⓑ hands used to hold animal steady during play.*
*   **Sitting Balance:** McKenna required touch cues to initiate stand → sit using walker and mod physical Ⓐ for postural stability during transition from side sit → cross-legged sit. She demonstrated adequate sitting balance to play for 5 minutes, requiring tactile cues twice to right herself from a lateral tilt.*

A: *Improved Ⓑ coordination and increased use of Ⓛ hand as functional assist now ~ 60% of the time indicates progress since last week. Decreased postural control necessitates CGA to maintain upright position when engrossed in an activity. She would benefit from continued skilled occupational therapist for activities, which challenge postural support to gain protective responses, body righting, and vestibular integration to ↑ her Ⓘ during play.*

P: *McKenna will be seen weekly for 7 weeks to continue strengthening postural support to ↑ her Ⓘ in play activities, promote Ⓑ hand use, and ↑ use of the Ⓛ hand as a functional assist during ADL and play activities.*

   Amy D., OTR/L

CONTACT NOTE: PUBLIC SCHOOL

S: *Kylee did not use verbal language to communicate, but did echo words spoken to her.*

O: *Kylee participated in OT session in classroom to work on fine motor skills to prepare for scissors use and improve prehension patterns for writing. Kylee initially presented with aversive behaviors (e.g., pulling away, facial grimacing) when asked to touch the various supplies for today's activity. After 5 minutes of brushing to decrease tactile sensitivity, Kylee worked on palmar pinch and tripod grasp prehension patterns using a "Fruit Loop" bracelet activity for 20 minutes. Kylee used tongs (in preparation for scissors use) to pull 15 Fruit Loops out of a cup one at a time. Then using a palmar pinch, she placed each Fruit Loop over a pipe cleaner. Five verbal cues were required for task completion.*

A: *Delayed fine motor skill milestones limit client's success with classroom tasks. Improved manipulation and positioning of tongs this date is an indicator that proper scissors use will be attained soon. Good attention to task for entire 25 minutes demonstrates good progress toward being able to participate with peers without sensory breaks. Kylee would benefit from continued OT intervention to address educationally-relevant fine motor skill development.*

P: *Continue prehension activities 3x/wk using a variety of media in 20- to 30-minute intervals until proper scissors use goal is achieved.*

   Durwood T., OTR/L

CONTACT NOTE: PROSTHETIC ADAPTATION

S: *Client expressed pleasure with adaptations to prosthetic leg fasteners made this date, stating "this will work."*

O: *Client participated in OT session in rehab gym for adaptations necessary to don/doff prosthesis. Client sit ↔ stand modified Ⓘ from w/c while keeping one hand on walker for support. Client positioned prosthetic leg and attempted to fasten straps. Client needed mod Ⓐ in fastening of straps, Ⓘ in undoing of straps to doff prosthesis. Adaptations of prosthetic leg harness completed this date.*

A: *Inability to don prosthesis Ⓘ currently limits Ⓘ with dressing, toileting, and functional mobility for IADLs. Ability to position prosthesis correctly and fasten straps indicates good progress toward stated goals. Client would benefit from additional skilled instruction in use of pulley-like fasteners installed this date on prosthesis to allow one-handed closure.*

P: *Pt. to be seen one more session prior to discharge home tomorrow for skilled instruction in donning prosthesis.*

Alissah D., OTR/L

Contact Note: Safety

S: *Client reports ↓ activity tolerance and ↑ shortness of breath with exertion. Client reports feeling ok about asking nursing for Ⓐ c̄ dressing, but has urgent incontinence and cannot always wait for Ⓐ to manage O_2 tubing to toilet.*

O: *Client participated in OT session in room to assess safety during toileting.*
Cognition: WFL; no deficits
Functional Mobility: Client uses walker, has difficulty managing O_2 tubing, requires SBA for safety.
Upper Extremity Strength: WNL; client fatigues c̄ use of UE.
ADLs: CGA for clothing management c̄ toileting. Mobility during toileting and dressing requires min Ⓐ for O_2 tubing management and safety. Client dresses with mod Ⓐ due to ↓ activity tolerance, and needs to stop p̄ 5 minutes dressing activity.

A: *Client at risk for falls due to inability to manage O_2 cord during functional mobility to toilet. Intact cognition is good indication for potential to incorporate adaptive strategies into ADL routines. Client would benefit from adaptive equipment and techniques to toilet with ↑ Ⓘ as well as instruction in energy conservation techniques and ↑ activity tolerance for ADL tasks.*

P: *Client will be seen 2x/wk for 1 week to ↑ Ⓘ and safety in toileting.*

Paige B., OTR/L

Contact Note: Skilled Nursing Facility

S: *Resident reports she hopes to return home independently within 1 month. Resident reports difficulty fastening her back brace "because I can't remember if I'm supposed to fasten the Velcro first and then pull the side strings tight or the other way around." Resident able to verbalize 2 of 3 back precautions (no bending, no lifting) but unable to call third precaution (no twisting).*

O: *Resident participated in 45-minute session in her room to address increased independence with ADLs following recent lumbar laminectomy and fusion. She presented supine in bed upon OT's arrival; required min verbal cues for correct log roll technique to complete supine to sit transition.*
Upper Body Dressing: Resident donned bra and undershirt with set-up and required min Ⓐ to sequence steps of positioning and fastening corset-style back brace. She donned oversized button up shirt over brace with SBA.
Lower Body Dressing: Resident donned underwear and pants using reacher with SBA; min Ⓐ required to don socks using sock aid as she originally had device positioned incorrectly to thread sock on it.
Grooming: Resident completed sit to/from stand with SBA and ambulated to sink CGA without assistive device; completed grooming tasks standing at sink with min verbal cues to avoid bending and twisting when reaching for grooming items. Client educated to remember the "BLT" mnemonic: No Bending, No Lifting, No Twisting.

A: *Decreased ability to remember and adhere to back precautions and corset application limits resident's independence with dressing and grooming tasks. Ability to recall 2 of 3 back precautions from previous session indicates good progress toward goals. Client would benefit from visual reminders of back precautions and corset-donning sequence.*

P: *Resident will continue to receive OT services 5x/wk for 1 week to address independence with ADLs in preparation for discharge back to home environment. OT will post visual reminders of back precautions and corset instructions in resident's room.*

Jasmine H., OTR/L

CONTACT NOTE: SPLINT

S: Mr. J stated that the pain in his right wrist and thumb was "not as bad as it was 2 weeks ago." He reported that his splint is rubbing a calcium deposit on the dorsum of his hand and that he is not wearing the splint at work during the day. He also reported feeling pain during treatment with movement of the Ⓡ thumb and that ice and iontophoresis ↓ pain.

O: Mr. J arrived at clinic wearing Ⓡ forearm-based thumb spica splint. Upon removal of splint, wrist appeared slightly swollen.

Ⓡ UE AROM: Wrist flexion ~25%   Wrist extension <25%
                         Thumb flexion and extension ~25%

Mr. J tolerated ~3 minutes friction massage over abductor pollicis longus and extensor pollicis brevis tendons. Ice applied for 5 minutes; Mr. J instructed in using ice at home and at work to ↓ pain by ↓ inflammation of tendons. Splint reformed to eliminate rubbing on dorsum of hand, and Mr. J instructed in wearing schedule at work. HEP modified and Mr. J demonstrated new procedures correctly.

A: Swelling ↓ since last treatment session shows good progress. Wrist and thumb AROM are ~50% below functional limits due to pain upon movement. Limited AROM & pain are causing functional problems in the work environment. Ice and iontophoresis ↓ pain & therefore ↑ functional ability c̄ Ⓡ hand. Splint reconstruction will also contribute to ↓ pain. Mr. J would benefit from continued skilled occupational therapy to ↓ pain, ↑ AROM, ↑ ability to use Ⓡ hand at work.

P: Continue to see Mr. J 2x/wk for the following:
- Ice & iontophoresis to ↓ pain in Ⓡ hand and wrist.
- Friction massage to ↓ inflammation and ↑ AROM in Ⓡ wrist and thumb.
- Re-evaluation of splint for fit and use after reconstruction.
- Re-evaluation of effectiveness and compliance of HEP.
- To achieve goal of ↓ pain in Ⓡ wrist and hand for use in functional activity at work and home.

Mark S., OTR/L

REFERENCE

Shipp, M., & Havard, A. (2006). Documenting driver rehabilitation services and outcomes. In J. M. Pellerito, Jr. (Ed.), *Driver rehabilitation and community mobility.* St. Louis: Elsevier.

Appendix
Suggestions for Completing the Worksheets

In this appendix, we will offer suggestions for completing the worksheets throughout this manual. As a student or new therapist using this manual, you can work your way through the exercises and check your work against those in this appendix. Remember that your answer can be different and still be correct, as long as it contains the essential elements. As long as your information and protocol are correct, you should not sacrifice your own writing style to be more like someone else's.

COAST goals and SOAP notes are very difficult to write if there is no client or treatment session about which to write. Although there are many examples in this manual, there is no substitute for observing or working with actual clients. Only then will you be able to translate your treatment session onto paper in a meaningful way.

CHAPTER 4

WORKSHEET 4-1: AVOIDING COMMON DOCUMENTATION ERRORS

1. Pt. stated my head really hurts this morning.
   Pt. stated, "My head really hurts this morning."

2. Resident reported "her right hand is working better today."
   Resident reported her right hand is working better today.

3. Student used right hand to cut with scissors. Student then switches to left hand for coloring tasks. Student did not demonstrate consistent hand preference.
   Student used right hand to cut with scissors. Student then switched to left hand for coloring tasks. Student did not demonstrate consistent hand preference.

4. The client's expressed excitement about the upcoming visit to the mall.
   The clients expressed excitement about the upcoming visit to the mall.

5. An occupational therapy referral was recieved from the childs' teacher.
   An occupational therapy referral was received from the child's teacher.

6. The child was unable to button their coat.
   The child was unable to button her coat.

7. The resident's were all in the dinning room weighting for there meal.
   The residents were all in the dining room waiting for their meal.

Gateley CA, Borcherding S. *Documentation Manual for Occupational Therapy: Writing SOAP Notes, Fourth Edition* (pp 235-255).
© 2017 SLACK Incorporated

8. Client demonstrated appropriate social interaction by responding your welcome to another group member.
   Client demonstrated appropriate social interaction by responding "You're welcome" to another group member.

9. Pt. required moderate assistance to use dominate right hand in hygeine tasks.
   Pt. required moderate assistance to use dominant right hand in hygiene tasks.

10. Client does not demonstrate awareness of the affect of his mood on other member's of the group.
    Client does not demonstrate awareness of the effect of his mood on other members of the group.

11. Pt. expressed intrest in getting dressed. Pt. required verbal cues when doning pullover shirt to utilize adaptive tecknikues due to right rotary cup injury.
    Pt. expressed interest in getting dressed. Pt. required verbal cues when donning pullover shirt to utilize adaptive techniques due to right rotator cuff injury.

12. The ot noticed assymetry in the childs sitting posture. Parents reports that the client is unable to sit independantly.
    The OT noticed asymmetry in the child's sitting posture. Parents reported that the client is unable to sit independently.

13. The OTR preformed a Cognitive Test on the client.
    The OTR performed a cognitive test on the client.

14. The Doctor called to check on the Patients status.
    The doctor called to check on the patient's status.

15. Client demonstrated poor judgement by attempting to stand up without their walker.
    Client demonstrated poor judgment by attempting to stand up without his walker.

16. Pt. had right arm imobilized due to a clavical fracture.
    Pt. had right arm immobilized due to a clavicle fracture.

17. Client required several breif rest brakes during ADL's.
    Client required several brief rest breaks during ADLs.

18. The clinic employs three otr's and two ota's.
    The clinic employs three OTRs and two OTAs.

19. The students principle stated Jimmy is disruptive at school.
    The student's principal stated, "Jimmy is disruptive at school."

20. A child at this age should be able to dress themselves.
    A child at this age should be able to dress herself.

21. The childrens' mother has difficulty keeping all they're appointment's.
    The children's mother has difficulty keeping all their appointments.

22. Client needed a visual aide to help them learn how to preform self-catherization.
    Client needed a visual aid to help him learn how to perform self-catheterization.

WORKSHEET 4-2: USING ABBREVIATIONS

1. Client C/O pain in Ⓡ MCP joint p̄ ~15 min PROM.
   Client complained of pain in the right metacarpophalangeal joint after approximately 15 minutes of passive range of motion.

2. Pt. A&Ox4.
   The client was alert and oriented to person, place, time, and situation.

3. Client transferred w/c → mat c̄ sliding board & max Ⓐ x2.
   Client transferred from his wheelchair to the mat using a sliding board and maximum assistance of two people.

4. 1° dx Ⓛ BKA, 2° dx COPD, CHF, DM, & PVD.
   Primary diagnosis is left below-the-knee amputation. Secondary diagnoses are chronic obstructive pulmonary disease, congestive heart failure, diabetes mellitus, and peripheral vascular disease.

5. Pt. is S/P Ⓡ THR. Orders received for OT 2x/day for ADLs & IADLs, TTWB Ⓡ LE.
   Patient is status post right total hip replacement. Orders received for occupational therapy two times per day for activities of daily living and instrumental activities of daily living. Toe-touch weightbearing restriction for right lower extremity.

6. Client has thirty degrees of passive range of motion in the left distal interphalangeal joint, which is within functional limits.
   30° PROM in Ⓛ DIP is WFL.

7. Client is able to put on her socks with standby assistance, but requires moderate assistance with putting on and taking off left shoe.
   Client dons socks SBA but requires mod Ⓐ to don & doff Ⓛ shoe.

8. The client requires contact guard assistance for balance during her morning dressing, which she performs while sitting on the edge of her bed.
   CGA required for balance for AM dressing EOB.

9. The patient participated in a bedside evaluation of activities of daily living. She was able to perform bed mobility with moderate assistance, but she needed maximum assistance to put on her adult undergarment. She was able to go from a supine position to a sitting position with minimum assistance and from a sitting position to a standing position with moderate assistance.
   Pt. participated in bedside ADL eval. Mod Ⓐ for bed mobility, max Ⓐ to don undergarment. Supine → sit min Ⓐ and sit → stand mod Ⓐ.

10. The resident came to the occupational therapy clinic via wheelchair escort. The resident was observed to lean toward his left. The resident needed verbal cues and minimum assistance in positioning his body in the wheelchair to maintain midline orientation and symmetrical posture. The resident transferred from his wheelchair to the toilet with moderate assistance of one person to help him keep his balance using a standing pivot transfer. He needed verbal cues and visual feedback from a mirror to maintain upright posture.
    Resident to OT via w/c escort. Resident leans Ⓛ and needs verbal cues, visual feedback from mirror, and min physical Ⓐ to maintain symmetrical posture in midline. Standing pivot transfer w/c → toilet mod Ⓐ for balance.

11. The veteran participated in an evaluation in his room to determine relevant client factors. The veteran's short-term memory was three out of three for immediate recall, one out of three after 1 minute, and zero out of three with verbal cues after 5 minutes. The left upper extremity shoulder flexion was a grade of 4, shoulder extension was a grade of 4, elbow flexion was a grade of 4, elbow extension was a grade of 4, wrist flexion was a grade of 4 minus, wrist extension was a grade of 4 minus, and grip strength was 8 pounds. The left upper extremity light touch was intact. The right upper extremity muscle grades and sensation were within functional limits.
    Veteran participated in eval. of client factors seated in w/c. Short-term memory 3/3 immediate recall, 1/3 after 1 minute, 0/3 c̄ verbal cues p̄ 5 min. Ⓛ shoulder and elbow strength grade 4, wrist strength 4-, grip strength 8#. Light touch intact. Ⓡ UE strength and sensation WFL.

Chapter 5

Worksheet 5-1: Identifying the Contributing Factors

1. Area of Occupation = Work
   Consumer is unable to sustain employment longer than 2 weeks due to:
   - *Use of inflammatory language at work*
   - *Aggressive behaviors on the job*
   - *Need for frequent redirection to task*
   - *Drug-seeking behaviors at work*
   - *Inability to plan and sequence a task*
   - *Inattention to social cues and personal hygiene*
   - *Arriving late 3 to 4 times weekly following nightly alcohol use*
   - *Lack of reliable daycare*

2. Area of Occupation = ADLs
   Veteran needs 1½ hours to complete grooming tasks due to:
   - *Motor planning deficits*
   - *SOB on exertion and need for frequent rest breaks to regain O_2 saturation*
   - *< 5 minutes activity tolerance before needing rest breaks*
   - *Inability to sequence the task*
   - *Slowness in locating items needed for grooming due to low vision*
   - *Intention tremors and rigidity 2° Parkinson disease*
   - *Decreased fine motor manipulation in Ⓛ UE*
   - *Muscle weakness and limited AROM in Ⓑ UEs*

3. Area of Occupation = Education
   Child is unable to complete grade-appropriate written worksheets due to:
   - *Increased tone in Ⓑ hands 2° to cerebral palsy*
   - *Attention span < 2 minutes for seated classroom tasks due to sensory-seeking behaviors*
   - *Mod verbal cues required to sequence multi-step directions*
   - *Deficits in figure-ground visual perceptual skills*
   - *Difficulty holding pencil due to multiple joint contractures related to juvenile rheumatoid arthritis*
   - *Visual motor deficits*

Worksheet 5-2: Writing Functional Problem Statements

1. The client has an acquired injury to his brain. As a result, he is not able to pay attention to task for very long at a time, and he is having trouble completing his morning routine. Usually he can pay attention to what he is doing for about 2 minutes, and needs to be redirected back to the task after that.

   < 3 minute attention span 2° ABI interferes with ability to complete ADL tasks

   or

   Client requires verbal cues to stay on task after ~2 minutes of ADL tasks.

2. The child is having trouble in school because she has difficulty staying within the lines when she is writing. She habitually grips her pencil in a gross grasp, although with help (someone's hand placed over hers) she can hold it with her thumb and two fingers.

   Child needs HOH Ⓐ to hold pencil in tripod pinch for writing tasks at school.

   or

   Inability to maintain tripod pinch unassisted limits child's ability to stay within the lines during writing tasks at school.

3. The resident is not very cognitively aware. About 40% of the time, she has trouble figuring out what to do first if she has to complete a self-care task, and she doesn't remember what she has just been told.

   Resident needs mod verbal cues in ADL tasks due to ↓ ability to sequence steps of task.

   or

   Memory and sequencing deficits result in safety concerns during ADL tasks.

4. Mr. J has recently sustained a Ⓡ CVA. His Ⓛ arm is flaccid and he forgets that it is there. He needs physical and verbal help with ADL tasks about 60% of the time.

   Client requires max Ⓐ to dress upper body due to flaccid Ⓛ UE and Ⓛ side neglect.

   or

   Flaccidity in Ⓛ UE & Ⓛ UE neglect result in max Ⓐ for grooming and hygiene.

5. The consumer has had trouble finding a job. His appearance is unkempt and he has a strong body odor, neither of which seem troubling to him.

   Inattention to personal hygiene interferes with consumer's ability to find employment.

   or

   Consumer has difficulty finding employment due to unkempt appearance and inattention to personal hygiene.

6. The client is unable to transfer safely w/c ↔ toilet without someone to remind him that he needs to follow his total hip precautions.

   Client requires SBA w/c ↔ toilet due to unfamiliarity with hip precautions.

   or

   Unfamiliarity with hip precautions results in need for SBA to follow hip precautions when toileting following recent THR.

CHAPTER 6

WORKSHEET 6-1: CHOOSING GOALS FOR MEDICAL NECESSITY

- **Problem:** Client unable to perform sewing due to 2+/5 strength in Ⓡ hand musculature.
  - **LTG:** Client will perform embroidery Ⓘ for 20 minutes within 8 weeks.
  - **STG:** To ↑ performance of embroidery, client will use needle continuously for 5 minutes within 2 weeks.

Other possible problem statements:

- **Problem:** *Client unable to handle small items needed for grooming due to 2+ strength in Ⓡ hand musculature.*
  - **LTG:** *Client will complete grooming activities Ⓘ within 1 month.*
  - **STG:** *Client will remove lid from toothpaste with min verbal cues for adaptive technique within 2 weeks.*
- **Problem:** *Client unable to write > 5 minutes due to 2+ strength in her Ⓡ hand musculature.*
  - **LTG:** *Client will write for 15 minutes with one rest break using adaptive pencil grip within 1 month.*
  - **STG:** *Client will sign first name within 1 week using adaptive pencil grip.*
- **Problem:** *Client unable to fasten ½" buttons due to 2+ strength in Ⓡ hand.*
  - **LTG:** *Client will fasten all buttons on shirt independently.*
  - **STG:** *Within 1 week, client will fasten 3 buttons on shirt using button hook with min Ⓐ.*

WORKSHEET 6-2: EVALUATING GOAL STATEMENTS

1. By the time of discharge in 2 weeks, client will dress himself with min Ⓐ for balance using a sock aid and reacher while sitting in w/c.

   This goal has all of the necessary COAST components.

2. Client will tolerate 10 minutes of treatment daily.

   This goal lacks an occupation, an assistance level, and a time frame. In addition, the behavior (tolerating treatment) is not useful because it is not something that the client needs to do after discharge. *Client will complete 10 minutes of grooming/hygiene activity with SBA and no rest break within 1 week.*

3. Client will demonstrate increased coping skills when communicating with her daughter within 2 weeks.

   "Coping skills" is far too broad. The coping skill(s) in question need to be specified as well as a way to measure those skills. For example: *By next group session, client will verbalize 2 anger management strategies that can be used when she experiences frustration during interaction with family members.*

4. Client will demonstrate 15 minutes of activity tolerance without rest breaks using Ⓑ UEs to complete ADL tasks before breakfast each morning.

   This goal lacks an assistance level and a time frame, and it needs to be turned around to focus on the occupation rather than the specific condition. *By September 27th, client will complete basic ADLs with supervision in < 15 minutes without rest breaks each morning before breakfast.*

5. OT will teach lower body dressing using a reacher, dressing stick, and sock aid within 3 treatment sessions.

   Most importantly, this goal is not client-centered. *Client will complete lower body dressing with SBA using reacher, dressing stick, and sock aid within 3 treatment sessions.* **(Remember, what the occupational therapist does is the intervention, not the goal.)**

6. Patient will demonstrate ability to balance his checkbook.

   This goal lacks an assistance level, a specific condition, and a time frame. *Within 4 weeks, patient will balance checkbook with modified independence using calculator with no mathematical errors.*

WORKSHEET 6-3: WRITING CLIENT-CENTERED, OCCUPATION-BASED, MEASURABLE GOALS

1. Ayana is not able to attend to task for more than a few minutes, which makes IADL activities difficult for her. Since she likes to cook and plans to return to cooking after discharge, you have been working with her in the kitchen. You would like to see her able to attend to a task for 10 minutes by the time she is discharged next week. Write a goal that addresses Ayana's attention span during cooking.
   Client will complete cooking activity with supervision, maintaining attention to task at least 10 minutes without redirection within 1 week.
   or
   Within 3 treatment sessions, client will complete cooking activity with supervision, attending to task at least 10 minutes with 2 or fewer verbal cues for redirection.

2. Now write a goal for Ayana to be able to follow directions so that she can read the back of a boxed meal, and eventually a recipe, when she is cooking.
   Client will complete a cooking activity c̄ min Ⓐ to follow 3-step written direction within 3 treatment sessions.
   or
   Client will follow simple recipe independently within 1 week.

3. Scott is having trouble dressing himself after his stroke. You have been teaching him an over-the-head method for putting on his shirt, and have given him a buttonhook to use. Write a dressing goal for Scott.
   Client will don shirt with modified Ⓘ using over-the-head method and a button hook within 2 tx sessions.
   or
   After skilled instruction, client will dress upper body with modified independence using one-handed techniques and adaptive equipment within 1 week.

4. Nikki is very weak, and she wants to be able to go back to work as a receptionist. She also wants to be able to care for her 4-month-old child. Write a goal that addresses her activity tolerance during an occupation-based activity.
   Client will complete simulated infant-bathing activity with SBA, standing for at least 10 minutes, by discharge in 2 weeks.
   or
   Within 1 week, client independently will complete seated work-simulation tasks using computer, telephone, and desk-top office supplies for 20 minutes without rest breaks.

5. Demarco wants to live independently in the community, but lacks basic money management skills. Write a goal for Demarco to improve his money management skills.
   Client will make change Ⓘ from $1.00 correctly 3/3 tries within 2 weeks.
   or
   With minimal verbal cues, client will select ads from the newspaper for an apartment that rents for less than 1/3 of his regular monthly income within 3 weeks.

6. Tiffany has become increasingly more depressed over the past several weeks and was admitted after a suicide attempt. You estimate that you will have her in group for 1 week. You would like to see her mood change in that week. Write an occupation-based goal that will indicate an improved mood.
   Within 1 week, client will follow her daily schedule spontaneously, as demonstrated by attending at least 3 scheduled activities per day.
   or
   Client will verbalize an interest in at least one future activity spontaneously within the next 2 days.

CHAPTER 7

WORKSHEET 7-1: WRITING CONCISE, COHERENT "S" STATEMENTS

1. Mrs. P is recovering from a total hip replacement. During a treatment session, she makes the following statements:
   - "I used that dressing stick and sock aid like you showed me to get dressed without bending down this morning."
   - "My hip doesn't hurt when I stand up or sit down, especially with that new toilet seat you got for me."
   - "It's getting easier for me to get dressed now."
   - "My daughter said they delivered all that bathroom equipment to her house yesterday."

S: *Client reports using adaptive equipment to don pants and socks while maintaining hip precautions without difficulty. She has not c/o pain with transfers using raised toilet seat. Bathroom equipment ordered by OT last week has been delivered to daughter's home.*

2. Tanner is a 14 year old recently admitted to an inpatient adolescent psychiatric unit following an unsuccessful suicide attempt by overdose with his mother's sleeping pills. During a group session, he makes the following comments:
   - "I have nothing to live for."
   - "I don't have any friends."
   - "My family would be better off without me anyway."
   - "The teachers at my school all hate me."
   - "Maybe next time I should do it right and just use a gun!"

S: *Client reports a lack of self-worth in both family and school situations and states that he does not have any friends. He continues to express suicidal ideation and suggested that he may use a gun in a future suicide attempt.*

WORKSHEET 7-2: CHOOSING A SUBJECTIVE STATEMENT

1. Client was very cooperative and engaged in social conversation throughout the tx session.
   Even though the client may have been cooperative, and even though it may have been important in this treatment session, it is an assessment of the situation, and does not belong in the "S" category of the note. The client's social conversation might be important in some situations. However, there is a better choice for this particular note.

2. Client remarked that her grandson will be coming to visit later in the week, and that she will be very glad to see him.
   In this instance, a pending visit by the client's grandson is not really relevant to the treatment session or to how the client sees her progress. It might be important in another situation. For example, if the client was planning to go live with her grandson after discharge, it might be very relevant and might be a topic the occupational therapist wanted to explore further with the client.

3. Client reports that she feels "pretty good" today.
   Feeling "pretty good" today might be important because it might show progress or a change in her condition. In this case, however, it is not the best choice.

4. Client says she has difficulty moving Ⓡ UE, although she does not know why it will not move. She reports, "It really doesn't hurt. It's just tight."
   The client's comments about her upper extremity seem most pertinent to this treatment session. Use of the Ⓡ UE is relevant in all aspects of this treatment session.

5. Nursing staff report client is incontinent at night.
   This information should be documented in the nursing notes. The subjective section of the note is generally used to document the client's views rather than views of the staff, except in rare instances. For example, if nursing staff had reported a safety concern with the client's ability to transfer to the toilet that was inconsistent with client report or occupational therapist observation, then that information would be relevant to this session. There is a better choice for this note.

CHAPTER 8

WORKSHEET 8-1: USING CATEGORIES

O: Child participated in 60-minute OT session at daycare to address feeding skills and reach/grasp/release during play. Child demonstrated strong Ⓡ hand preference, flexed position of Ⓛ UE, and did not spontaneously initiate use of Ⓛ UE as a functional assist during self-care or play. With min Ⓐ for facilitation of extension at elbow, child demonstrated ability to use Ⓛ UE to reach, grasp, and release 5 objects with 1-2 verbal cues per object and restriction of Ⓡ UE movement. Child was able to feed self with modified Ⓘ c̄ ~50% spillage, but demonstrated significant limitations in chewing action p̄ ~3 rotary chews & swallowing ~90% of food s̄ chewing. Child required verbal cues throughout session to maintain attention to task. Child wore soft spica thumb splint for entire session.

Some or all of the following categories might be used to make this note easier to read:
- Ⓛ UE use or reach/grasp/release
- Feeding
- Attention/attention to task/attention span
- Splint

Depending on the categories selected, the note might read like this:

O: *Child participated in 60-minute OT session at daycare to address functional use of Ⓛ UE during play and self-care. Child demonstrated strong Ⓡ hand preference, flexed position of Ⓛ UE, and did not spontaneously initiate use of Ⓛ UE as a functional assist during self-care or play. Child wore a Ⓛ soft spica thumb splint throughout tx session to facilitate functional grasp patterns.*
Reach/Grasp/Release: With min Ⓐ for facilitation of elbow, child demonstrated ability to use Ⓛ UE to reach, grasp, and release 5 objects with 1-2 verbal cues per object and restriction of Ⓡ UE movement.
Feeding: Child was able to feed self with modified Ⓘ with ~50% spillage, but demonstrated significant limitation in chewing actions with ~3 rotary chews and swallowing ~90% of the food without chewing.
Attention: Child required verbal cues throughout the session to maintain attention to task.

WORKSHEET 8-2: BEING MORE CONCISE

O: Pt. participated in 60-minute OT session bedside to complete morning ADL routine. Pt. presented with decreased standing balance and safety awareness. Pt. ambulated ~36 inches to shower c̄ SBA for safety. Pt. instructed to complete shower while sitting. Pt. performed shower c̄ SBA to manage IV line. Pt. able to wash upper and lower body with SBA and dry entire body with SBA after completing shower. Pt. required ~20 minutes to complete shower. Pt. then ambulated ~36 inches to chair and sat. Pt. needed verbal cues to remain seated while donning underwear and pants. Pt. able to dress upper body modified Ⓘ and lower body p̄ verbal cues for sitting. Pt. demonstrated good sitting balance, but needed SBA for standing balance. Following shower, client stated he would like to take a nap and was assisted back to bed.

A more concise note might read:

O: *Pt. participated in 60-minute OT session bedside for skilled instruction in self-care activities. Pt. presented with decreased standing balance and safety awareness. Ambulated ~3 ft. to/from shower c̄ SBA to manage IV line while ambulating and showering for 20 minutes. Client showered c̄ SBA and completed upper body dressing modified Ⓘ and lower body dressing c̄ verbal cues to sit for safety. Client demonstrated good sitting balance but required SBA for standing balance. Client returned to bed c̄ SBA at end of session.*

Or

O: *Client participated in 60-minute OT session in room for skilled instruction in safe showering and dressing. Pt. presented with decreased standing balance and safety awareness. Client ambulated ~3' SBA for balance. After verbal cues to sit, client showered for 20 min c̄ SBA to manage IV lines. Client donned shirt modified Ⓘ seated; client required verbal cues to remain seated when threading underwear and pants over feet.*

Worksheet 8-3: Being Specific About Assist Levels

1. Client completed supine → sit with min Ⓐ; bed → w/c with mod Ⓐ.
   - *Client completed supine → sit with min Ⓐ to initiate activity; bed → w/c with mod Ⓐ for balance.*
   - *Client completed supine → sit with min Ⓐ to pull up using trapeze; bed → w/c with mod Ⓐ to lift body weight.*
   - *Client completed supine → sit with min Ⓐ to sequence movement; bed → w/c with mod Ⓐ for postural control.*
2. Client required SBA in transferring w/c ↔ toilet.
   - *Client required SBA for proper hand placement in transferring w/c ↔ toilet.*
   - *Client required SBA for sequencing in transferring w/c ↔ toilet.*
3. Client retrieved garments from low drawers with min Ⓐ.
   - *Client retrieved garments from low drawers with min Ⓐ to grasp drawer handles.*
   - *Client retrieved garments from low drawers with min Ⓐ to release trigger on reacher.*
   - *Client retrieved garments from low drawers with min Ⓐ to judge HALO placement in space.*
4. Client required max Ⓐ to brush hair.
   - *Client required max Ⓐ to reach back of head when brushing hair.*
   - *Client required max Ⓐ to flex Ⓡ shoulder past 35° when brushing hair.*
5. Client completed dressing, toileting, and hygiene with min Ⓐ.
   - *Client completed dressing, toileting, and hygiene with min Ⓐ to reach feet.*
   - *Client completed dressing, toileting, and hygiene with min Ⓐ for activities requiring fine motor dexterity.*
   - *Client completed dressing, toileting, and hygiene with min Ⓐ to adhere to hip precautions.*

Worksheet 8-4: De-Emphasizing the Treatment Media

1. Client played catch using Ⓑ UEs to facilitate grasp and release patterns.
   Client worked on functional grasp/release patterns needed to manipulate household objects.

2. Resident put dirt into pot to halfway point, added seedling, and filled remainder of pot with dirt transferred by cup. Resident completed 3 more pots while standing 8 minutes before requiring a 5-minute rest. Resident resumed standing position to water completed pots for approximately 5 minutes.
   Resident demonstrated standing tolerance of 13 minutes during leisure activity with a 5-minute break after 8 minutes to increase standing needed for ADL tasks.

3. Client painted some sun catchers in crafts group to be able to see that she could do something successfully.
   Client completed a series of quick-success projects to increase self-esteem.

4. Pt. cut out magazine pictures that indicated her emotions and glued them onto construction paper.
   Client indicated her emotions through identification of pictures that represented those emotions.

5. Child picks up beans with tweezers and placed in pill bottle to work on tripod grasp in preparation for handwriting.
   In prep for handwriting, child demonstrated sustained tripod grasp for 5 minutes using tweezers to grasp/release small objects

Chapter 9

Worksheet 9-1: Writing About Problems in the Assessment

1. Client demonstrated difficulty with laundry and cooking tasks due to memory and sequencing deficits.
   Memory & sequencing deficits cause difficulty c̄ home management tasks.
2. Decreased level of arousal noted during morning dressing activities, requiring redirection to task.
   ↓ level of arousal limits client's ability to complete basic ADL tasks.

3. Client unable to follow hip precautions during morning dressing due to memory deficits.
   Memory deficits interfere c̄ client's ability to incorporate hip precautions into basic self-care tasks.
   or
   Memory deficits limit pt.'s ability to follow hip precautions while dressing.

4. Client problem solved poorly while performing lower body dressing, as evidenced by multiple attempts required to button pants and don socks successfully.
   ↓ problem solving limits client's ability to dress herself s̄ Ⓐ and raises safety concerns in all ADL areas.

WORKSHEET 9-2: JUSTIFYING CONTINUED TREATMENT

Yes   Evaluation of a client
No   The practice of coordination and self-care skills on a daily basis
Yes   Establishing measurable, behavioral, objective, and individualized goals
Yes   Developing intervention plans designed to meet established goals
Yes   Analyzing and modifying functional activities through the provision of adaptive equipment or techniques
Yes   Determining that the modified tasks are safe and effective
No   Routine exercise and strengthening programs
Yes   Teaching the client to use the breathing techniques he has learned while performing ADLs
Yes   Providing individualized instruction to the client, family, or caregiver
Yes   Modifying the intervention plan based on a re-evaluation
No   Donning/doffing of a client's resting hand splint on a regular schedule throughout the day
Yes   Providing specialized instruction to eliminate limitations in a functional activity
Yes   Developing a home program and instructing caregivers
Yes   Making changes in the environment
Yes   Teaching compensatory skills
No   Gait training
Yes   Adding instruction in lower body dressing techniques to a current ADL program
No   Presenting informational handouts without having the client perform the activity
Yes   Teaching adaptive techniques such as one-handed shoe tying

WORKSHEET 9-3: WRITING THE ASSESSMENT—ELLIE'S DEVELOPMENT

A: *Infant's inability to right head, roll, or push up to prone Ⓘ limits ability to engage in age-appropriate play skills and developmental exploration. Infant's decreased activity tolerance also limits her ability to engage in developmental play activities. Ability to maintain facilitated positions and decrease in need for oxygen indicate progress. Visual tracking and scanning by turning head indicates visual awareness and orientation and shows good potential for increased interaction with environment. Infant would benefit from continued facilitation of functional mobility during play as well as increasing strength and endurance through activities that stimulate normal development.*
    or

A: *Decreased postural control and need for facilitation of weight shift limits infant's ability to perform early mobility skills needed for play. Limited mobility combined with her tolerance for less than 20 minutes of activity and the need for frequent rest breaks limit her ability to explore her environment and reach developmental milestones at a typical age. Ability to perform transitional movements with facilitation, orientation to black and white design, and ability to track in horizontal plane show good progress and potential for future developmental gains. Infant would benefit from continued OT services to stimulate developmental skills and from parent education in a home program.*

WORKSHEET 9-4: WRITING THE ASSESSMENT—MS. D'S SOCIAL SKILLS

1. What problems do you see in the above "S" and "O"?
   - **Unkempt appearance**
   - **Interrupts when others are talking**
   - **Does not stay on topic of conversation**

2. What areas of occupation do these problems affect?
   - **Social participation**
3. What evidence of progress and/or potential do you see?
   - **Engages in conversation**
   - **States that she understands purpose of the group**
   - **Willingness to attend and participate in group**
   - **Spontaneously shared thoughts and ideas**
4. What would this client benefit from?
   - **Groups that focus on conversational skills**
   - **Skilled instruction in attending to social cues**
   - **ADL activities stressing hygiene and appearance**
5. Write a complete assessment statement for this note.

A: *Client's unkempt appearance, interrupting behaviors, and need for redirection to topic of conversation interfere with her ability to engage in social participation with peers. Her expressed interest in groups and her willingness to engage in conversation and share her ideas show good potential to develop relationships and to express herself verbally in place of acting out. Client would benefit from participating in groups where conversational skills are stressed, from further facilitation of attention to social cues, and from instruction in ADLs stressing hygiene and appearance.*

CHAPTER 10

WORKSHEET 10-1: COMPLETING THE PLAN FOR ELLIE

P: *Infant to be seen 2x per week for 30 minutes each visit for 3 months for stimulation of normal developmental sequences and facilitation of appropriate movement patterns during play and exploratory activities. Design and modification of home program for parents also planned.*

or

P: *Child will be seen in home twice weekly for 3 months for activities that encourage postural control needed for play and environmental exploration. Sessions to include parent education targeted at facilitating infant's development. Plan to formally reassess infant's developmental level using standardized testing in 3 months.*

WORKSHEET 10-2: COMPLETING THE PLAN FOR MS. D

P: *Client to be seen daily for the next week to ↑ skills needed for social participation in a variety of contexts. Focus will be on development of conversational skills including not interrupting others and staying on topic.*

or

P: *Client to continue social skills group 3x/wk for 1 wk to improve conversational skills. Client will also be given individual feedback daily on her attention to appearance and social cues.*

CHAPTER 11

WORKSHEET 11-1: WRITING PROBLEM STATEMENTS

1. Pt. unable to dress LE Ⓘ due to trunk instability.
   - **Tell what assist level is needed rather than saying unable to dress Ⓘ.**
   - **Say "lower body" rather than LE, since the client is dressing more than just the extremity.**
   - **If there is one particular part of the task that requires assistance, specify that. For example: Trunk instability results in client needing mod Ⓐ to maintain balance while dressing lower body.**

2. Child doesn't tolerate very much classroom activity due to ↓ activity tolerance.
   - **Specify how much "very much" is.**
   - **Tell what kind of classroom activity. For example:** ↓ *activity tolerance results in child being able to tolerate less than 30 minutes of desk work.*
3. Consumer acts out.
   - **Specify what is meant by "acts out."**
   - **Specify what area of occupation is problematic because of the acting out.**
   - **Specify the contributing factor that is responsible for the acting out. For example:**
     - *Inappropriate verbal and physical actions result in difficulty sustaining friendships.*
     - *Consumer's self-injurious behavior of cutting and burning extremities when upset affects relationship with spouse and is an ongoing safety concern.*

WORKSHEET 11-2: WRITING COAST GOALS

1. Client will make a clock independently using the appropriate materials by anticipated discharge in 1 week.
   Client will demonstrate ability to grasp/place/release objects of various sizes needed for IADL activities by assembling a clock Ⓘ by anticipated discharge in 1 week.

   or

   Client will demonstrate ability to follow written directions for IADL tasks by assembling a clock from written instructions Ⓘ within 1 week.

2. Consumer will stay in his chair without reminders and spend at least 30 minutes lacing the leather billfold during the 45-minute craft group session within 2 weeks.
   Within 2 weeks, client will demonstrate attention to task needed to qualify for sheltered workshop program by staying in his chair without reminders and attending to craft project 30 minutes or more.

WORKSHEET 11-3: SOAPING YOUR NOTE

O Client supine → sit in bed Ⓘ.
O Client moved kitchen items from counter to cabinet Ⓘ using Ⓛ hand.
A Decreased coordination, strength, sensation, and proprioception in Ⓛ hand create safety risks in home management tasks.
S Client reports that his fingers are stiff this morning and that he is having trouble handling small items like buttons.
A ↑ of 15 minutes in activity tolerance for UE activities permits client to prepare a light meal Ⓘ.
O Child participated in 60-minute eval. of hand function in OT clinic.
A Decreased proprioception and motor planning limit Ⓘ in upper body dressing.
P Continue retrograde massage to Ⓡ hand for edema control.
A Correct identification of inappropriate positioning 100% of time indicates memory WFL.
S Client reports that she cannot remember hip precautions.
A Veteran would benefit from further instruction to incorporate total hip precautions into lower body dressing, bathing, and toileting.
A Client's improvement with repetition indicates good potential for successful access of augmentative communication device using eye gaze.
O Client did not make eye contact during group session.
O Client wrote check for correct amount to pay electric bill with 2 verbal cues.
A Client's request to take breaks demonstrates awareness of her limitations in endurance.
O Client completed weight shifts of trunk x 10 in each of anterior, posterior, left, and right lateral directions in preparation for standing to perform IADLs.
A 3+ muscle grade of Ⓡ wrist extension this week shows good progress toward goals.
P Continue OT 3x/wk for 2 weeks to address cognitive impairments that affect safe performance of IADLs.
A Unkempt appearance in mock interview situation indicates poor judgment and self-concept.

Worksheet 11-4: Writing the "S"—Subjective

S: *Client reports arthritis in Ⓡ shoulder and Ⓛ knee, pain on weightbearing. Pain at Ⓡ BKA site 8/10. During transfer, client requested specific adjustments such as sliding board placement, proximity to bed, and approaching from Ⓡ side. Fatigue reported after transfer.*

or

S: *Pt. reports significant arthritis in Ⓡ shoulder and Ⓛ knee, and prefers to approach transfers from Ⓡ side. Pt. reports, "It hurts to stand on my left leg." Pt. also stated w/c → bed sliding board transfers are the most difficult, and reported fatigue after transfer.*

or

S: *Client reports arthritis in Ⓡ shoulder and Ⓛ knee and pain weightbearing on Ⓛ LE. Pt. able to verbalize needs regarding transfer (placement of sliding board and approach from affected side). Client reports fatigue after transfer.*

Worksheet 11-5: "O"—Writing Good Opening Lines

1. Client seen in room for 45 minutes for self-care activities.
    - *Client participated in 45-minute OT session in room to increase Ⓘ in ADL activities. Client has total hip precautions and demonstrates memory deficits and decreased safety with walker during ADLs.*
    - *Client participated in 45-minute OT session in hospital room for education on use of adaptive equipment and toilet transfer during morning self-care activities. Client able to list hip precautions with verbal cues but does not consistently adhere to precautions during ADLs.*
2. Client seen at workshop for 1 hr. to work on job skills.
    - *Client participated in 1-hr. session at workshop to address skills needed for job task completion. Pt. has cognitive, sensory, and bilateral integration deficits.*
    - *Client participated in 1-hr. session at workshop to improve efficiency of package handling work task. Session focused on sequencing, bilateral coordination, concentration, and sensory awareness.*
3. Client seen bedside for 30 minutes for morning dressing.
    - *Client participated in 30-minute bedside session for morning dressing to improve safety and independence with ADLs to return home. Client exhibits ↓ balance, Ⓑ motor control, and functional mobility during ADLs.*
    - *Client participated in 30-minute bedside session to address balance and Ⓑ UE motor control during morning ADLs. Client uses manual w/c for positioning and mobility and demonstrates decreased safety during ADLs due to poor balance and Ⓑ UE coordination.*
4. Client seen in kitchen for 1 hr. to work on Ⓘ in cooking.
    - *Client participated in 1-hr. session in kitchen to address safety and independence during cooking tasks in prep for return home with limited caregiver supervision during the day. Client continues to exhibit decreased dynamic standing balance and inattention to affected Ⓛ UE.*
    - *Client participated in 1-hr. session in kitchen to work on safety during cooking tasks. Session focused on attention to affected Ⓛ UE positioning and dynamic standing balance.*

Worksheet 11-6: "O"—Being Specific About Assist Levels

No Client required max Ⓐ x 2 bed → bedside commode and bed → w/c; Ⓓ for pericare.
Yes Child required HOH Ⓐ **to stay in the lines** when following path with crayon.
Yes Client needed mod verbal cues **to participate in discussion** during life skills group.
No Resident needed min Ⓐ to don sock due to pain.

<h1 align="center">WORKSHEET 11-7: REVISING THE "O"</h1>

- An opening statement is needed, stating where, for how long, for what purpose the client was seen, and what the client's primary deficits are. One possibility is: *Client participated in 30-minute session in room for skilled instruction in compensatory dressing techniques and evaluation of splinting needs. Client presents with pain and limited function of dominant Ⓡ hand.*
- The categories could be reduced to three: toileting, dressing, and splinting evaluation.
- It would be helpful to know what part of the task required assistance.
- The UE and LE wording is not inclusive enough since the client is dressing the upper and lower body rather than just the extremities.
- Under "hand status," there is no functional component, and "index finger greatest amount" is not very informative.

WORKSHEET 11-8: DIFFERENTIATING BETWEEN OBSERVATIONS AND ASSESSMENTS

O Client is unable to don AFO and shoe Ⓘ for ambulation.

A Inability to don AFO and shoe Ⓘ prevent client from ambulating safely around the house for IADL performance to live alone.

A Decreased sensory tolerance limits the client's attention to task in the classroom.

O Client required verbal cues to stay on task due to decreased sensory tolerance.

O Client was unable to incorporate breathing and energy conservation techniques, requiring several prompts to complete task.

A Inability to incorporate breathing techniques and energy conservation techniques into basic ADL tasks s̄ verbal prompts limits her ability to live alone Ⓘ p̄ discharge.

1. Client demonstrated difficulty with laundry and cooking tasks due to memory and sequencing deficits.
   - *Decreased memory and sequencing abilities limit client's ability to perform IADLs such as laundry and cooking tasks.*
   - *Memory and sequencing deficits interfere with client's ability to perform IADLs such as laundry and cooking, and limit her ability to return to an Ⓘ living situation.*
   - *Deficits in memory and sequencing lead to difficulty with IADL tasks such as laundry and cooking tasks necessary for household management.*

2. Client unable to complete homemaking tasks or basic self-care activities independently due to decreased endurance and not following hip precautions.
   - *Decreased endurance and non-adherence to hip precautions limit client's ability to complete homemaking tasks and self-care activities Ⓘ and safely.*
   - *Failure to follow hip precautions and decreased endurance interfere with client's ability to complete homemaking tasks and decrease ability to successfully complete basic self-care activities Ⓘ and safely.*
   - *Decreased endurance and failure to follow hip precautions prevent client from performing homemaking and ADL tasks Ⓘ and safely.*

3. After the use of behavioral modification techniques, client displayed courteous behavior for the remainder of the treatment session.

   You could take a positive or negative approach to this one:
   - Positive:
     - *Client's ability to behave courteously with the aid of behavioral modification techniques indicates good potential for improving problem behaviors at school.*
     - *Positive response to behavioral modification techniques shows good potential to meet social participation goals.*
   - Negative:
     - *Need for behavioral modification techniques to elicit courteous behavior limits client's ability to interact appropriately with peers at school in social settings.*
     - *Need for instruction in behavior modification limits his ability to communicate with others effectively in social situations.*

Worksheet 11-9: Problems, Progress, and Rehab Potential

Problems: After reading through this note, several problems stood out for this occupational therapist:

- **Dynamic sitting balance**
- **Weight shifting**
- **Posture**
- **Transfers**

(The four above are related to safety and functional mobility.)

- **Decreased AROM in Ⓡ UE (mod Ⓐ to reach)**
- **Cognition**

On thinking a little further, the occupational therapist decided that the "cognition" problem might really be one of the following, because the patient does seem to understand the goal of the activity:

- **Short-term memory**
- **Motor planning**
- **Problem solving**
- **Initiation**

Finally, the occupational therapist decided that the problem with initiation is probably some combination of problem solving and motor planning deficits.

Progress/Rehab Potential:

The therapist then groups the problems according to the impact they have on the client's occupational performance. She decides that the first three cause difficulty with functional mobility and are of particular concern because they create safety issues. The motor planning and initiation problem is a concern in the area of self-care, as is the problem with decreased AROM of the Ⓡ UE. The need for continual instruction, whether it is a problem with short-term memory or with his ability to problem solve, is likely to require a lot of attention from a caregiver at home. The client does, however, understand why he is doing the task she has given him. As long as the goals are not set too high, he should be able to make good progress in rehabilitation. Her assessment and plan read as follows:

A: *Deficits in postural control, dynamic sitting balance, and weight shifting raise safety concerns when transferring. ↓ AROM and motor planning ability negatively affect ability to perform self-care tasks. Need for continual instruction for safety will necessitate a high level of caregiver assistance during ADL tasks. Client's ability to understand treatment goal indicates good rehab potential for goals established. Client would benefit from continued skilled instruction in activities to ↑ balance, safe functional mobility, and Ⓘ in ADL tasks.*

P: *Continue tx daily for 2 weeks for skilled instruction in self-care tasks and safe transfers during ADLs. Focus will be on improving level of independence to min Ⓐ or better to return home with caregiver assistance. Adaptive equipment needs for home will also be assessed.*

Another occupational therapist might assess the situation a little differently. For example:

A: *Deficits in motor planning, movement initiation, cognition, and muscle weakness in Ⓡ UE result in ↓ safety and independence in ADL tasks and functional mobility during ADLs. Ability to tolerate 3 minutes of activity at a time indicates progress over baseline of 1 minute activity tolerance. Client would benefit from skilled OT to increase balance, functional mobility, and grasp/release activities with involved UE to ↑ Ⓘ in self-care activities.*

P: *Continue tx bid for ½-hour sessions for 2 weeks to work on Ⓡ UE movement and cognitive retraining. Sessions will focus on improving independence in grooming, dressing, toileting, and bathing to work toward goal of returning home with spouse. Will consult with speech language pathologist regarding short-term memory strategies that can be incorporated during OT sessions.*

or

A: *Decreased functional use of Ⓡ UE, decreased sitting balance, and difficulty with sequencing and problem solving limit ability to perform ADLs. Increased shoulder flexion and motor planning since initial evaluation* *and increased understanding of treatment activities indicate good rehab potential. Client would benefit from continued skilled OT to increase functional AROM, exercises in grasp, exercises in weight shifting to improve dynamic sitting balance, and evaluation of both cognitive status and ability to initiate activity to increase ① in ADL tasks.*

P: *Continue bid for 30-minute sessions for 2 weeks to increase independence with ADLs. Initial sessions to address dynamic sitting balance and functional ® UE movement in preparation for ADL training.*

WORKSHEET 11-10: WRITING THE "A" AND "P"—THE SCHOOL NOTE

Problems:
- Decreased visual tracking and eye convergence
- Low muscle tone/upper body weakness
- Decreased bilateral coordination
- Impaired fine motor skills
- Poor handwriting
- UE weakness
- Proximal instability

Progress/Rehab Potential:
- Improvement in ability to form letters within lines
- 90% accuracy from memory of some letters
- Handwriting improvement

A: *Decreased upper body strength and proximal stability limit the child's ability to use his upper extremities in an accurate and coordinated manner in class. Lack of fine motor and bilateral coordination limit the child's accuracy in schoolwork (including handwriting, art, and play activities). Inaccuracy in visual tracking and eye convergence interfere with ability to form letters and numbers or to complete written work from a book or whiteboard at grade level. Lack of visual tracking and convergence skills also limit ability to perform age-appropriate games safely. Improvement in accuracy of letter formation since last note and ability to remember 6 letter shapes indicate good progress and good potential to meet IEP goals. Child would benefit from continued work on postural stability to support functional UE use, as well as from continued work on visual and motor skills needed for classroom activities.*

P: *Continue OT twice weekly for 30-minute sessions for remainder of school year to improve functional performance in educational activities. Sessions to focus on improving postural control, bilateral coordination, and oculomotor control. Will consult with classroom teacher regarding classwork modifications to accommodate oculomotor deficits.*

WORKSHEET 11-11: WRITING THE "A" AND "P"—MR. S'S COMMUNICATION SKILLS

Problems:
- Communication (changes subject rather than answer the question)
- Assertion (does not define, and states he does not wish to use)
- Nonresponsive to group role-play activity
- Sitting with head down and eyes closed during group
- Self-expression (verbal and nonverbal)

These behaviors limit his appropriate social participation and his likelihood of leaving the institution.

Progress/Rehab Potential:
- Neat appearance
- Attended group and was on time
- Remained for duration of group

A: *Poor ability to define assertive behavior and the statement that he prefers manipulation and aggression as relational skills limit Mr. S's ability to resolve conflicts and relate to others effectively, thus limiting his ability to function ① in a community setting. Lack of participation in group activity limits ability to explore alternate ways of communicating with others. Ability to manage time, willingness to remain in group until the end, and good dressing/grooming skills indicate good potential to meet stated goal of moving to next level of least restrictive environment. Client would benefit from group and individual OT sessions to address social communication skills*

P: *Client to participate in all regularly scheduled psychosocial skills groups for 1 month, in addition to weekly 1:1 session on unit to offer opportunities to relate effectively. Focus will be on increasing participation in group activities to improve effective communication skills with others.*

WORKSHEET 11-12: REVISING THE "ALMOST" NOTE

+ The "S" would be better if the therapist had asked pertinent questions, such as what the client's pain levels were.
+ The occupational therapist is mixing the "O" data and the "A" data.
+ There is nothing in the "O" to show that skilled occupational therapy is being provided. The list of observations of assist levels fails to provide the richness of skill used in treatment. The therapist erroneously puts some of that information in the "A" section, rather than assessing her data. In the "A" she tells us:
  Client Ⓘ in dressing EOB, but is min Ⓐ in dressing when standing with a walker. Ⓛ UE AROM is WFL but Ⓡ UE has deficits noted in shoulder flexion. Client needs SBA in bed mobility when rolling to unaffected side and min Ⓐ in sit → stand 2° ↓ UE strength. Client needs SBA for transfer to unaffected side in pivot transfer bed → w/c and min Ⓐ w/c → toilet.
+ Even if this information were moved into the "O," there is nothing to tell us what part of the task the assistance was for.
+ The therapist used a nonstandard abbreviation of "VCs." She means verbal cues, but since VC is a standard health term meaning *vital capacity*, it is inappropriate in its usage here.
+ The coordination deficits mentioned in the "A" section come out of the blue. There is no mention of coordination in the opening statement (*to work on dressing and functional mobility during ADLs*), nor is it mentioned anywhere else in the "O." Thus, the statement that coordination deficits are one of the problems noted and the statement that the client would benefit from coordination exercises are unsubstantiated. Remember not to introduce any new information in the "A" section of your note.
+ There is no real assessment of the meaning of the data found in the "S" and the "O." There is a short list of problem areas, but no assessment of their impact on the ability to engage in meaningful occupation, and no assessment of the rehab potential shown by the client's willingness to "*do whatever it takes to get out of the hospital.*"
+ The best thing for this therapist to do is to rewrite the "O" section, providing a more comprehensive picture of the treatment session. Then she needs to assess her data based on her observations. There needs to be an indication of how the observed data affect the occupational performance of the client, before the statements about what the client would benefit from.
+ Depending on the assessment she makes, the plan to work on balance may be appropriate, but it is likely to be only one of the things to be addressed.

CHAPTER 12

WORKSHEET 12-1: CHOOSING INTERVENTION STRATEGIES

STG (Objective)	Intervention	Type of Intervention
Client will be independent in managing financial affairs within 3 weeks.	1. *Complete worksheets with basic math skills (add, subtract, multiply, divide).*	1. *Preparatory task*
	2. *Role play to make change correctly.*	2. *Activity*
	3. *Set-up task for writing checks to pay fabricated bills.*	3. *Activity*
	4. *Practice comparison shopping online using an electronic tablet.*	4. *Activity*
	5. *Set up task of writing out a budget.*	5. *Activity*

STG (Objective)	Intervention	Type of Intervention
Client will be independent in managing financial affairs within 3 weeks.	6. *Set up task of balancing checkbook.*	6. *Activity*
	7. *Set up experience for deciding whether a given amount of money will be enough for living expenses once a set of fabricated bills has been paid.*	7. *Activity*
	8. *Have client make a purchase in the hospital cafeteria or gift shop.*	8. *Occupation*
	9. *Have family bring in credit card bill statements and client's checkbook so client can pay bills.*	9. *Occupation*

Worksheet 12-2: Writing the Assessment and Intervention Plan—The Case of Georgia S

A: ↓ *activity tolerance and standing balance, weakness in* Ⓑ *shoulder flexion/abduction, and* ↓ *problem-solving skills result in* ↓ *safety and* Ⓘ *in dressing and grooming.* ↓ *standing balance impairs safe and* Ⓘ *functional mobility during ADLs. Weak grasp and pinch of* Ⓡ *hand and* ↓ *coordination impairs fine motor ADL tasks including donning sock and brushing teeth. Rehab potential is good for returning home with caregiver assistance. Client would benefit from continued occupational therapy to increase activity tolerance, dynamic standing balance, and safety for ADL tasks.*

P: *Pt. to be seen bid for 45-minute sessions for 3 weeks to* ↑ Ⓘ *in self-care activities. Client will be instructed in adaptive equipment/techniques. Interventions will also focus on* ↑ *activity tolerance, standing balance, and* Ⓘ *in functional mobility for ADLs, and* ↑ Ⓡ *hand strength to complete dressing and toileting* Ⓘ.

Strengths: Ⓘ *in self-care prior to cerebrovascular accident; able to ambulate* c̄ *walker; intact sensation except* Ⓡ *hand stereognosis; all UE AROM WNL or WFL*

Functional Problem Statement #1: *Impaired problem solving,* ↓ *coordination,* ↓ *stereognosis, and* ↓ *standing balance impair ability to perform self-care tasks* Ⓘ.

Long-Term Goal #1: *Client will complete all dressing and grooming tasks with modified* Ⓘ *using walker for task set-up by anticipated discharge on 7/03/17.*

STG (Objective)	Intervention
STG #1: *Client will don/doff gown and robe with min* Ⓐ *and verbal cues by 6/17/17.*	1. *Instruct client in upper body dressing techniques and have client demonstrate over-the-head and button-up methods, first in sitting, then progress to standing.* 2. *Provide tactile cues to use alternative techniques.* 3. *Have client problem solve next step of dressing or grooming tasks in sequence using visual aid and then verbal cues as needed. Ask client what to do next or why this is not working now.* 4. *Engage client in reaching activities that provide a graded challenge to balance.* 5. *Engage client in activities that* ↑ *AROM and fine motor tasks such as buttoning and zipping that are graded for level of difficulty in coordination.*
STG #2: *By 6/24/17, client will complete grooming tasks standing at sink for at least 10 minutes with CGA for balance and one 30-sec rest break.*	1. *Educate client on identifying signs of fatigue. Plan rest breaks as needed to* ↓ *fatigue.* 2. *Perform tabletop activities including self-care tasks with time increasing as tolerated.* 3. *Perform deep breathing exercises and instruct in energy conservation techniques.* 4. *Instruct client in therapy putty exercises to be performed in room in between OT sessions to increase grip and pinch strength.* 5. *Gradually introduce standing components during morning ADLs such as standing to retrieve clothes from closet, standing to complete one grooming task.*

Functional Problem Statement #2: *Fatigue during ADLs and* ↓ *dynamic balance during toileting raise safety concern for being home alone during the day.*

Long-Term Goal #2: *By discharge on 7/03/17, client will perform toileting with modified independence using a walker and bedside commode.*

STG (Objective)	Intervention
STG #1: *In 1 week, client will transfer safely* ↔ *3-in-1 commode for toileting with min* Ⓐ *to manage clothing and no more than 2 verbal cues.*	1. *Instruct client in safe transfer techniques; reinforce compliance when transferring* ↔ *bed, armchairs, commode, and mat for therapeutic activities, strengthening exercises, toileting, or dressing activities.* 2. *Provide* Ⓡ *UE strengthening and AROM through reaching and weight-bearing activities such as reaching at sink for grooming and dressing items in graded challenging positions, pushing up from armchair and bedside commode, and table top activities of interest that require alternating support on one arm while actively reaching with the other.*
STG #2: *In 2 weeks, client will transfer safely* ↔ *3-in-1 commode for toileting with SBA to manage clothing and no more than 1 verbal cue.*	1. *Continue with transfer education and practice.* 2. *Interview client and daughter regarding home environment; explore and discuss equipment use & placement in home; discuss support services needed if discharge to home is warranted.* 3. *Schedule a home visit for assessment of client's ability to manage in home environment.*

Discharge Plan: *To home if environmental adaptations and support of caregiver and/or agency services are available. If client is not* Ⓘ *in self-care activities by 7/03/11, the recommendation will be to discharge to a skilled nursing facility for 2-3 weeks until self-care goals are met.*

Worksheet 12-3: Planning Interventions Using Groups—Heather's Suicide Attempt

Problem #1: *Exacerbation of depressive symptoms resulting in a suicide attempt.*

LTG #1: *By anticipated discharge in 4 days, Heather will demonstrate improved self-esteem by verbally identifying strengths, caring for her appearance, making eye contact when interacting with others, and developing a plan for coping with suicidal thoughts.*

	Intervention
Goals Group	1. *Listen attentively to Heather when she shares her goal.* 2. *Offer eye contact and offer Heather the opportunity to make eye contact in return before cueing her.* 3. *Help Heather identify the relationship between her values and her daily goals (i.e., a goal to wash her hair if related to valuing a neat and clean appearance).* 4. *Help Heather break down larger goals (such as "be happy") into smaller accomplishable and measurable increments.* 5. *Show respect for Heather's choices.* 6. *Provide feedback on Heather's successes in meeting her daily goals.* 7. *Facilitate goal choices that show increased self-esteem.* 8. *Compliment Heather on her appearance when any part of her appearance shows more attention to her self-care.* 9. *Facilitate goal choices that involve taking care of herself.*
Stress Management Group	1. *Welcome Heather by greeting her warmly, sitting by her, or smiling.* 2. *Offer opportunities to identify strengths through visualization and imagery.* 3. *Help Heather identify stresses that led her to recent suicide attempt.* 4. *Help Heather identify stresses that occur frequently.* 5. *Help Heather identify physical and behavioral changes that occur when she experiences stress.*

Stress Management Group	6. *Help Heather identify both successful and unsuccessful stress relief strategies that she has used in the past.* 7. *Brainstorm ways of handling stressful situations that seem overwhelming before those situations become life-threatening.* 8. *Use positive affirmations.* 9. *Provide practice for a variety of stress management strategies.* 10. *Develop a plan for managing stress when feeling overwhelmed.*
IADL Group	1. *Identify strengths about each person through group discussion, art activities (draw your best quality, personality collage, etc.), and games.* 2. *Use a peer feedback activity that gives group members opportunities to identify and recognize each other's strengths.* 3. *Offer quick success projects, such as putting together jewelry, making bookmarks, or completing small kits.* 4. *Ask Heather for her ideas about how best to use the group time.* 5. *Note aspects of Heather's work that are executed with competence.* 6. *In a group that is all women, learn to apply make-up or style hair.*

Problem #2: *Stress related to recent role changes result in Heather's inability to concentrate and make decisions for her daily life.*

LTG #2: *Heather will apply a decision-making strategy to her two most important current life decisions by discharge in 4 days.*

INTERVENTION	
Goals Group	1. *Identify a small accomplishment goal for the day.* 2. *Help Heather identify what is realistic to accomplish in 1 day.* 3. *Help Heather make her goal measurable.* 4. *Write that goal on a card for Heather to carry with her throughout the day.* 5. *Make a verbal contract with Heather to accomplish her goal.* 6. *Teach the relationship between setting daily goals and making larger life decisions.* 7. *Follow-up daily on Heather's goal for the day.* 8. *Encourage Heather to make goals related to major life stressors.*
Stress Management Group	1. *Help Heather identify triggers in her environment that cause a stress reaction.* 2. *Help Heather identify negative thoughts that increase her stress level. Instruct Heather on how to replace them with more positive and realistic thoughts.* 3. *Help Heather bring her thoughts to the present moment and to come back into the present moment when she drifts into the past and future.* 4. *Use movement, such as stretching or progressive relaxation, to help Heather focus on the task at hand.*
IADL Group	1. *Ask Heather what strategies she uses to focus her mind.* 2. *Plan group topics around Heather's current issues, such as: ways of getting to sleep, overcoming loneliness, and feeling worthwhile.* 3. *Use a cognitively stimulating activity to help Heather focus.* 4. *Instruct Heather on a problem-solving strategy and practice applying it to sample problems.* 5. *Brainstorm strategies for making good decisions and rank these in effectiveness.* 6. *Ask Heather to identify one major decision needing to be made, and list pros/cons of each possible course of action.* 7. *Role play a decision-making situation.* 8. *Use games that require decision making.* 9. *Adapt tasks so that Heather will be able to concentrate on a task long enough to complete it.*

Problem #3: *Inability to manage anger constructively resulting in behaviors that damage self, relationships, and property.*

LTG #3: *By anticipated discharge in 4 days, Heather independently will identify potential anger triggers, identify her physical reactions to being angry, and develop a plan to prevent escalation and destructive behaviors.*

INTERVENTION	
Goals Group	1. *Use active listening to help Heather identify feelings related to her goals.* 2. *Ask Heather about daily incidents involving anger and encourage goals for useful solutions if incidents arise.*
Stress Management Group	1. *Use stress management techniques that focus on body sensations.* 2. *Teach Heather to focus on the breath to bring her to the present moment, to relax, and to enhance sleep.* 3. *Invite Heather to identify and express feelings that arise during the exercises.* 4. *Use sounds and recordings that activate the parasympathetic nervous system.* 5. *Identify strategies for restful sleep and encourage her to practice these at night.*
IADL Group	1. *Teach anger management strategies.* 2. *Help Heather identify potential anger-provoking situations.* 3. *Help Heather identify early physical signs of escalating anger.* 4. *Help Heather develop a plan for what to do when she notices her anger beginning to escalate.* 5. *Help Heather identify safe outlets for anger to prevent it from escalating.* 6. *Instruct Heather on constructive ways to communicate her anger to others.* 7. *Help Heather identify feelings that arise during the group.* 8. *Use sounds and language to elicit feelings.* 9. *Use art activities to explore and express feelings.* 10. *Identify stressors that trigger anger through group discussion, adapted games, or art.* 11. *Role play situations around anger and frustration.* 12. *Identify social supports (friends, family, support groups, crisis lines) to use when angry.* 13. *Teach and role play problem solving.* 14. *Coach Heather as she practices managing anger with phone calls and visitors.* 15. *Teach the use of an "anger continuum" to recognize varying degrees and experiences of anger.*

Index